Second Edition

Dimensions of Family Life

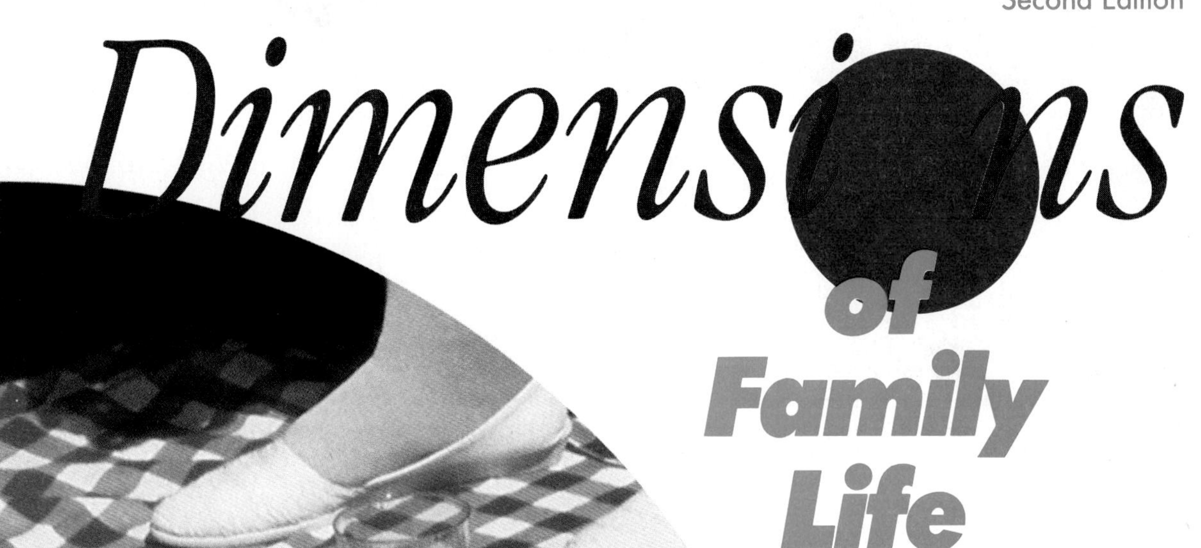

Stephen R. Jorgensen, Ph.D.
Associate Dean
College of Home Economics
Professor, Department of Human Development and Family Studies
Texas Tech University

Gail H. Henderson, Ph.D.
School and Community Relations Specialist
Eastland Vocational School District
Groveport, Ohio

OF01BA
PUBLISHED BY
SOUTH-WESTERN PUBLISHING CO.
CINCINNATI, OH WEST CHICAGO, IL
DALLAS, TX LIVERMORE, CA

Content Consultants

Dr. Joan K. Comeau
Project Coordinator
Minnesota Curriculum Services Center
Work and Family Institute
White Bear, Minnesota

Dr. J. Ross Eshleman
Professor
Department of Sociology
Wayne State University
Detroit, Michigan

Dr. Richard K. Kerckhoff
Professor
Department of Child Development and Family Studies
Purdue University
West Lafayette, Indiana

Dr. Sharon Alexander
Consultant
Charlotte, North Carolina

Photo Credits

Cover Photo: © Michael Weisbrot

For permission to reproduce the chapter-opener photographs indicated, acknowledgment is made to the following:

Chapter 2: Brent Petersen/The Stock Market
Chapter 4: Henley & Savage/The Stock Market
Chapter 5: Sybil Shackman/Monkmeyer Press
Chapter 8: Mike Kagan/Monkmeyer Press
Chapter 9: Courtesy of Apple Computer, Inc.
Chapter 10: H. Armstrong Roberts
Chapter 13: Hansen/Bavaria/H. Armstrong Roberts
Chapter 15: James Kulander/Monkmeyer Press
Chapter 17: Sandy Roessler/The Stock Market

ISBN: 0-538-60093-4
Library of Congress Catalog Number: 88-63430

2 3 4 5 6 7 8 Ki 6 5 4 3 2 1 0 9
Printed in the United States of America

contents

Part Four

Exploring Family Life • 209

Spotlight on Issues

preface

We hear much today about advanced technology, computer-controlled activities, and impersonal things being important in our daily lives rather than people. There is some concern that technology will create a society in which personal and family relationships are not significant. This concern may be unfounded. Futurists such as John Naisbitt (author of the influential *Megatrends: Ten Directions for Transforming Our Lives*) indicate that high tech will eventually be balanced by "high touch," or better interpersonal relationships. Increased technological impact will need to be offset by improved and expanded human relationships. Families remain a chief provider of such relationships. Now, more than ever, positive interpersonal and family relationships are necessary for an individual's well-being. Being able to understand yourself, relate to others, and function positively in your present and future families are important responsibilities. These topics are given special attention in this text.

Another noteworthy area explored in this textbook concerns the role of work in our family interaction. In more and more families, all of the adults are workers outside of the home. Work—whether it be schoolwork, work for wages, or voluntary work for personal fulfillment—is common today for many family members. Therefore, developing the ability to balance the worlds of work and family is becoming necessary for all family members. The degree of success in creating this balance is often a factor in the happiness and well-being of individuals and families today.

Dimensions of Family Life is about you as a person. It is also about the way people grow and develop in the context of family life. The self is examined in Part One, *Establishing a Personal Identity* and in Part Two, *Forming Interpersonal Relationships*. Parts Three and Four, *Exploring Human Development* and *Exploring Family Life*, focus on patterns of growth and development of people as individuals and as members of different types of family groups. Work and its implications for families are covered in Part Five, *Combining Work and Family.* Part Six, *Enhancing Family Functioning*, presents information to help families manage and strengthen themselves. Critical life skills are presented throughout the text.

This book has many special features:

- Clear learning goals
- Definitions and applications of all key words and concepts
- Carefully controlled reading level
- Personalized case studies
- Spotlights on issues that today's families may face
- A conversational writing style
- A comprehensive index
- Many colorful illustrations that reinforce concepts and stimulate exploration
- A useful, complete glossary
- End-of-chapter guideline questions highlighting review, consideration, and application of the content

A separate Student Activity Guide, Teacher's Manual and Key, and testing diskettes (MicroExam) for use with the IBM PC and Apple computers (II Plus, IIe, IIc, and IIGS) are available. These materials elaborate on the concepts in the text by providing additional activities and experiences for the student as well as important guidelines for the teacher.

The dimensions of your life—yourself, your family, and your work—are meaningful now and in your future. This book can help you discover, explore, and make decisions about these dimensions.

meet the authors

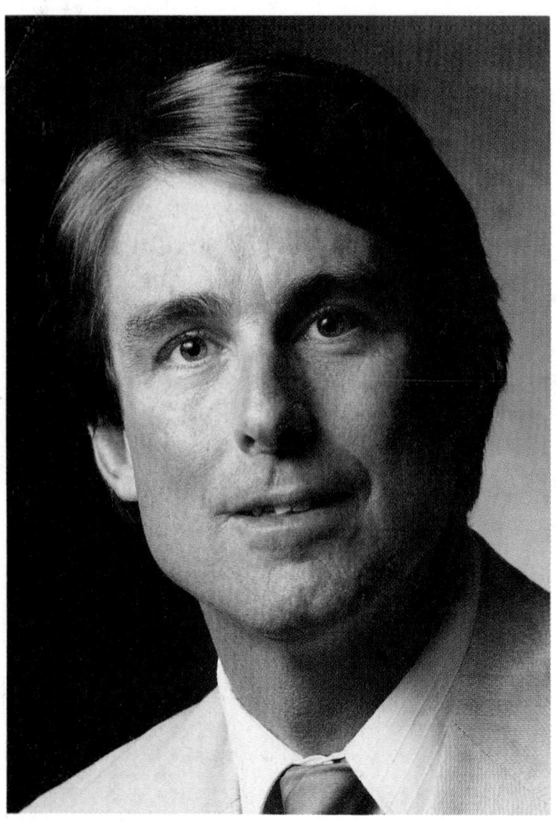

My name is Stephen R. Jorgensen. I currently serve as Associate Dean for the College of Home Economics at Texas Tech University, which is located in Lubbock, Texas. I am also Professor of Human Development and Family Studies and teach many college courses in the areas of marriage, family relations, and human development. I first became interested in this field of study when I was a student at the University of Minnesota in the early 1970s. I was granted the Ph.D degree in family sociology at Minnesota in 1976. Before that, I was granted the Bachelor of Arts degree in Spanish and Sociology by Hamline University in St. Paul, Minnesota. In a sense, I also have my own "marriage and family laboratory." I have been married to my wife Julie for 18 years and have three children—Jesse, Erik, and Brett. Their contribution to my own "human development" is worth far more than words can describe.

I have a strong belief in the critical importance of families for the well-being of individual people and of society as a whole. My belief is based on 16 years of research and study of the role that families play in our society and in societies all over the world. When families are strong and meet the needs of individual members for love, support, and nurturance, societies are strong and people are productive citizens. I hope that when you read this book, you too will develop a fresh application for the important role that marriage, parenthood, and other family relationships play in all of our lives. You are making a wise decision in taking this opportunity to learn about these issues at this early stage in your lifetime.

Steve Jorgensen

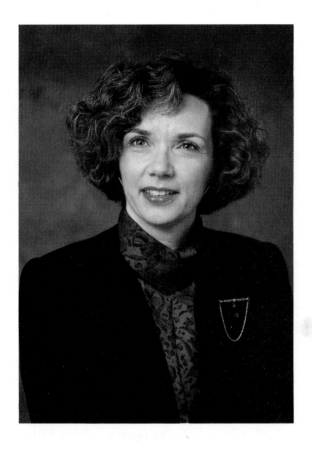

My name is Gail Henderson. I live in Columbus, Ohio, with my husband, who is a college professor, and two daughters—one in college and one in high school. My formal education includes degrees in home economics, human ecology, and education. I have taught family life classes in high school, at the college level, and in adult programs. I am presently a supervisor in a career center where I work with vocational teachers to assist them in strengthening and promoting their programs and keeping current in their subject matter and teaching skills.

Nearly all of my work experiences have focused on family relationships. I believe that families are integral parts of people's lives. I feel strongly that families, in all their varieties of shapes and sizes, will continue to be the centerpoint around which our lives rotate. This rotation is not always peaceful and calm; sometimes it can be confusing, frustrating, and uncomfortable. Parents and children disagree, spouses argue, and siblings fight. Yet I firmly believe that the family provides a central pivot point for most people's lives. I also believe that family life can be strengthened and that logical, caring decisions can help individuals and families add positive, meaningful dimensions to their lives.

My beliefs and ideas are supported by factual information, research, and study. I hope you will enjoy learning about these dimensions of life.

Gail Henderson

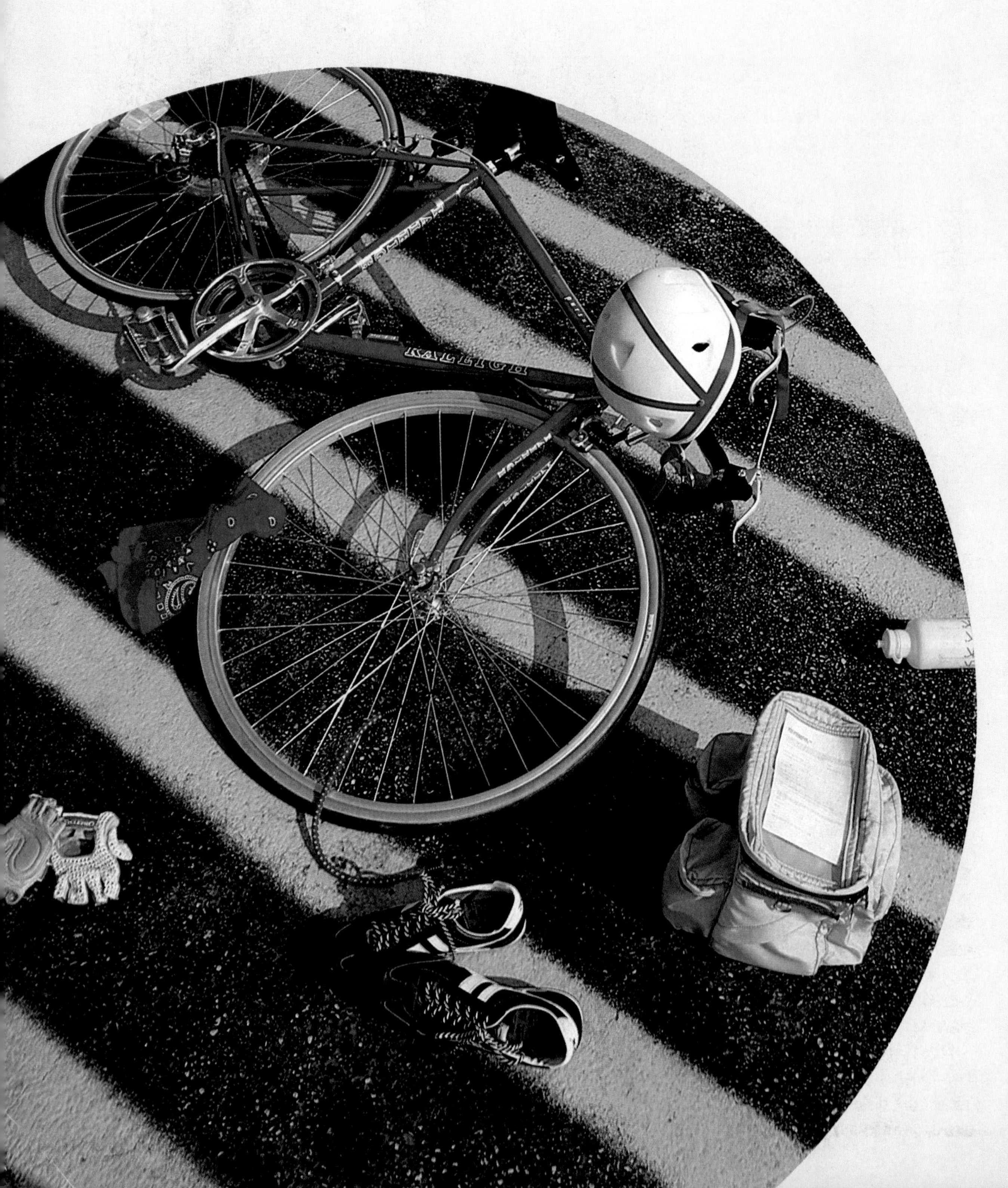

part one

Establishing a Personal Identity

Establishing a personal identity is the first step in forming positive and meaningful relationships with others. Interpersonal relationships involve you. You have the power to influence other people in these relationships; likewise, you are influenced by others. The better you know yourself, the better the likelihood of gaining and maintaining strong relationships with family members and friends.

Establishing a personal identity begins with assessing and strengthening your self-concept. You are unique. There is only one *you*—complete with strengths and weaknesses, virtues and faults! Exploring and assessing your own definition of self can help you to pinpoint areas in which you feel most and least secure. You have the ability to strengthen the weaker areas.

What is your personal potential as a human being? What is possible for you to achieve in life? In what ways can you contribute to others? Knowing yourself and knowing your basic human needs can help you strive to become the best you can possibly be. This striving is an important part of establishing your personal identity.

Awareness of your self-concept and human needs can help you form your personal values and goals. These personalized values and goals are a necessary part of making decisions that influence you and other people.

This part includes chapters on assessing and strengthening self-concept, becoming a fully functioning person, forming values, and making decisions. Understanding and applying these topics will help you to know yourself and assist you in forming healthy, functional interpersonal relationships.

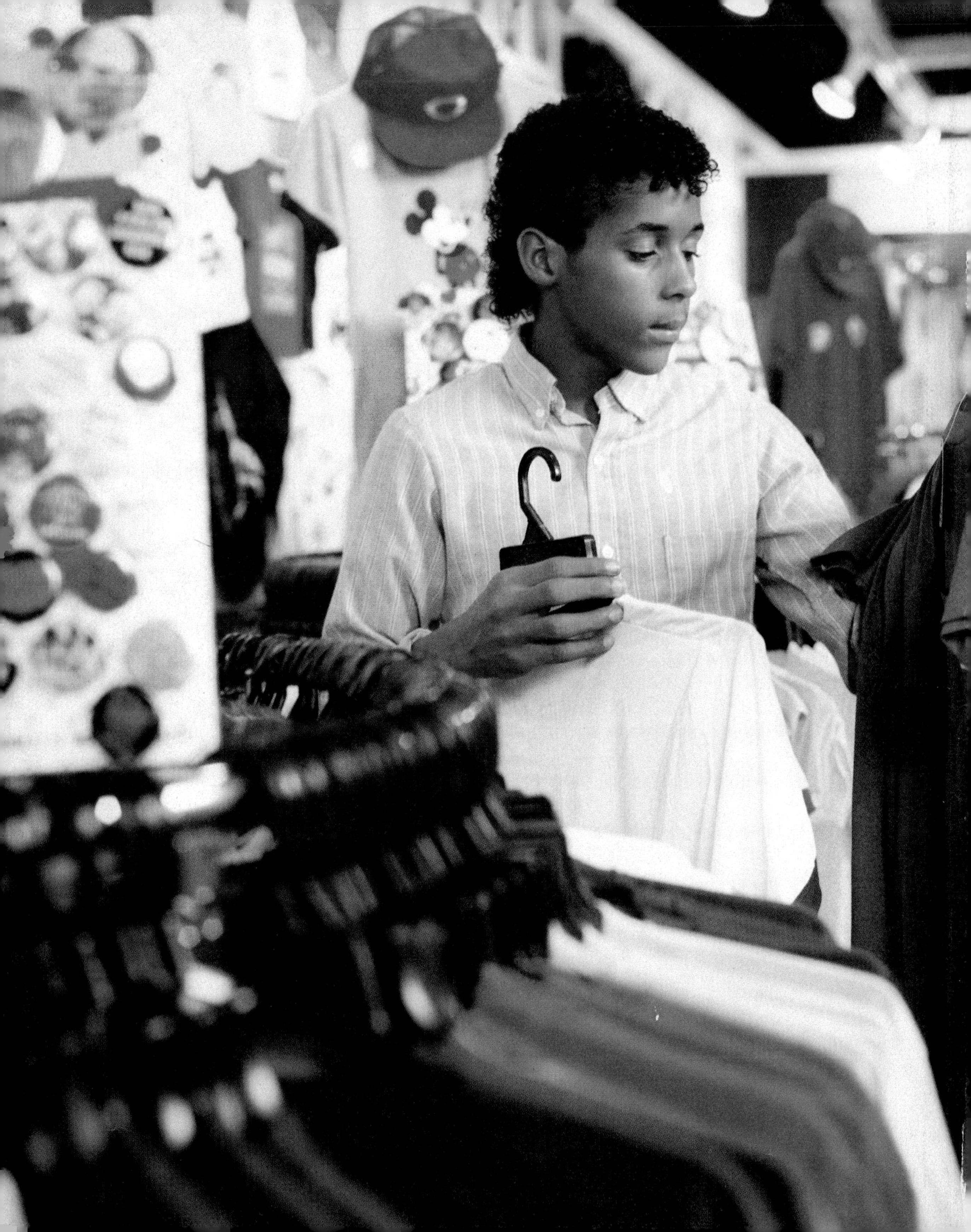

one

ASSESSING AND STRENGTHENING SELF-CONCEPT

This chapter provides information that will help you to:

- Understand the formation of the self-concept.
- Realize roadblocks to self-concept exploration.
- Explore your self-concept.
- Assess your self-concept.
- Strengthen your self-concept.

Knock,knock.
Who's there?
I don't know.
I don't know who?
I don't know who either.

This knock-knock joke describes how we sometimes feel about ourselves. Even when we see ourselves in a mirror, we may hardly recognize ourselves (Figure 1-1). It is often difficult to know who we really are or to know the person inside us. At other times we have a good awareness of who we are. This knowledge may cause feelings of pride, pleasure, anger, shame, or many other reactions.

Figure 1-1

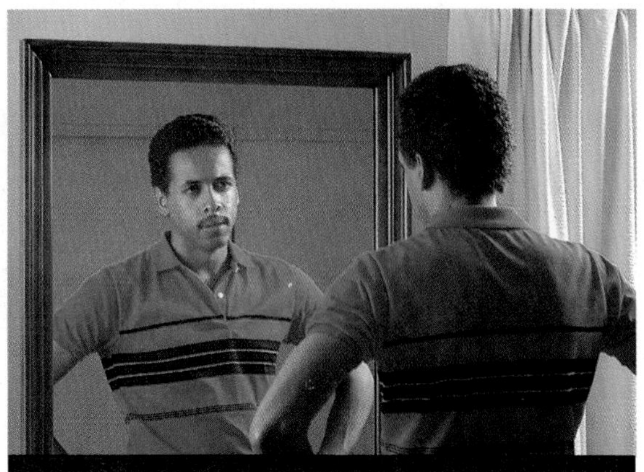

When we look in the mirror, who do we see? Do your friends see what you see?

The set of ideas about one's own unique being is called the **self-concept**. Self-concept includes beliefs, values, and feelings about our own strengths and weaknesses—the total awareness of one's worth as a person. This chapter focuses on the self-concept and the vital role these definitions of self play in building and maintaining all family and interpersonal relationships. It also emphasizes exploring, assessing, and strengthening self-concept.

EXPLORING SELF-CONCEPT

Self-concept is involved in nearly all aspects of human life. Exploring the formation of self-concept, its relationship to personality, and the roadblocks to realizing one's own definition of self is helpful in understanding why we feel and behave as we do.

Formation of Self-Concept

It would be interesting if everyone could receive a positive self-concept immunization. Perhaps we could receive one basic shot at infancy. Then as we grew older, we could get periodic self-concept booster shots to help protect us from experiences in everyday life that lower our self-concepts. Of course, such shots do not exist. But if they were available, the infancy immunization would be necessary since the formation of self-concept begins at a very early age.

We know that **cultural learning** is the major factor in influencing individual self-concept. Cultural learning is the sum of the effect that our society, culture, and environment has on individuals. Young children are dependent on their families and spend long periods of time in the home environment. Therefore, the family plays an important role in the child's cultural learning. Consider a child who is always attended to, talked to, encouraged to be part of the family's activities, praised, loved, and made to feel worthwhile. In contrast consider a child who is not attended to, who is excluded from family decision making and activities, criticized, and seldom loved or made to feel worthwhile.

Which child do you think would develop the higher self-concept?

Clearly families, as part of society and culture, affect the self-concept of children. But self-concept continues to be shaped throughout the life cycle by other forces as well. The expectations held by your family, school, community, country, and even the world will likely affect your self-concept. For example, if your school, community, or family emphasize excelling at sports and physical activities (and if your abilities are not in this area), your self-concept will probably be diminished. On the other hand, if your family, school, and community appreciate and praise achievement in many areas, and if people are considered worthy despite their limitations, then a positive self-concept will be more readily developed, as shown in Figure 1-2. Cultures and subcultures that emphasize competition and give praise only to the winner of the competition may foster a negative self-concept for those who are not winners. Cultures and subcultures that emphasize the self-worth of all people foster positive self-concepts.

Figure 1-2

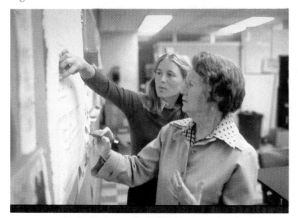

A teacher often influences a student's positive self-concept by recognizing abilities and limitations.
VISTA PHOTO/ELLIOT SMITH

Unique experiences also help shape self-concept. Figure 1-3 presents some of these experiences. Each time individuals encounter a rewarding or deflating experience, it can influence or modify their self-concept. Experiences that provide the awareness that you can achieve, you have worth, others have similar difficulties, and you are normal, offer the opportunity for improving your definition of self. Experiences leading to feelings that you can't achieve, you're worthless, and you're the only one with such difficulties, foster low concepts of self.

An interesting example of unique experiences can be found within a person's own family. Have you ever known two siblings (brothers and/or sisters) so different that you can't believe they are from the same family? One person is confident, willing to try, outgoing, and fully believes in his or her self-worth. The other person is self-doubting, lacks confidence, is timid, and convinced of his or her own unworthiness. How can these two people be siblings? The answer lies in each person's unique experiences. Despite the fact that these people have the same parents and have lived in the same house and community, they have unique family experiences. For example, one came into the family as an only child. Later this child played the role of older sibling and met the expectations of being the older child in this particular family. The second child came into a formed family of three people and took the expected role of the younger child. The experiences of these two siblings were unique even though they were in the same family. The resultant self-concepts and personalities will also be unique.

Figure 1-3

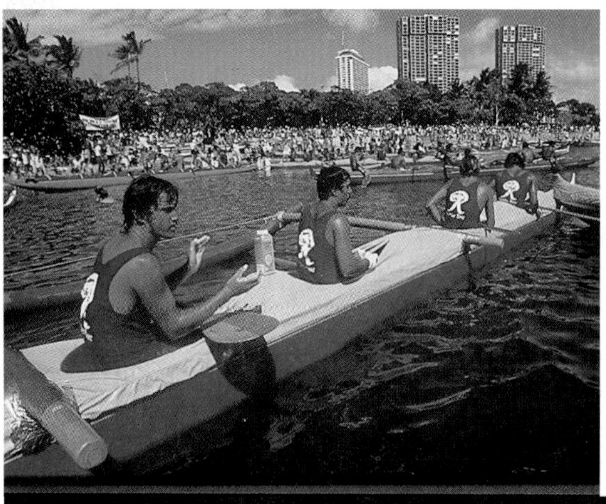

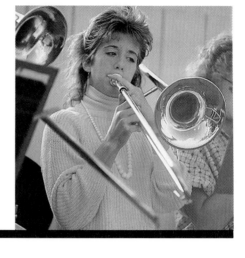

Unique experiences shape self-concept.

Hawaii Visitors Bureau

Peter Glass/Monkmeyer Press

Research has also shown that we are born with certain **personality predispositions** or tendencies to behave in a certain way toward other people. You have probably noticed how some babies seem to be naturally easy to warm up to, while others are often fussy, irritable, and unhappy. The "easy to warm up to" baby is more likely to have positive interactions with parents, siblings, and other people. Such babies are viewed as cuddly and cute. They are held and talked to affectionately. They respond to their caretakers in ways that ensure continued nurturance (Figure 1-4).

The "difficult" baby, on the other hand, may generate quite different responses. Fussiness or frequent temper tantrums may frustrate a parent and try the patience of others in the household. Therefore, the "difficult" baby may be held and cuddled less often. Difficult babies are not as likely to hear positive things, like "What a *good baby* you are!" Such responses from others, then, may lead to a more positive self-concept for the "easy to warm up to" baby than for the "difficult" baby.

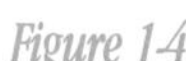

Figure 1-4

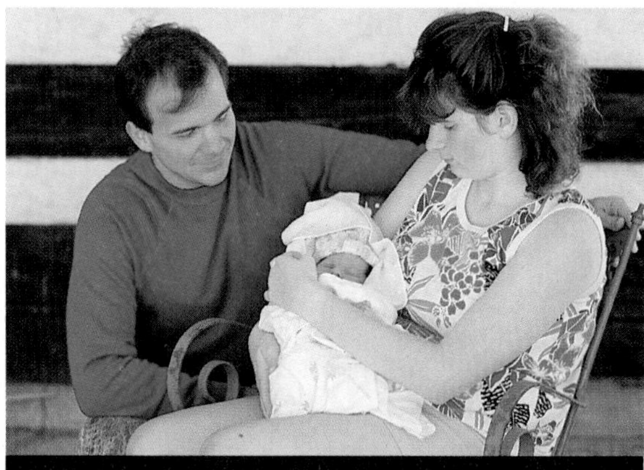

Positive interaction between an infant and parents can produce a happy, good-natured child.

Hence, while our unique experiences and cultural learning have a strong impact on our self-concept, these experiences, combined with our personality predispositions, shape self-concept as we grow older. In the example of the two siblings, it is likely that they were born with different personality predispositions. The blending of their family experiences with these traits, then, led to one being more secure and out-going, and to the other being more shy and insecure.

Personality

What is personality? During adolescence and young adulthood there is much discussion about personality. "He has a great personality." "Her personality is zero." "Neither of them has any personality." What does all this mean?

Personality is the visible pattern of an individual's characteristics and behavior. It is not separate from a person's self-concept: it is the expression of one's self-concept. When a person has a positive self-concept it is usually expressed in a bright, pleasant disposition or personality. The personality we display is important because people react positively to a pleasant person. This tends to increase one's positive feeling of self. Thus, one's self-concept is strengthened by interactions with others (Figure 1-5).

Figure 1-5

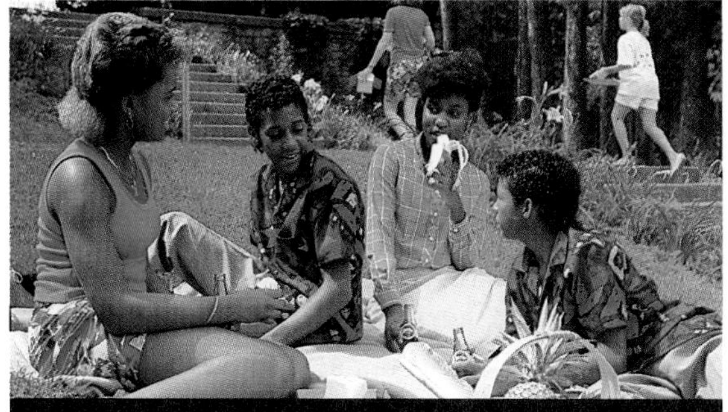

Interactions with others affect one's self-concept.

Personality, then, if it reflects your true feelings of self, is an indicator of your feelings about yourself as well as a strengthener of these feelings.

Roadblocks to Self-Exploration

It is sometimes difficult to explore how we really feel about our self-worth. There are often roadblocks or barriers that prevent us from seeing our true selves. The roles we play can cover or mask who we really are. The expected student behavior, the role expected on the job, and the responses given to family members can hide our true feelings and prevent us from being aware of who we are (Figure 1-6).

In addition, people become influenced by **external evaluations**. That is, people tend to rate themselves on the basis of outside rewards rather than rewards within themselves. Good grades, driving an expensive car, wearing the right clothes, and winning awards often are the most important indicators we use to evaluate ourselves. We begin to rely

Figure 1-6

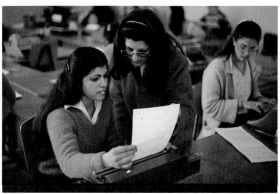

We often play expected roles as students in the classroom.
UNRWA Photo

on these evaluations to determine our worth rather than using our inner feelings about ourselves.

Our real self, hidden by roles and external evaluation, can be compared to the construction of a rose, as illustrated in Figure 1-7. Inside is the real center of the rose (or the self), the real "me," with layers of petals surrounding the center. The layers represent the roles we play and the external evaluations we apply to ourselves. Yet, the layers (and the roles) are a significant part of the rose (self). It is sometimes hard to find the real person at the center of these roles.

It can be threatening to reveal our real self. The "outer show" may be more acceptable than the "inner know." An individual who shows many outward signs of confidence, assertiveness, and strength may be more pleased with this self than with the true inner feelings of insecurity, meekness, and dissatisfaction. It takes courage to explore and assess your definition of self, particularly when these definitions are inconsistent with what we think others expect or think of us.

Figure 1-7

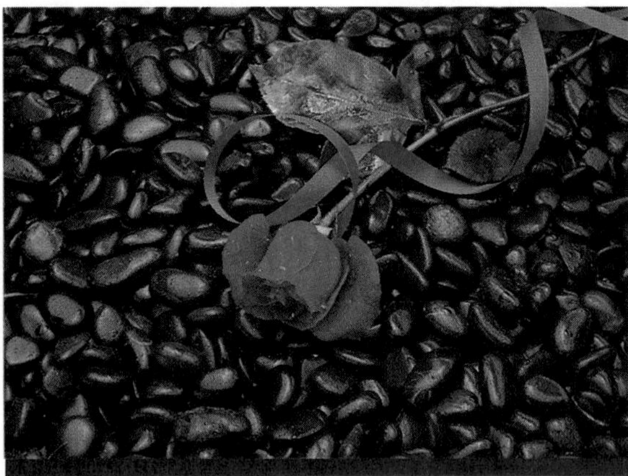

Our real self-concept is sometimes hidden by the many outer roles we play: brother or sister, son or daughter, student, athlete, employee, boyfriend or girlfriend, musician, church member, club leader, neighbor, camper, etc.

ASSESSING SELF-CONCEPT

If it takes so much courage and it's so difficult, why bother to assess your self-concept? Martin Buber, the philosopher, said, "Every person born into the world represents something new, something that never existed before, something original and unique." Buber also said that it is everyone's duty to know these uniquenesses and that everyone should fulfill their potential in the world. A responsibility to humankind is Buber's reasoning for assessing self-concept.

Another reason for learning more about our self-concept is that, to some degree, nearly all human relationships are based on our definition of self. Until we can define who we are, it is difficult to extend ourselves to others. This point will be discussed further in Part Two, "Forming Interpersonal Relationships."

The quest for knowing more about ourselves is continuous because our individual selves change and grow. Periodic rests in which we assess our feelings about ourselves are essential if we want to build the best possible relationships with others.

A major reason for assessment of self-concept is found in Shakespeare's *Hamlet:* ". . . to thine own self be true." No matter what definition of self you reveal to teachers, classmates, or parents, you must be honest with yourself if you are to gain from the self-assessment practices. Exercise this self-honesty as you read and think about Figure 1-8, the Personal Trait Checklist and Figure

1-9, Assessment of Personal Strengths and Weaknesses.

The Personal Trait Checklist and the Assessment of Personal Strengths and Weaknesses should help you gain some awareness of yourself. You may be pleased or discouraged about your findings. (If you are discouraged, remember that you can't change your behavior until you're aware of it. So you've made a big step already!)

Figure 1-8

Personal Trait Checklist

	Agree	Disagree
1. I worry a lot	_____	_____
2. I always finish things that I start	_____	_____
3. I like being female (male)	_____	_____
4. I'm an interesting person to be with	_____	_____
5. I don't like the way I look	_____	_____
6. I don't seem to have any ambition	_____	_____
7. Sometimes I let my anger get the best of me	_____	_____
8. I handle most of my problems pretty well	_____	_____
9. I generally find it hard to get along with people	_____	_____
10. I'm basically a healthy person	_____	_____
11. I tend to get jealous easily	_____	_____
12. People can depend on me	_____	_____
13. I'm more comfortable when someone tells me what to do	_____	_____
14. Criticism tends to upset me	_____	_____
15. I solve problems easily	_____	_____
16. I feel reasonably confident about myself	_____	_____
17. I tend to be afraid of meeting new people	_____	_____
18. I give in easily	_____	_____
19. I'm basically smart	_____	_____
20. I don't care what happens to me	_____	_____
21. I feel left out a lot of the time	_____	_____
22. When I make up my mind, I stick to it	_____	_____
23. I'm a nervous person	_____	_____
24. I'm a helpful person	_____	_____

Figure 1-9

Assessment of Personal Strengths and Weaknesses

1. My best trait is __________.
2. People care about me when __________.
3. I am helpful to others when I __________.
4. I like to spend my time __________.
5. I am hurtful to others when I __________.
6. I like myself when __________.
7. The first thing people notice about me is __________.
8. My worst trait is __________.
9. I am happiest when __________.
10. I am basically unkind when __________.
11. What I want most from a friendship is __________.
12. What I like best about myself is __________.
13. I dislike myself when __________.
14. A friendship is __________.
15. If I could change one of my habits it would be __________.
16. What I like least about myself is __________.
17. I feel I am not smart because __________.
18. I am unhappiest when __________.
19. I feel I am smart because __________.

Many of the points in these activities reflect or imply the influence of others. Other people—especially those we care most about—are a mirror for us. They reflect our behavior back to us. This is known as the "looking-glass self." If your friends, for example, make you feel accepted and wanted and treat you as if you are worthwhile, you will see yourself as adequate, competent, lovable, and worthwhile. In essence, your friends are a mirror in which you can see your own image.

The important role others play in knowing our true self becomes even more clear when we describe characteristics we desire in ourselves. Most of these desired characteristics require interactions with other humans. Generosity, helpfulness, love, kindness, affection, and possessing a sense of humor are some of the characteristics that require interaction with other human beings.

A tool to get a clearer feeling of various aspects of our self-concept is **Johari's Window**. This tool, illustrated in Figure 1-10,

	Known to Self	Not Known to Self
Known to Others	Public Self	Unaware Self
Not Known to Others	Private Self	Potential Self

Figure 1-10
Johari's Window is a tool for assessing your self-concept.

helps us to reveal four specific parts or arenas of our self-concept or personality in relation to how much we reveal to others: a public self, a private self, an unaware self, and a potential self. As you see from the diagram, the **public self** is known to both yourself and others. Such parts of your personality would be totally nonthreatening. For example, you want to be in the school play and you have made this known to others.

The **unaware self** is known to others but not known to you. This is a blind area to you. Examples include the fact that you have a pleasing singing voice or that you make others feel important because you listen attentively when they speak. Others may be aware of these qualities in you, while you are not.

A third area is the **private self**. It is known to you but not known to others. You may feel too threatened to reveal this self because it may reveal weaknesses in you, and thereby, leave you vulnerable to criticisms from others. Examples include the fact that you're terrified of storms, or that you are secretly afraid that no one will want to have a serious relationship with you. No one should be *forced* to reveal aspects of the private self. The private self provides safety for you. However, as relationships with others become more comfortable, individuals more willingly share their feelings and move toward the public arena.

The fourth area is the **potential self** which is unknown to both yourself and others. For example, you may possess skills in making people feel comfortable and at ease, but, because you have not tried to do these things yourself, you and others have no way of knowing that you possess these skills. Ideally the potential self may become known to the self and to others. Try to think of one aspect of yourself you could put in your personal Johari's Window.

Realize that you will only be able to complete the public self and the private self boxes. A friend, parent, or other person will need to complete your unaware self. (This will then need to move to the public self arena because you will become aware of it.) Your potential self will remain blank. Chapter 2, "Becoming a Fully Functioning Person," will reveal some things in the potential self arena.

Self-concept is an encompassing and important aspect of our interpersonal lives and our relationships with others. Exploring and assessing our own definition of self is difficult but beneficial. Having gained awareness of ourselves we can work to strengthen and build a more positive self-concept.

STRENGTHENING SELF-CONCEPT

Exploring and assessing self-concept have shown you that self-concepts can be positive or negative. Differences between positive and negative self-concepts can be seen in the comparisons shown below.

Fortunately self-concept is not a permanent thing like eye color or blood type. Self-concept can be altered. A person with poor or low-level feelings *can* change those feelings. For example, you can build and strengthen your self-concept by doing something creative as shown in Figure 1-11. *You* can raise your self-concept, but no one can raise it for you. Teachers will often say that students need to improve their self-concept. In other words, teachers want to provide the experiences and opportunities for others to feel better about themselves. But the individuals themselves must alter their own self-concept.

Improvement of your self-concept can occur through conscious action. Your definition of self can be made more positive by accepting yourself, highlighting your strengths, changing what can be changed, and encouraging continuous self-growth. For example, through exercise you can improve your aerobic capacity, raise your energy level, tone your muscles, and become more alert as shown in Figure 1-12.

Acceptance of Self

Recognizing strengths and weaknesses and accepting them as part of you is the first step

Characteristics of a Positive Self-Concept	Characteristics of a Negative Self-Concept
Belief that you are a worthwhile person.	Belief that you are not a worthwhile person.
Consideration of your possibilities and potentials.	Consideration of your limits and lack of potentials.
Emphasis on individual strengths.	Emphasis on individual weaknesses.
Formation of a positive picture of yourself.	Formation of a negative picture of yourself.
Exploration of options to make wise decisions.	Failure to explore options to make wise decisions.

Figure 1-11

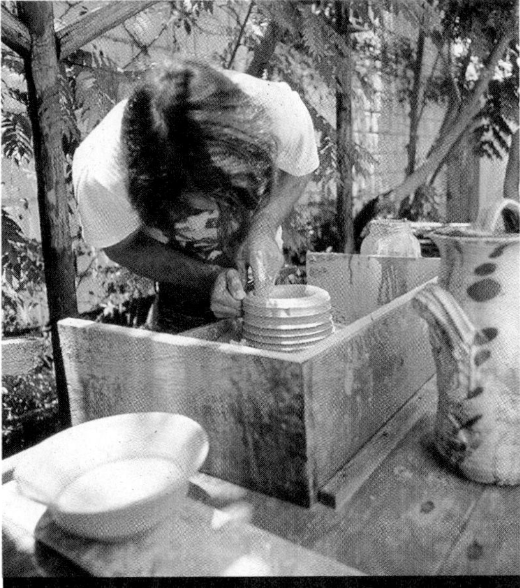

Doing something creative or trying something new builds and strengthens self-concept.
Florida Department of Commerce
Division of Tourism

Figure 1-12

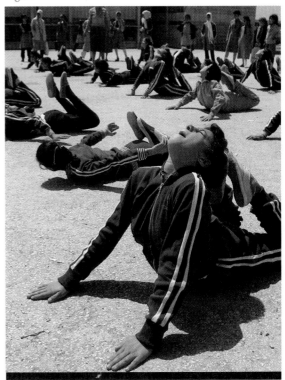

An aerobics class can change what needs to be changed—self-concept!
UNRWA Photo

in strengthening self-concept. This basic advice sounds easier than it is. It may be difficult to conclude that you may not be the best-looking student in the school. It may take courage to say that you do not have the artistic talent you would like to have. It may be a personal struggle to conclude that you will not receive a college scholarship. Nothing is easy about learning to live with a limitation. Yet, wasting time and energy on unchangeable characteristics is foolish.

The acceptance of self provides solid groundwork for forming relationships with others. Learning that we can't change all our characteristics helps to prevent us from trying to change the characteristics of others with whom we form close relationships. Thus, we can improve our ability to accept others for who they are, rather than expecting them to change to what *we* would like them to be.

Highlighting Strengths

Emphasizing those areas of our personality in which we have excellence can improve our definition of self and thus strengthen our personality. On the Personal Trait Checklist that you completed, you may have concentrated on the negative aspects of yourself and totally overlooked the positive qualities that you possess. We need to be more willing to look for these strengths and focus on our accomplishments. Several mechanisms can be developed that can encourage us to see these strengths. Try keeping a "Log of Strengths." This is a notebook or diary in which you can record those positive accomplishments that you may overlook generally in your daily activities. Search diligently for these strengths. Something as simple as a good attendance record in school is often overlooked by people, yet it is a very important quality to have when seeking a job. Other examples are promptness, assisting others, keeping your word, refraining from gossip, or the ability to remember and recall things. By keeping a log of strengths in which we record such examples, we begin to see a long list of things we *can* do and do well. Share and trade the log of strengths with friends, classmates, parents, and teachers, and ask them to add comments about strengths you possess. You will soon see that these highlighted strengths add up quickly.

Another way to highlight our strengths is to review memorabilia or items that we choose to keep to remind us of pleasant situations. A collection of your personal memorabilia will probably show that you have saved and cherished those items that show some of your accomplishments. These items might be certificates commending your efforts, various awards, remembrances from neighbors and friends, and photos and other items that recall past experiences. Reviewing such items points out those areas in which we have strengths and accomplishments and in which we can continue to accomplish in the future.

Another technique to highlight strengths is to work in small groups to point out individuals' positive features. Each person writes his or her name on a sheet of paper. The papers are passed among the group members who write the strengths and positive personality features of each individual. When the papers are returned, individuals are often surprised at some of the strengths others reveal about them.

Change What Can Be Changed

We discussed earlier that acceptance of self is necessary to strengthen self-concept. It is essential to accept those aspects of personality that can't be changed. At the same time, it is essential to determine those areas of our self-concepts that are weak but can be strengthened. An example of changing what can be changed relates to body structure. Though we may not be able to alter our basic inherited body structure, we can alter our attitude about our bodies. By focusing on building a healthy, physically fit body, regardless of body structure, we can change what can be changed.

We learned earlier that personality predispositions, cultural learning, and unique experiences were major factors in self-concept formation. It is difficult for us to alter basic personality traits and the cultural learning that we have experienced since infancy. However, we can add many experiences that could enhance and strengthen our self-concept. Look at the sample experience chart below (Figure 1-13). This chart points out many experiences that might strengthen self-concept. What experiences have helped to strengthen your self-concept?

Figure 1-13

Experience Chart

1. Watch the night sky from a planetarium.
2. Collect funds for a civic cause.
3. Scan the newspaper for upcoming activities or meetings you would enjoy.
4. Sit in the waiting room of a hospital just to observe.
5. Beautify your community.
6. Write to your representative in Congress.
7. Try out for a play or musical presentation.
8. Offer assistance to a neighbor.
9. Get up before dawn to watch the sunrise.
10. Spend some volunteer time at a nursing home.
11. Assist in a political campaign.
12. Listen to an older relative trace your family history.
13. Accompany an aging person to a park.
14. Publicly support a cause by making a speech or public appearance.
15. Visit an art museum.
16. Join a physical fitness group.
17. Plant a vegetable garden.
18. Enroll in an art or craft class.
19. Observe people caring for animals at a fair, a pet show, or the zoo.
20. Study extra hard for an important test in school.

Continuous Self-Growth

Exploring, assessing, and strengthening self-concept is an ongoing process. Throughout life, individuals must strive to understand who they are and how they want to lead their lives. Results of this continuous striving produce self-growth—changing and growing in order to be the best person one can be. Self-growth will be explored in Chapter 2.

WRAPPING IT UP

The total set of beliefs, values, and feelings about one's own strengths and weaknesses is the ***self-concept***. The self-concept is a vital building block for establishing meaningful interpersonal relationships with family members, friends, and other people in our lives. Positive self-concepts promote healthy personal development and satisfying relationships with others. Negative self-concepts, on the other hand, are barriers to our growth as individuals and reduce our chances of building strong relationships with other people. *Personality* is the pattern of an individual's visible characteristics and behavior; it is the expression of one's self-concept that others can see.

The formation of one's self-concept and personality is based largely on a process of *cultural learning*. It is also based on one's inborn tendencies to behave in a certain way, known as *personality predispositions*. Experiences in our families, in school, and with our friends shape our self-concepts. Self-concepts are more positive when others treat us with respect, praise, and love. Self-concepts are more negative when others criticize us and treat us as if we have little value and cannot achieve. Positive self-concepts lead to more pleasant personalities and interactions with others. Such interactions, in turn, strengthen the positive self-concept in a cycle of reinforcement.

It is important that we explore and come to understand our self-concepts. Often we hide our "true selves" from others and from ourselves by hiding behind roles that we play. We also tend to judge ourselves on the basis of external factors—such as possessions, grades, and awards—which may not be a good reflection of who we really are inside. In assessing our self-concept, we must try to accept those limitations that cannot be changed. We should also search for our personal strengths and try to build upon them. Other aspects of our personality and self-concept are weak and can be improved if we are willing to make the effort. Searching for ways to improve weak areas is a life-long process. It is a difficult task to assess and improve our self-concepts. It is also a beneficial and rewarding experience to be able to strengthen and build a more positive self-concept.

Exploring Dimensions of Chapter One

For Review

1• On a separate piece of paper, answer true or false to the following statements:

a. Once a negative self-concept has been formed there is nothing you can do to change it.

b. The roles we play sometimes hide or mask our self-concept.

c. External evaluations are ratings that people give themselves based on outside rewards.

d. The potential self is the part of the self-concept of which both you and others are aware.

e. Personality has little relationship with the self-concept.
f. Self-concept depends entirely on how our family members treat us.

2. For each statement above that you said is "False," write down an explanation for why it is false. Then, write a substitute statement that is true.
3. Can you raise the self-concept of someone else? Explain your answer.
4. Why might it by difficult to explore your self-concept?

For Consideration

1. Write a paragraph explaining how self-concept can affect relationships with others.
2. If parents and other adults help formulate children's self-concept, might children affect adults' self-concepts? Discuss situations in which young people affect their parents' self-concepts, their teachers' self-concepts, aging people's self-concepts. Consider both positive and negative self-concepts.
3. List ten phrases that are common to people with high self-concepts. How many are part of your normal vocabulary? How many can you adopt to help remind yourself that you are a worthwhile person?

For Application

1. After determining some of your strengths and weaknesses, promise yourself you will find ways to work on your weaknesses and to continue to develop your areas of strength in order to raise your total self-concept.
2. List some of your favorite television, movie, and fictional characters. Discuss whether these characters are generally good or bad or whether they have a variety of personality characteristics. Is the good character only good? Does the bad character have only negative traits? Do characters seem more real when they have both positive and negative traits? Why might writers and directors create characters in which we see only one side of the characters' personalities?
3. List some theme songs for high self-concept people and for low self-concept people. People with high self-concepts, for example, sing "Everything's Coming Up Roses," "If My Friends Could See Me Now," and "Fame." Low self-concept people might sing "I Got a Right to Sing the Blues," "Rainy Days and Mondays," and "A Day Late and a Dollar Short." Can songs or the attitudes they produce affect people's feelings about themselves? Try some experiments in class to see if music can have an effect on our feelings.

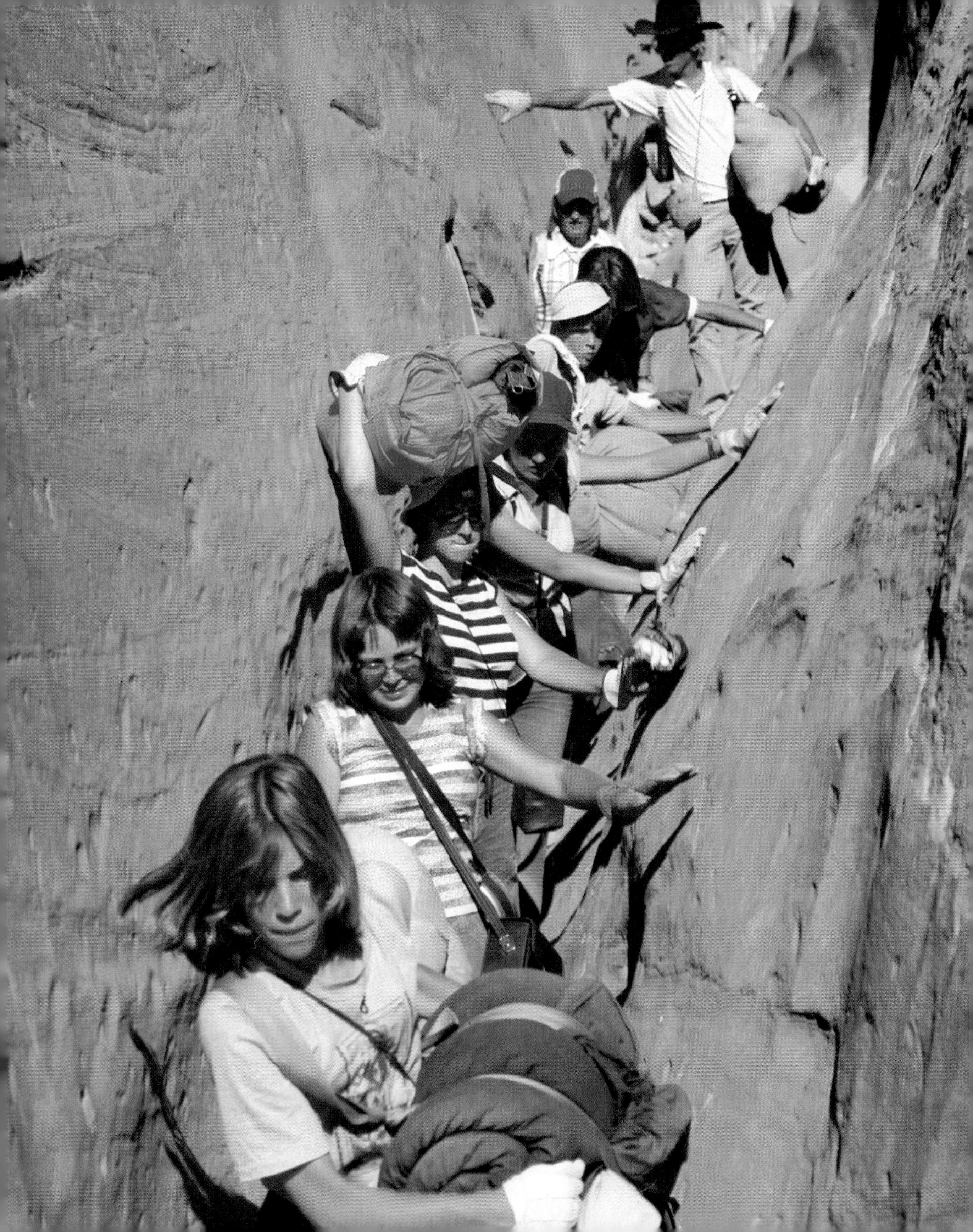

two

BECOMING A FULLY FUNCTIONING PERSON

This chapter provides information that will help you to:

- Identify the five basic human needs.
- Explain how these needs form a hierarchy.
- Describe a fully functioning person.
- Identify behaviors and characteristics that can lead people to function more fully.

Beth Heiden was the 1979 Women's World Speed Skating Champion. She was expected to excel at the 1980 Winter Olympics. The news media predicted that she would win several gold medals. Instead, Beth won only one bronze medal.

She experienced a high level of stress and frustration which were magnified by the press. The competition and pressure of the Olympics and the demanding news media appeared to be too much for Beth. She was led from the awards platform sobbing. But, Beth used this experience to help her develop and strengthen her potential. "It was a learning experience. I learned a lot about myself and it toughened me," she said after the Olympics. Beth refused offers for commercial endorsements in which she could have earned large sums of money. She said she was too involved with her engineering studies. She began training as a racing cyclist by riding 40 to 50 miles a day. She entered more than 20 races. In the summer of 1980, she won the Women's World Cycling Championship in France. Beth is also involved in cross-country skiing. As a collegiate competitor, Beth was named to the U.S. Ski Team's "talent pool."

We cannot all be like Beth Heiden. Yet, we all have talents, skills, and abilities that we could be using in many ways. Too often these talents lie dormant, or we use only a small portion of our potential.

CASE IN POINT

Susan has a definite skill in organizing, planning, and management. She has successfully managed several community money-making activities and has shown leadership capabilities in school and church activities. But Susan will not expand these talents. She will not run for a public office, nor will she consider a job in a management field.

Pete has always been able to make people laugh. He used his quick wit and ability to mimic throughout his school years to get laughs from students and teachers and often to help a group overcome a tense situation. Pete has never used this skill in skits, plays, or in acting. He has never auditioned for any theatrical presentations where his natural talents could be developed even further.

Susan and Pete are not alone in using fewer of their skills and personal resources than they are capable of doing. Psychologists estimate that humans use only a relatively small amount of their potential abilities. It is difficult to determine the personal waste of talent as well as the possible loss to humanity because of unused potential. Consider the world problems of crime, limited resources, disease, and social unrest that might be solved if humans used only half of their potential!

Psychologist Carl Rogers used the term **fully functioning individuals** to describe people who want to develop themselves as far as their potential allows.

Why do so few of us use our talents fully? Why aren't more people considered fully functioning individuals? What blocks or prevents humans from being fully functioning?

HUMAN NEEDS

All human beings have basic human needs. One of these basic needs is the need to be fully functioning. However, other needs must be met before a person can meet the need to be fully functioning.

Psychologist Abraham Maslow described five basic human needs that follow in a particular order called a hierarchy of needs.

A hierarchy, as shown in Figure 2-1, can be thought of as levels of mountain climbing. Humans must fulfill each level before going on to the next level. Maslow and others feel that many people spend so much effort and energy meeting the early level needs that they may never get to the level of fully functioning—what Maslow termed "self-actualization."

As you consider these needs, be aware that all persons, regardless of culture or background, have the same basic needs. However, they will fulfill their needs in different ways. For example, all humans need physical shelter. But depending on the climate and socially accepted standards, people may live in elaborate condominiums, in tents, or in caves. The need is the same, but the means for meeting the need will differ.

Physical Needs

The physical needs are the most basic of human needs. They are the things your body needs in order to maintain good health. Physical needs include food, water, shelter, clothing, sleep, and exercise.

CASE IN POINT

Phil works after school and on weekends in a men's clothing store. His hours were increased last week because of the holiday season. Phil's school schedule is heavy because he is carrying an extra course load in order to graduate early. Phil also is taking an evening computer course at the community college so he can earn college credit. Phil is finding that his schedule does not allow him enough time for necessary sleep and rest. He can't concentrate in class, he is sluggish at work, and he nearly had an accident driving home last night. Phil's unmet physical need for relaxation and sleep prevents him from successfully carrying out his daily activities.

Karen was disgusted with herself for being overweight. Once again she found it nearly impossible to fasten her skirt because she was three pounds over her previous week's weight. She decided that grapefruit and black coffee for breakfast and cottage cheese and coffee for dinner would eliminate her weight problem quickly. After two days on this diet, Karen

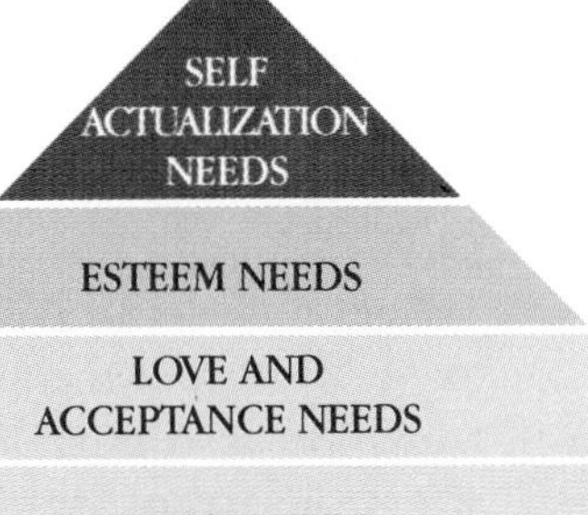

Figure 2-1
The five basic human needs form Maslow's hierarchy. Physical and safety needs, the most essential, must be met before other needs can be considered.

noticed that her hands were shaking while writing in class. She had difficulty concentrating. She also found that she could not participate fully at chorus practice. Her knees became so weak that she thought she was going to fall down. Karen's physical need for food is demanding her body's attention. She will not be able to attend to her other needs until she meets this physical need for food.

Figure 2-2

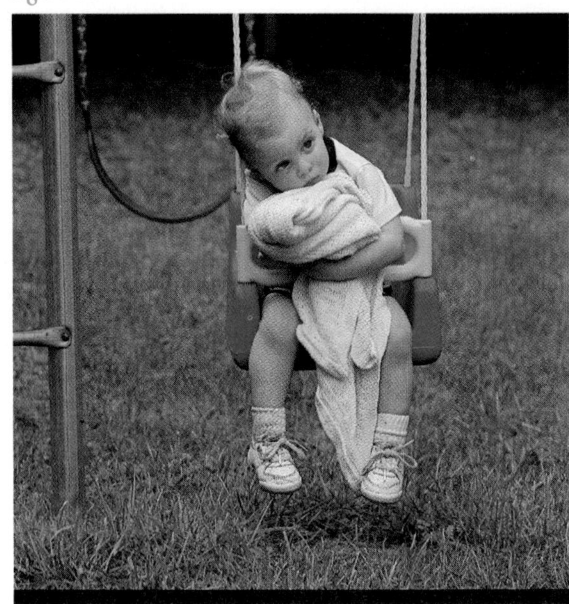

An infant's blanket provides comfort and feelings of security.

Safety Needs

Humans need to feel safe from crime and violence. They need to feel secure in their environment and protected from financial difficulties. The means for meeting safety needs may differ by age and by culture. An infant feels secure when clutching a blanket (Figure 2-2). A preschooler feels secure with a stuffed toy. A senior citizen feels more secure when pension checks are received promptly. A sheep farmer is more secure with watch dogs to guard against coyotes. And you may feel more secure when attending a dance at your own school where you know more people than at a neighboring school where you feel like a stranger. Until safety and security needs are met, it is impossible to develop abilities and personality or to excel in any other aspect of life.

Love and Acceptance Needs

People have a need for love, affection, and acceptance. They need to feel needed and accepted by others. Being a friend, being a family member, being a community and group participant helps meet this need.

The ways to meet love and acceptance needs alter as one grows older. Small children receive nearly all their love and acceptance needs from their parents and/or other caregivers. As children grow, they begin to gain acceptance from their friends, or peers. In the elementary school years, children often form small groups of "best" friends (Figure 2-3) or form clubs with special names and special meeting places. These activities satisfy the need for affection and belonging.

Family love and close friendships continue to be important through the teen years. Most teenagers also begin to meet their love and affection needs through members of the opposite sex. This doesn't necessarily mean that all teens have strong attachments or date steadily. It means that teens begin to look for the attention of members of the opposite sex

Figure 2-3

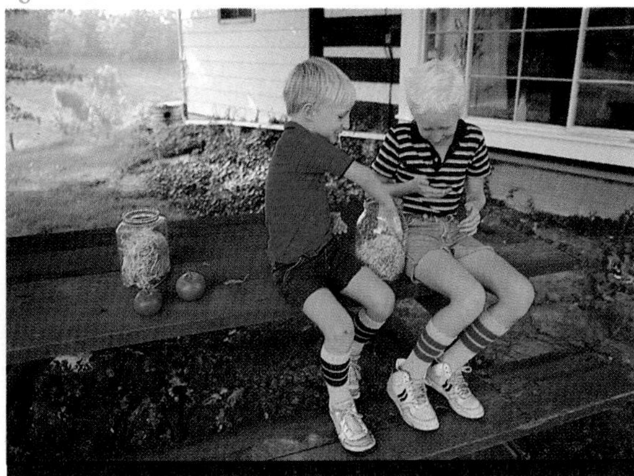

Best friends fulfill the need for acceptance and love.

to meet their love, affection, and acceptance needs.

The need for love often leads to serious commitment and marriage. Through all stages of life, humans need to receive and give love, affection, and acceptance.

CASE IN POINT

Mr. Carlson, the sour town librarian, was known for his unwillingness to smile or give a pleasant response. When a group of students presented him with a birthday cake, his unfriendly behavior changed to appreciation, joy, and affection for the students. The students' acceptance and friendliness helped to meet Mr. Carlson's need for love and acceptance.

Esteem Needs

The esteem need is the human need to feel important and of worth—that is, to feel valued. When you feel that others respect and approve of you, you feel esteem and respect for yourself. You feel good about yourself. Esteem is closely related to self-concept, which was discussed in Chapter 1. A positive self-concept also brings about esteem. When your esteem needs are met, you are less threatened and you can more readily appreciate and respect others.

Esteem needs are met in different ways for different people. Some of your friends meet their esteem need by excelling in sports, such as tennis, swimming, or skiing (Figure 2-4). Other friends may use dramatics and public speaking to meet their esteem needs. You may know people who find helping others either as an employee or as a volunteer to be a rewarding experience that fulfills their need to feel worthwhile.

Figure 2-4

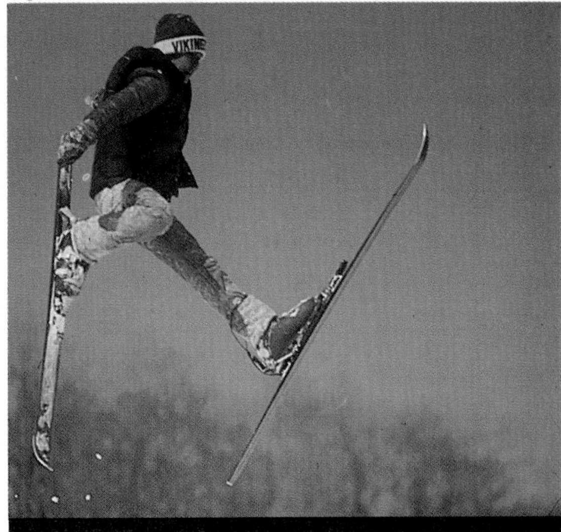

Some people meet esteem needs by excelling in sports. The exhilaration skiers feel when executing difficult maneuvers gives them the confidence to pursue other life challenges.
Indiana Dept. of Commerce

When your esteem needs have been met you have the confidence to continue to develop your own personality—to become what you want to be.

Self-Actualization Needs

Self-actualization needs are the highest level of human needs. All the previously mentioned needs must be met, at least in part, before you can be a self-actualized individual.

Self-actualized people are reaching toward their full potential: all talents have been used toward the goal of becoming the most effective human beings they can be. Self-actualized people have the confidence to express their beliefs and to stick to them. They are not afraid of change. In fact, self-actualized people often seek to create changes in the lives of people in order to make them better. Self-actualized people get involved in projects and activities devoted to helping others. They feel strong enough about themselves to reach out to others. Do you know community members, a teacher at your school, a relative or friend whom you consider fully functioning, or self-actualized? These are unique human beings who are functioning at high levels.

STRIVING TO BECOME MORE FULLY FUNCTIONING

We have said that the five basic needs compose a hierarchy, or a step-like process. The lower, most primary needs must be met before you can meet higher level needs. For example, people cannot become fully functioning when they are continuously worrying about where they will get their next meal. Persons who continuously fear for their personal safety cannot meet their need for self-confidence and esteem. Excessive time spent on meeting the more basic needs prevents efforts to meet higher level needs.

In our society most people have their primary needs (physical needs and safety needs) met most of the time. But, according to scientists, few of us use more than a tiny portion of our potential. How can we begin to use and develop more of our potential? What behaviors or actions help us move toward becoming a more fully functioning individual?

Psychologists have indicated several behaviors and attitudes that are typical of the self-actualized person. As these traits are discussed, assess yourself. Do you exhibit these behaviors? Could you begin to develop these traits? Can you see long- and short-term benefits for you and society if you could begin to develop such characteristics?

Acceptance of Self and Others

Acceptance of self and others is necessary to become fully functioning. Having a clear knowledge and acceptance of personal strengths and weaknesses is a key characteristic of those who have developed toward their full potential. Fully functioning people have a positive feeling toward others. They appreciate the worth of all human beings even though they may not accept particular behavior and actions of all persons. Acceptance of limits or flaws in ourselves, our friends, and our loved ones is essential for good mental health (Figure 2-5).

Spotlight on issues

Taking Action

The words proactive and reactive describe personal action or behavior. **Proactive** behavior is characterized by action initiated to make things happen. **Reactive** behavior is action taken in response to an event. People in leadership roles often possess proactive behavior; likewise, followers usually exhibit reactive behavior. Seeking out and creating new opportunities is proactive behavior. Responding to available opportunities is reactive behavior.

We need both proactive and reactive people. Good leaders as well as good followers are necessary. For example, planners and instigators need those who can successfully implement their ideas.

Seldom is a family member totally reactive or proactive. Most of us experience some part of our lives in which we are proactive, and some part in which we are reactive. At times, proactive behavior is desirable and should be encouraged. There are also many instances when such behavior is inappropriate. Here, reactive behavior may be more proper. On different occasions different kinds of behavior are welcomed and others are discouraged.

Personal behavior that is both proactive and reactive is probably the most healthful behavior for family members and people in general. Fully functioning individuals need to experience some behavior in which they act, display leadership, and make things happen. Personal behavior involving little proactive or reactive behavior is probably the least healthful behavior for people. Those who fail to act or react but instead accept all situations placed before them can become mentally unstable. Some of the most desperate and unfortunate people are those who feel they have no control and no means to change their lives. They seem unable to find a positive way to act or react to the situations in which they find themselves. Gaining control of at least some part of your life can help you to move toward a more positive existence.

Figure 2-5

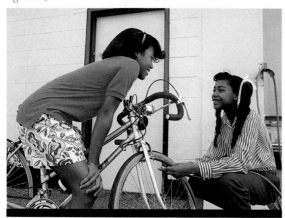

Acceptance of ourselves and others is essential to becoming fully functioning people.

CASE IN POINT

Sarah's mother is an alcoholic. Throughout her early teen years Sarah had difficulty accepting her mother's condition. Sarah did all she could to change her mother's behavior. But in doing so, Sarah has left much of her own potential undeveloped. As Sarah grows older she realizes that even though she'll help her mother if she can, she must accept her mother's condition and not let it prevent her own development.

Sometimes as people enter a serious relationship, they have difficulty accepting certain characteristics or behaviors of their partner. Therefore, they want to change or alter their partner's behavior. Such changes seldom work. It is basically healthier for both persons if acceptance without judgment can be a part of the relationship.

Seeking New Experiences

Fully functioning persons are involved in new ideas and activities. They are not only willing to try new experiences but they seek out opportunities to experience new situations. They function as *proactors* rather than as reactors. If the experience is not totally successful, they do not feel defeated. Having experienced the situation is often the reward for the fully functioning person.

CASE IN POINT

Becky wanted to take riding lessons. She had never been on a horse or even been close to one, but riding was something she had always wanted to do. Becky saved her money and signed up for a series of six lessons. Though she may never become an expert rider, Becky had a great time, learned a lot about horses, and met some really interesting people.

Todd is not as eager for new experiences as Becky. When Todd's friend asked him to go to a Russian art show at the downtown museum, Todd laughed and said he wasn't interested. After some persuading, Todd went along with his friend and found he really enjoyed the exhibit. He also liked the other museum displays and wondered why he had never come to the museum before. Todd enjoyed this new experience. As his personality develops, Todd may learn to purposefully seek situations that allow him to experience new ideas, sights, and relationships. Todd may become a **proactor** rather than just a **reactor**.

Some people have difficulty seeking new experiences and trying new things. It is often easier to maintain the **status quo**—a Latin term meaning the existing state of affairs. It takes less energy and less courage to stay just as we are rather than change. Unfortunately few exciting, challenging things happen when we maintain the status quo. Opportunity for stimulating thoughts and the creation of new goals can be increased when we seek new experiences.

Eliminating Psychological Crutches

A psychological crutch is a device people use to prevent themselves from developing more fully. These crutches are excuses given to others and to ourselves for why we can't or why we won't be able to do a particular thing.

The crutch we verbalize usually has a different meaning behind it. Consider these commonly used crutches and their real meaning:

In many cases we believe the psychological crutch and we do not give thought to the real feeling behind what we say.

CASE IN POINT

Louise has a handicapped brother. Louise's family shares in the time needed to take care of the child. Louise uses the necessity for extra care as a crutch to limit her own development. Louise didn't audition for the chorus in the school musical. She told her friends, "I would really like to audition, but I just can't. I have to take care of my brother." What Louise really meant was, "I'm afraid to risk trying. I may fail. My brother provides a good excuse for me." Louise is limiting her own experiences and development while she uses her brother's handicap as a crutch.

Stated Crutch	Real Meaning
"I just don't have the time."	"I'm not willing to make the time or to give up something else."
"My parents won't let me."	"I've never asked them, but it makes a good excuse since I'm afraid to do it."
"I'm not good at that."	"I've no idea whether or not I could do it, but I'm afraid to take the risk of failing."
"That's stupid! Who would want to do that?"	"I'd really like to try but I'm afraid I'll fail, so I'll ridicule the whole idea."
"I don't have the skill to do that."	"I've never tried anything like that, and I'm afraid I would look like a fool."
"Only brainy (or dumb, or city, or country, or other groupings of people) kids do that."	"I'm afraid I'll be associated with people who make me uncomfortable. It's too big a risk for me."
"My boyfriend (girlfriend) wouldn't let me."	"He or she might laugh or make fun of the idea especially if I fail."

Spotlight on issues

Getting Help

No man is an island.
John Donne

Fully functioning or self-actualized people are self-sufficient, confident, and responsible individuals who are capable of taking care of themselves. In most cases, this is true. However, from time to time even the most fully functioning person needs help solving a problem or reaching a goal. No matter who we are, each of us depends to some degree on others to help us through tough times.

Recognizing when you need help and where to turn to get help are important life skills to have. At what point does a person say, "This problem is too much for me to handle. I think I need help!"? First, you must realize that seeking help is not a sign of personal weakness. Rather, seeking help is a sign that you are able to recognize your limitations (an important quality in Chapter 1). It means that you realize that you need more than just yourself to get you through the problem. Usually a person should seek help when personal resources are not sufficient to handle a situation or solve a problem. Such resources as time, money, skills, and knowledge may not be enough for you at certain times. Consider the following examples:

Jesse is studying for an important algebra test. He needs a high score to earn an "A" for the year. Naturally, he is very nervous. As he reads his math book the night before the test, Jesse realizes that he just doesn't understand a new section on equations. He gets very nervous and starts to panic. Soon he begins to confuse other things he thought he already knew. Jesse needs help. What can he do?

Missy was saving money for a school trip to Hawaii. She had worked hard to save the $750 needed for this special trip. One month before the trip, Missy's friend, Sheila, asked Missy if she could borrow $150 to buy some new clothes that were on sale. Sheila promised to pay Missy back in one week. Missy waited until the last minute to ask Sheila to pay her back. Much to Missy's disappointment, Sheila told her that she couldn't pay her back. It now looked as if Missy could not go on the school trip. Missy was angry and hurt. She needed help, but where should she turn?

Picture yourself in Jesse's or Missy's situation. Jesse lacked the resources of knowledge (to understand the tough section on equations) and time (the test was the next morning). Missy lacked the resources of money to go on the school trip to Hawaii. Both Jesse and Missy were capable individuals who had many of the qualities of fully functioning people. Yet, they both had genuine needs for help. What would you have done if you were in Jesse's or Missy's position?

In order to get help, it is important to know the places or people to whom you can turn. Your family members (brothers, sisters, parents), friends, teachers, school counselors and coaches, and a variety of community agencies are often excellent "extra resources" that a person has for getting help. Fortunately for Jesse, he telephoned his algebra classmate Rob. Jesse knew that Rob was a good student and would be able to help Jesse understand the equations. Missy went to her parents for help. They agreed to loan money to Missy so she could go on the trip. She agreed to pay back the loan in the six weeks following her return. Both Jesse's and Missy's parents were pleased to help, and Jesse and Missy both realized that someday they too might be able to help others by serving as "extra resources."

In addition to parents and friends, your own community has "extra resources" for special problems. These might include churches and synagogues, counseling agencies, police departments, and health clinics. The following is a list of special problems that some teenagers might face. Each involves a situation where help is needed. Where in your community could a person go to get help for each of these problems?

1• A person with a drug or alcohol problem.
2• A girl whose father is touching her in sexually inappropriate ways.
3• A friend who says that he feels like killing himself.
4• A boy whose father beats up on his mother, causing her physical injury.
5• A friend who thinks she might be pregnant.

Spotlight on issues

Drug and Alcohol Abuse

The use of harmful drugs and alcohol is usually related to a desire to prove independence or to belong. A negative self-concept is often related to use of harmful substances. These individuals lack respect for their own bodies, so they do not believe that using drugs or alcohol will really harm them. Drug and alcohol use is also related to friends and/or family members who influence decisions by examples, threats, antagonisms, or pressure.

People who become involved with drugs and alcohol believe that they can control their use and that they will never become physically addicted. They drift into drug and alcohol use without much thought about the consequences. Others who have considered the issues and chosen not to use drugs or alcohol feel that peer pressure is too strong, and that they do not have the strength to withstand the urgings of their friends.

Many people rationalize their use of drugs and alcohol. You've probably heard some of the following rationalizations.

"**My parents drink. It's only natural that I drink, too.**"

Your parent's drinking habits may be a role model, but do you do everything that your parents do? If your parents drink to excess, their drinking has probably had a negative effect on you as well as on themselves. Their use of alcohol may be the best rationale *not* to drink.

"**Abuse of drugs or alcohol is a personal issue. It's no one else's business.**"

Wrong! There are too many instances where the use of drugs or alcohol affects other people. Crime and traffic accidents are dramatically linked to drugs and alcohol. Industry also suffers from substance abuse by employees. For example, industry loses millions of dollars annually to alcohol-related employee problems. Friendships are lost and families are damaged by drug and alcohol abuse. Clearly, abuse of drugs or alcohol affects other people—often those most important to us.

"**Marijuana isn't addictive.**"

Some researchers say that marijuana isn't physically addicting. However, many people develop an emotional or psychological dependency on marijuana that is as strong as a physical addiction.

"I have to go along with my friends. Otherwise, I'll be left out."

Perhaps, but if your friends won't accept your personal values and behavior, maybe you need a new set of friends. A friend accepts you for who you are; a friend doesn't force or pressure you to go against your beliefs.

"Women seldom become alcoholics or drug abusers."

Wrong! Sexual equality exists in substance abuse. Females abuse drugs and alcohol as frequently as males.

Having Multiple Interests

Fully functioning people have many interests. They are interested in their occupation or career and many related areas. They are also aware and involved in fields far different from their occupations. For example, Senator Howard Baker, who was President Reagan's White House Chief of Staff, is also a photographer and has published several books on photography. This area is quite different from his career as a national public leader. Fully functioning individuals seem to continually build new interests by adding areas of interest in both their work and their hobbies as they move through the life cycle (Figure 2-6).

Figure 2-6

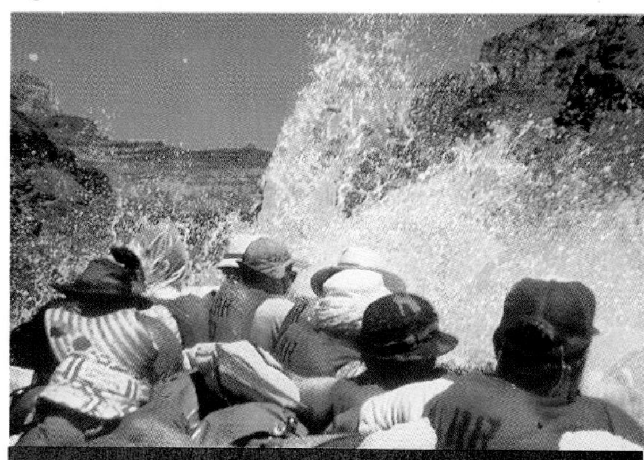

Fully functioning people develop areas of interest outside of their work and homes.

Arizona Tourist Bureau

Sometimes adolescents worry about how they can develop their career or occupational area when they have many interests or fields of involvement. You may wonder how all of your interests will fit into your life. Can a prospective veterinarian play the French horn for fun? Can an accountant enjoy and excel in sailing? Will a welder be able to continue with oil painting? Fully functioning people would answer, "Yes." They would encourage continuing all these interests. Vocations (the occupations in which people are regularly employed) and avocations (hobbies or vocations for enjoyment) are the means by which humans develop their potential to the maximum for the good of themselves and society.

Persons who are fully functional have assessed and strengthened their self-concepts. They accept themselves and others, they seek new experiences, they eliminate psychological crutches, and they have multiple interests. These behaviors and attitudes allow fully functioning persons to explore their values, establish personal goals, and have deliberate ways of making decisions. Chapter 3 will be helpful in exploring and developing values, goals, and decision-making skills.

WRAPPING IT UP

People who strive to develop themselves as far as their potential allows are known as *fully functioning individuals*. Such people are successful in meeting the basic needs that all humans have. These needs form a hierarchy and include needs for physical comfort, safety, love and acceptance, and esteem. Self-actualization needs are the highest of all human needs on the hierarchy. Self-actualizing people are confident in their own abilities. They are involved in activities. They help others and they accept the strengths and weaknesses in themselves and in others. Self-actualizing people also seek out new experiences. They have multiple interests and invite change in their lives.

A positive self-concept is essential in order to move up the needs hierarchy to the self-actualizing level. A positive self-concept promotes one's ability to satisfy needs for love, acceptance, and esteem. In turn, having these needs fulfilled enhances self-concept in a cycle of reinforcement. Fully functioning people also engage in *proactive* behavior as well as *reactive* behavior. They are able to distinguish those situations where each type of behavior is appropriate.

An important characteristic of fully functioning people is that they know when they need help. They are also aware of places to go and people to turn to when help is required. Getting help is necessary when a person lacks the resources to meet a need or solve a problem. Thus, fully functioning people are dependent upon others to help them meet their needs and strengthen their self-concepts.

Exploring Dimensions of Chapter Two

For Review

1• List the five basic human needs.
2• Explain why the first level needs are important.
3• Describe a fully functioning person.
4• Write a brief description of four basic approaches that can help people become more fully functioning.

For Consideration

1• In small groups discuss which of the five basic needs are being met in the following behaviors:

a. John's father came home and announced that he'd been promoted to supervisor.
b. George makes sure he changes his socks whenever his feet are wet and cold.
c. Pete gave Jo Ann a heart-shaped locket.
d. Rose uses dental floss after each meal.
e. Kelly looks through the newspaper to find her name listed in the "honor roll."
f. Randall plays first-chair violin in the school orchestra; he is the only teenager in the civic orchestra; and he continually strives to play better and better.
g. Sue waited for Elaine and Kate so they could walk home together after last night's meeting.

2• In small groups, discuss crutches that you have heard others use. What crutches do you use? What can you do to stop using these excuses?

For Application

1• With the help of your teacher, choose a volunteer project to work on for a four-week period. You might help in a nursing home, a nursery school, at a food pantry, as an elementary school aide, or in a relocation center. After four weeks, present an explanation to the class of the needs you saw being met in the volunteer program. Where were these needs on Maslow's hierarchy?

2• Start an "I Can" notebook. Become aware of all those areas in which you have skills and abilities. No skill is too small to list. Now ask several family members to make a list of your skills and abilities. (Don't let them see your list.) Do the same with several of your friends. Continually add to your own list. After a week, analyze the lists. Were some of these talents a surprise to you? Did other people list abilities you were not aware of? Which of the abilities and skills would you like to develop?

3• Interview at least two people to determine the degree to which they possess the characteristics of fully functioning persons. You will need to be able to explain the characteristics in order for the interviewees to respond. Determine their reaction to these characteristics, some examples of how they carry out these characteristics, and whether they would like to develop the characteristics more fully. Now interview yourself by asking yourself the same questions. Write a brief review of your feelings.

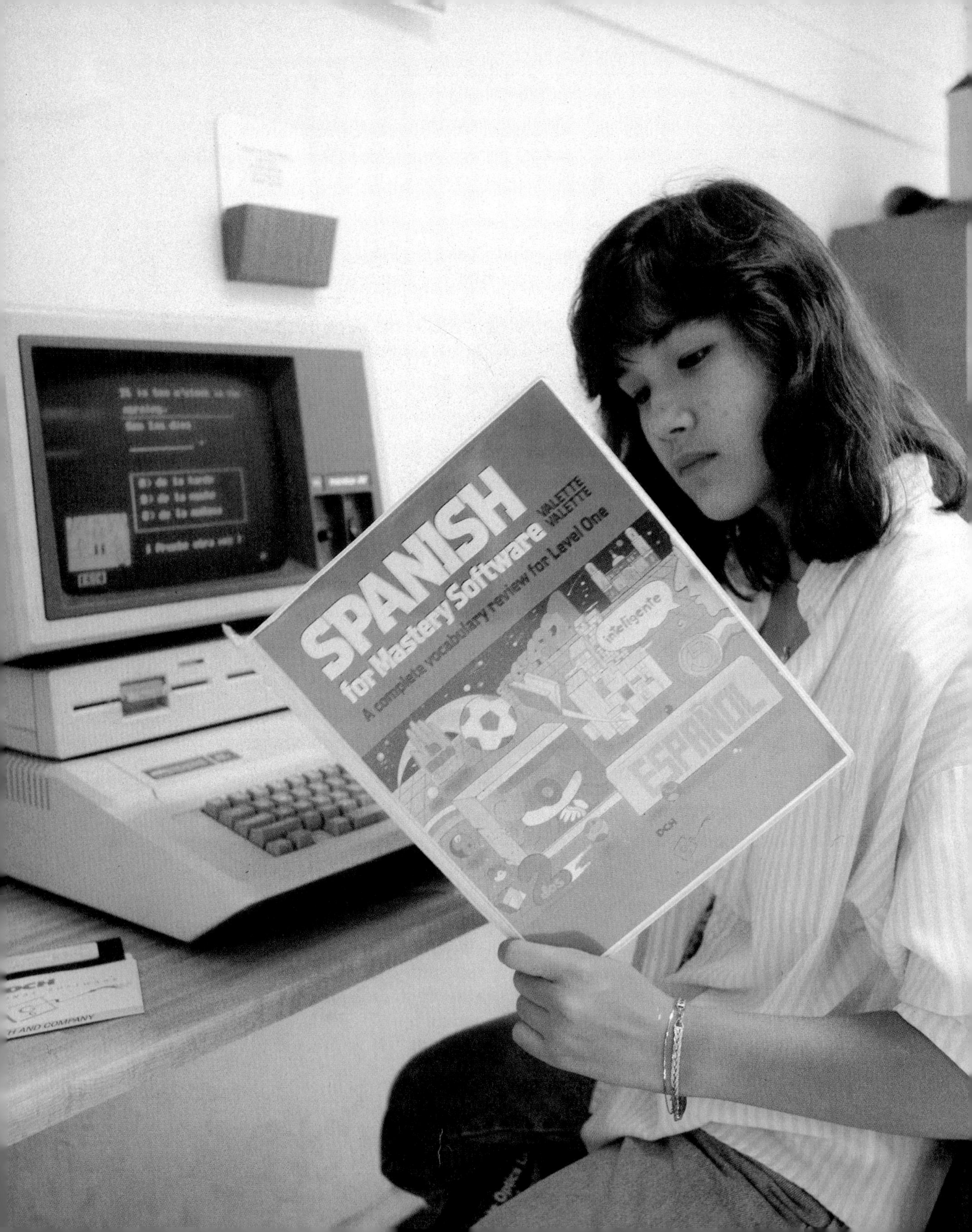
SPANISH
VALETTE
VALETTE
for Mastery Software
A complete vocabulary review for Level One
inteligente
DCH

three

FORMING VALUES AND MAKING DECISIONS

This chapter provides information that will help you to:

- Recognize types and sources of personal values.
- Determine personal values.
- Apply the valuing process.
- Establish and clarify personal goals.
- Apply the decision-making process.
- Analyze the relationship among values, goals, and decision making.

Life is filled with decisions to be made. In order to make these decisions, we must know ourselves. We must know what we consider important, what we are willing to strive for, and how to weigh all these factors to come to a definite plan of action. Does this sound tough? You bet it's tough! But it's also exciting and challenging (Figure 3-1).

Figure 3-1

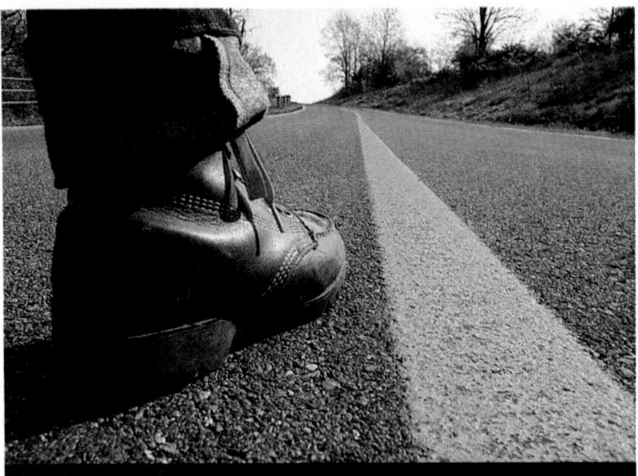

A goal is an aim toward which effort is directed. Saving money for the future is an important goal to set.

EXPLORING VALUES

In order to explore our personal values, we must understand the various kinds of values, the sources of our values, the alternation of values over time, and the valuing process.

What Are Values?

A **value** is a belief or feeling that someone or something is worthwhile. Values define what is of worth, what is considered beneficial, and what is considered harmful. Values can be thought of as standards or yardsticks to guide your actions, judgments, and attitudes.

It is unlikely that all your values are the same as all of anyone else's values. Values differ because people differ. You may value classical music, good grades, and membership in many clubs and groups. A friend of yours may not highly value any of these things. Instead, your friend may place a high value on leisure time, a large savings account, and physical fitness. It's clear that individuals value many things, but they have **priorities** in their values. That is, some things have a higher value than others.

Values are important because they inspire the setting of goals and supply a framework for decision making. That is, values provide reasons for action. Individuals' values determine how their resources (time, talent, energy, and money) will be used (Figure 3-2). The following situation demonstrates the importance of values in daily living. This message was given on the public address system in Grant High School:

> **Attention Seniors:** Orders for graduation invitations can now be placed with Miss Simpson in Room 180.
>
> The guidance office has information on several part-time jobs. Anyone who is interested should see Mr. Alvarez.
>
> Committees are being formed for the Senior Valentine's Day Dance. Those who want to serve on one of the committees should see Sue Goldstein.
>
> Volunteers are needed to help with Student Government Day. People interested in meeting and talking with local government representatives should sign up in their homerooms.

The ways in which any senior student responds to these announcements will be determined by values. Values placed on education and completion of high school will be reflected in the students' action related to the invitations (family values may also be evident here). Students who place a high value

Figure 3-2

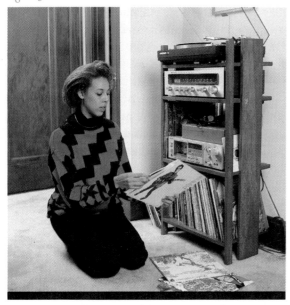

Your values determine how you spend your time—perhaps by listening to music.

on earning money are more likely to follow up on the part-time job posting than students who do not place high value on income or job experience. Leadership in school is a value that may encourage some students to volunteer for the dance committee. Those who value public service and participation in public action will be more likely to sign up for the student government activity than those who have public action and service as a lower-level value. Values determine action!

Sometimes values and facts become confused. A value is a statement of personal or group beliefs or feelings. A value is often stated in "should," "ought," or "supposed to" form. Facts state what actually is. Facts are established by careful observation and measurement. Problems arise when someone states a personal value which is interpreted as a fact or vice versa. You might accept certain statements as fact because they have been part of your behavior for a long time. These statements may actually be values you have formed. Consider the following statements and determine if they are fact or value.

- Houseplants make a home more cheerful and more comfortable.
- Houseplants are used to decorate many homes.
- Everyone should support the heart fund.
- Nearly everyone in Edgemont supported the heart fund this year.
- Children below age 12 should not watch television after 10:00 p.m.
- Television programs after 10:00 p.m. are more violent than programs shown at earlier times.
- The best time to buy ski equipment is at the end of winter.
- The most economical time to buy ski equipment is at the end of winter.

In each of the above examples, the value was stated first and the fact was stated second. The first statement of each example expresses how someone feels or thinks. The second statement of each example expresses something that can be shown or proven.

Values are continuously in operation. Few things that we think, do, or feel are value-free. By knowing more about values and understanding our own values, we can function better in our daily lives.

Kinds of Values

There are various kinds of values and ways to categorize them. Knowledge of the different kinds of values is helpful in exploring your own values and understanding why you think and act as you do.

Values can be categorized in at least three basic groups: moral values, aesthetic values, and material values. They can also be categorized as intrinsic or extrinsic, universal or group specific.

Moral values are based on what an individual considers to be right or wrong. Moral values are thoughts or codes to live by in relation to kindness to self and others. For example, one's moral values would come into play in the following situation.

CASE IN POINT

One evening, you are with a group of friends at a roadside park. Several people, including a friend of yours, are drinking beer and have become intoxicated. Another carload of friends arrives with more beer. These people suggest that the whole group stay longer because "the party has just begun."

Individuals would respond to this situation in different ways. However, it is clear that moral values play a major role in how each individual responds.

Aesthetic values reflect your feelings about what has beauty in nature and life. Aesthetic values reveal your appreciation for the way things look, sound, feel, taste, and smell.

One need not be an artist to have aesthetic values. Nearly everyone values things aesthetically to some degree. You may prefer one room in your house because it is lighter or brighter, or because it is darker and cozier. Perhaps you like to walk home on certain streets where the buildings are more attractive and the shrubs and flowers are pleasant. You may prefer the soft splashing of a brook in the park to the loud hammering of the factory around the corner. These preferences are based on aesthetic values.

Material values are reflected in the posessions we treasure. Material items are usually purchased and can vary from motorcycles to moccasins, from neckties to cookbooks (Figure 3-3), from sportscars to stereos. The items can be as permanent as a house or as temporary as a candy bar. Material values also vary in terms of quality and cost. One person may value having many books or

Figure 3-3

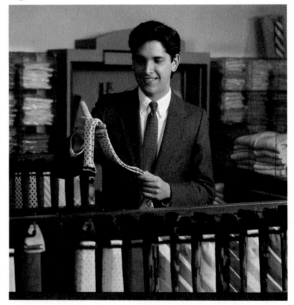

Your material and aesthetic values determine what you consider to be important in your life. Buying a certain necktie for a job interview reveals your aesthetic and material values as well as those efforts required to achieve a goal.

records regardless of the kind or quality of each. Other people may value specific and costly books or records.

Values can also be intrinsic and extrinsic. **Intrinsic values** are those that have worth to us in their own right. That is, intrinsic values are the ends and not the means. Examples of intrinsic values are valuing a lovely antique simply because you enjoy having it, or valuing a friendship simply because you enjoy being with a particular person. The antique and the friendship are intrinsic values.

Extrinsic values are means or ways to gain other values or desired results. They are not ends in themselves. If the antique is valued because of its material worth (that is, if it is a means to gain money), then it is an extrinsic value. If the friendship is valued because there might be some other benefit (for example, the friendship will get you into the right crowd or enable you to join a particular club), then it is an extrinsic value. Sometimes values are extrinsic *and* intrinsic—the value may be an end in itself as well as a means to the end. For example, one can simply enjoy writing newspaper articles and, at the same time, value the reader's praise of the news articles.

By considering the intrinsic or extrinsic worth of a value, you can gain clarity on what and why you value certain things and act as you do. Consider the following questions. Do you value high grades for the knowledge and skill they represent (intrinsic), or because high grades may help you get into college (extrinsic), or because your parents pay you for good grades (extrinsic)? Do you spend time and energy on your wardrobe because you enjoy feeling and looking good (intrinsic), or because you want to gain the approval and admiration of others (extrinsic)? Do you value the Art Club because you enjoy expressing yourself in a particular art form (intrinsic), or do you value the Art Club because it is a prestigious organization that sponsors several parties (extrinsic)?

Realize that intrinsic and extrinsic values are not necessarily good or bad. The more you consider why you value particular things and people, the better you will be able to determine your best behavior.

Values can be considered in terms of how widely they are accepted. **Universal values** are those on which most, if not all, people can agree. These include equality, justice, brotherhood, and respect for self and others. **Group specific values** are those that differ from society to society, from group to group, and from subgroup to subgroup. Examples of group specific values include the importance of time, proper behavior in public, type of foods, eating habits, and appropriate behavior for children. There are fewer universal values, and they are more general than group specific values.

Source of Values

Values come from our environment. The **environment** is made up of conditions that influence the life of an individual. We develop values from many different aspects of our environment. Families, peer groups, mass media (television, radio, and newspapers), other people, and experiences guide our value development over time. Our values are developed both consciously and subconsciously.

VALUES DEVELOPED FROM THE FAMILY • Families demonstrate and display a set of values to the youngest of children. As children grow, they learn what is important and what is valued by family members.

Behaviors and attitudes displayed in the home setting usually set a stage for learning particular values. This will be evident in behavior and attitudes of children. For example, honesty and truth may not be highly valued in a home in which truthfulness is not a major priority. Parents who say they are busy when they don't wish to take part in community affairs, or parents who readily cheat on income tax and insurance forms, are teaching the values of dishonesty and untruthfulness to their children.

Religion, a primary source of values, is usually determined by the family. Levels of religious involvement, choice of religious affiliation, and general attitudes and beliefs about religion are nearly always determined by family members.

Families provide the main source of values until children enter school, when teachers and classmates become important sources of values. However, even with these new and influential values, children move through school and enter young adulthood being strongly influenced by family values.

VALUES DEVELOPED FROM PEERS • As discussed above, the peer group (friends and other people who are about the same age) become an important source of value development from the time children enter school. Peer groups tend to become increasingly important during the early adolescent period (ages 11–13). In this time period, peer values have great strength.

Though many peer values may coincide with family values, some values of family and peer group may conflict. It is possible to have an overall value shared by both family and peers. Yet, the means for valuing or way to carry out the value may be different. Dressing well or having a good appearance may be a value in both family and peer group. However, the means for carrying out this value may be quite different. For example, your family may think dressing well includes wearing a certain type of clothing or hairstyle. But your peer group may think dressing well includes wearing a totally different type of clothing or hairstyle than your family would prefer.

VALUES DEVELOPED FROM THE MEDIA • The media—television, radio, newspapers, books, magazines, and films—are influential in developing values (Figure 3-4). The ideas, attitudes, and behaviors reflected in the media influence values that may differ from values of familiar groups such as family and peers. The different values can conflict or coordinate

Figure 3-4

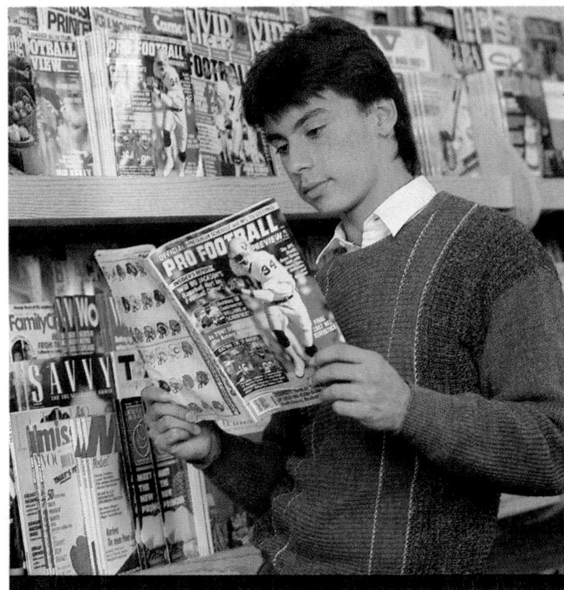

Values can be influenced by the media.

with other values. Consider the following examples from the media and determine the possible values that they may be showing. Consider also if these values are in conflict with your own family and peer values.

- Laura, a main character on an afternoon soap opera, decides to tell her father that she smashed his car and took $30 from the glove compartment.
- A popular movie depicts two teenagers setting fire to buildings as they drive across the country. They are chased by police, but are never caught.
- A weekly television series highlights life with a "macho" male and a "dumb" blonde who find themselves in various humorous situations.
- A new book portrays the plight of Japanese Americans placed in detention camps in California during World War II.
- A television commercial depicts a teenage boy who is sad because he has few friends. He gets a new stereo set and suddenly has many friends who say, "This is cool, Jeff!" "Can you have a party next week, Jeff?" "Hey, you're okay, Jeff."
- A front page news article describes the border-crossing escape of a family in South America that is fleeing the tyranny and injustice of the government.

Some people feel that the media have too much influence on developing values—especially the values of young people. How do you feel about this?

VALUES DEVELOPED FROM OTHER PERSONS AND EXPERIENCES • Neighbors, religious leaders, teachers, community leaders, and employers influence values. Experiences, both locally and in a wider range, are also likely to develop values. A particular teacher, club leader, a camping experience, or the opportunity to act in a drama may have been or will be very influential in developing your values.

Sometimes a single incident can establish a value that lasts for life. Consider Susan's situation.

CASE IN POINT

When Susan was 14, she had the opportunity to visit and observe a center for retarded children. She was amazed at what the students accomplished when given time, patience, and well-trained teachers. Over a period of two years, Susan read about handicapped persons and observed similar situations. She developed a value for the ability and worth of all human beings regardless of handicaps. Susan currently has a summer job teaching swimming to handicapped children, and she has plans to study physical therapy after graduating from high school.

Not only do you develop values from sources, but you are the source of other people's values. You may be the role model for others without realizing it. You may be serving as a pattern of behavior for others. This is particularly important when you interact with younger siblings, children of your own, or young people in the community. Your attitudes and behavior are strong forces in establishing values in others.

Alteration of Values over Time

As you consider the values you possess and those you are beginning to form, you may realize that values change over time. As people mature and move from one stage of life to another, the things and ideas they value may change. It is also possible that the basic value may remain constant, but the means of reaching the value changes. For example, you may continue to value education, but you may no longer emphasize grades. Rather, you may see the importance of acquiring overall knowledge and skill.

The universal values (equality, justice, brotherhood) will likely remain with you throughout your life. Some of the group specific values will likely change over time.

The Valuing Process

Gaining or adopting a value for your own is not an instantaneous act. Rather, gaining a value is a process through which you determine the worth of an idea or thing. This valuing process contains three actions: choosing, prizing, and acting on (or living), your values. The most significant values, those having the most influence on your life, are those values that have been developed through this three-step valuing process.

CHOOSING VALUES • In order to have a true value, you must be able to choose freely from alternatives. You cannot choose a value if there is only one option. For example, your parents insist that you learn to play the piano and that you practice an hour every day. If you have no choice in deciding to play the piano or in choosing which instrument to play, then you probably will not develop a true value. Thus, if a value has been imposed on you by others, it will guide your behavior only superficially. The value will likely cease when you are not under the influence of those who imposed the value on you. (You will probably not continue to play the piano as an adult.) A value must be chosen.

PRIZING VALUES • Prizing or cherishing a value means that you hold it dear: it has a positive quality for you. You're also willing to publicly affirm your value choice. That is, you are willing to tell others of your value. You cannot be ashamed of a value you have chosen and still maintain it as your value.

LIVING OR ACTING OUT YOUR VALUES • In order for values to guide your life, they must be acted upon. The values you have chosen must be repeatedly evident in your life in order for them to be meaningful and important. Your life must be influenced when you live by or act out a true value.

How do you act on a value? You can seek more information by reading and learning more about the value. You might invest resources (time, money, and energy) on the value. You form a life pattern that reflects and gives evidence of the value.

A necessary part of living and acting out a value is considering the consequences of the means for living and acting a value. For example, you value work for the theater. If you live by this value by acting or working on many plays in the community, the consequence may be too little time spent on school or job. Likewise, if you value good clothing but your means for having this value is shoplifting, the consequences for yourself and others are inappropriate.

By putting together the three aspects of valuing—choosing, prizing, and living the value—the process of making a value becomes your own rather than simply a copy of what someone else does or says. The following case depicts the valuing process in action.

CASE IN POINT

Yoko values her experiences in Future Homemakers of America (FHA). She has chosen this club activity from an array of other school activities. She has given considerable thought to the consequences of possible alternatives before choosing FHA. Yoko prizes her membership in FHA. She's happy with the choice and willingly tells others about the benefits of the organization (fun, learning, opportunities for growth). Yoko lives and acts on her choice of organizations by being an active member. Though Yoko will not be an FHA member forever, she can continue to support the organization during her adult life.

Determining Our Own Values

Having discussed sources of values, kinds of values, and the process by which we adopt a value, it may seem that most people have a clear grasp of what they value. This is not true! Teenagers nearing adulthood are often confused with the many value choices available and the accompanying pressures from peers and adults. Parents and teachers may apply pressure in one direction, peers in another. What seems important today may seem unimportant tomorrow. Sometimes it seems easier to avoid thinking about value issues, such as politics, love, and self-respect. It's not easy to know just what is right for you.

Exploring values requires time and thought. You must weigh pros and cons, consider consequences, and gain information. It doesn't seem particularly easy, so why bother? Exploration of values is important for the following reasons.

1• When people know what they value and what is important to them, they are better able to face new situations.
2• The more people know about their values, the better they can understand themselves.
3• The more people understand their values, the better they will be able to make good choices and take appropriate action.
4• The more people understand their values, the less likely they will be to make decisions based on peer pressure, authority figures, and power advertising.
5• The more people understand their values, the more appropriate will be their individual goals.
6• The more people understand their values, the more critical they can be when determining what is right for them.
7• The more people understand their values, the more confident and enthusiastic they can generally be about their lives.

As you can see, knowing and understanding one's values is an important part of being a fully functioning person (as discussed in Chapter 2).

Several techniques can be used to clarify and understand our values. Consideration of the following points can clarify what you really value.

Compare what you believe with what you actually do. If you really believe in equality of the sexes but if you joke about and put down the opposite sex, your actions do not match your beliefs. Is your belief strong enough to act on or are you only giving lip service to the value?

Critically think about whether you believe in what you're doing. As you take part in experiences and activities, consider if this is something that you really feel good about. Keep an open mind when asking yourself these objective questions. Are you doing what you enjoy and what you feel is right for you? Or are you doing what your peers and others have told you to do?

Consider five major values you would hope your younger siblings, your child, or another younger person might develop. After listing the five values, consider how you would expect the persons to live by these values. For example, you might hope they value education. You hope they live by this value by studying hard, appreciating books as sources of knowledge and personal enrichment, and sharing their knowledge with others. By considering values you hope others will adopt, you can gain insight into your own values.

In addition to these general techniques used to clarify values, there are specific exercises that can be performed in groups or individually to clarify the values one possesses.

VALUE CONTINUUM • A **continuum** is a line that is marked to represent degrees or levels of certain characteristics or issues. As in Figure 3-5, the right side indicates a definite no; the left side indicates a definite yes. Select the point on the line that reflects your feeling as you consider these topics: the military draft, legalized abortion, welfare, euthanasia (mercy killing), capital punishment, mental health/group homes, and gun control.

PRIZED SITUATIONS • By considering activities and situations that we find pleasing, we sometimes see things we value that we had not previously considered. List several activities that were the absolute best for you this past year, whether they were exciting things or quiet special moments. After determining these high spots, consider characteristics about these special times. Who were you with? Were you alone? What season of the year was it? What was the weather like? Did the activities involve many material things? What were you doing, and what kind of feeling did it bring to you? Now consider some prized situations that haven't occurred but that you would like to have happen. Consider the same points that are listed above in these imaginary situations.

Determining our personal values by means of the valuing process and various value clarifying techniques is a significant and necessary step in forming personal goals. You'll see the importance of values as you proceed to the next section.

Figure 3-5

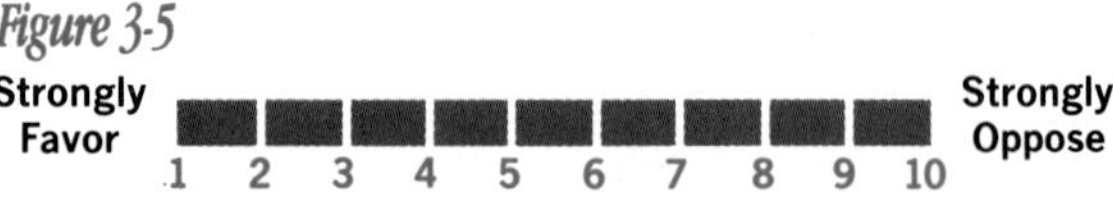

Topics or issues can be placed on this values continuum according to your level of feeling.

UNDERSTANDING GOALS

Before setting goals, it is important first to understand the meaning of the word "goals."

Defining Goals

A **goal** is an end or aim toward which effort is directed. A goal may be something we want to do or experience, something we want to achieve or attain, or a way of life we want to follow. Goals are set in order to help gain the things or experiences that are important and have value.

There is a strong interrelationship among self-concept, values, and goals. Values help determine goals we set for ourselves (Figure 3-6). We value those things that help us reach our goals. A positive self-concept guides the determining of our values and encourages high and positive goal setting.

Figure 3-6

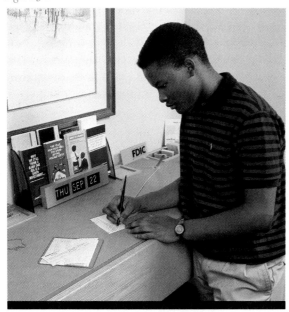

If one values going to college, then saving money for college becomes a goal. Goals and values are closely related.

Goals are influenced by family, peers, experiences, and other aspects of our environment. This influence occurs in two ways. Family, peers, experiences, and other aspects influence values: these values direct goals. Thus, goals are influenced *indirectly* by our family, friends, and other aspects of our environment.

Families, peers, experiences, and other aspects of our environment can also influence goals *directly* by setting patterns of behavior related to goals. Some parents, for example, set high goals such as graduating from college (Figure 3-7) for themselves and their children. Some teachers urge students to raise their goals higher. Peers and the media may stress greater striving and a "Yes, I can" attitude. Such direct influences will foster high and positive goals. Conversely, parents, peers, teachers, and other aspects or influences that do not set specific goals or have limited goals may set a pattern or create an example for low-level and negative goals.

Goals can be categorized by time span. Most people have both long-term and short-term goals. A **long-term goal** is a goal that is to be achieved over a long period of time. Such goals cannot be acquired quickly. To become head nurse in the pediatric wing or to develop a close relationship with the people in the community may be long-term goals.

A **short-term goal** is one that can be achieved quickly. Examples include: cutting the grass tomorrow, getting an A on an English exam, or mailing all the Christmas cards by Friday.

Goals can also be categorized by the segment or sphere of your life they represent. Goals can be clustered as family/home goals, social goals, educational/school goals, religious/spiritual goals, achievement/recognition goals, career goals, and physical/health goals.

List at least one goal you have in each of the spheres of life listed above. Determine if these are long-term or short-term goals.

Figure 3-7

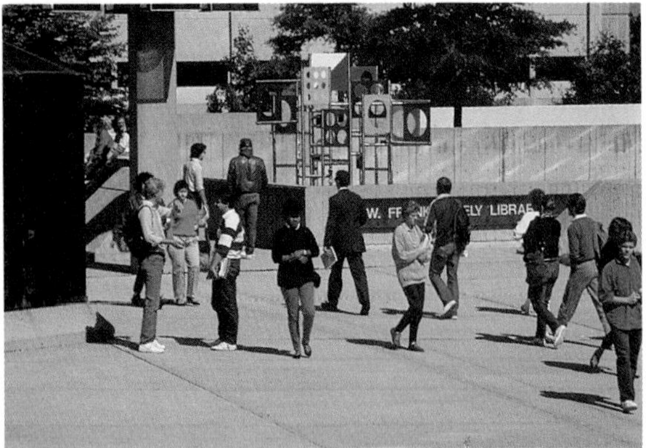
Joe Ruh

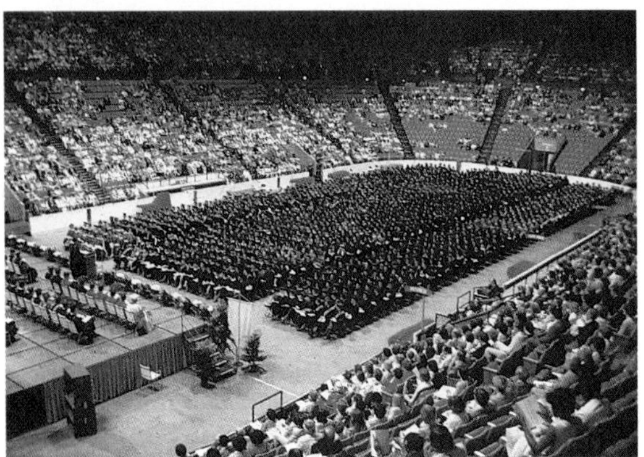
Indiana University—Purdue University at Indianapolis

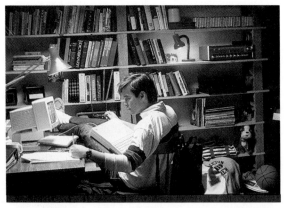
Values direct goals.
Courtesy of Apple Computers, Inc.

Setting Goals

A well-stated goal is like a map that shows not only the final destination but also the road to take to reach the final destination. In setting personal goals (or creating personal maps), self-concept and values must be considered. These are the foundation for goal setting. The setting or stating of the goal can now take place.

In setting a goal ask yourself where you want to go and where you want to end up. You must answer these questions personally. No one can provide the answers for you. Parents, teachers, and others can provide guidelines to help you think through a particular goal. But ultimately you must decide on your own goals just as you must strive to reach those goals in ways consistent with your definition of self and the values important to you.

STATE YOUR GOALS CLEARLY • Writing or clearly stating a goal can help you clarify what you really think. As you put your goal on paper, you begin to see the end result more clearly. Describing your goal as thoroughly as possible to a friend or on tape can also help you to state your goal definitely.

STATE YOUR GOALS POSITIVELY • Your goal should help you see the end point you wish to achieve. Stating an end point negatively prevents seeing the desired outcome. Imagine that your goal is to improve your appearance. Negatively stated, this goal is, "I will not be so sloppy." This goal doesn't allow a vision of what the outcome will be, it only states what the outcome *won't* be. Phrase your goal as, "I will become better groomed by wearing cleaner, neater clothes." This allows a visual picture of how the end goal will appear.

GOALS SHOULD BE PERSONAL • Since everyone has unique self-concepts and values, everyone will have different goals. Goals cannot be copied; they must fit individual needs. Goals that your parents, peers, or boss have set for you are not your goals unless you have accepted them for your own. Finding your own personal goals is a developmental process that changes with stages in your life. As a small child you may have adopted the goals set by your parents. You may have wanted to become a teacher, an accountant, or whatever your parents indicated you should strive for. As you grew older, you may have adopted goals of older siblings and friends. Later, you may have borrowed goals from your peers. In young adulthood new goals may emerge.

GOALS SHOULD BE REALISTIC • A realistic goal is a goal toward which you are able and willing to work. If you have never worn ice skates, then a goal to win next year's national skating championship is unrealistic. If you've never spoken a foreign language, then a goal to speak another language fluently in several months is not realistic. Choosing realistic goals does not mean the goals should be insignificant. People need to strive for new achievements and stretch their abilities. At the same time, they need to use logic and good sense.

Consider the goals you created for the various spheres of life. Are these goals stated positively? Are they *your* goals? Are they realistic?

Clarifying Goals

Consider the following goals:

- To win the national rodeo competition
- To attend and perform with the church choir at the National Interdenominational Conference of Church Choirs in Denver next summer
- To travel to Ireland
- To do more to improve your community
- To lose weight
- To get along better with your parents
- To become manager and chief of your local bank within three years
- To become more patient
- To save more money
- To fight less with your brother and/or sister

All of these goals are things or experiences on which you are willing to expend resources, such as time, energy, and money. However, the goals vary in their degree of specificity. That is, some of the goals specifically state what end or outcome the person hopes to achieve. The goal of singing in national choir competition tells what, when, where, and with whom the goal will be accomplished. Other goals, such as the trip to Ireland, are less specific. When will the trip take place? Will the goal be reached alone or will others be involved? Where in Ireland will the traveling be done?

There is nothing wrong with having a general goal, such as visiting Ireland. General goals are necessary to see the overall direction of our values. However, if we really want to make progress in achieving that goal it must become more specific and exact. We need to know what we want to take place. A field goal kicker has a difficult time earning three points if thick fog covers the field and the goal posts are not visible. Likewise, it is difficult to reach a goal when the end point or aim is not clear and when guidelines are unavailable.

When goals are stated specifically, we get hints as to steps or subgoals that can help us reach the final goal. Consider how the goal of saving more money is altered and clarified to state action that can begin immediately.

- To save more money.
- To save $15 each week.
- To save $15 each week from my paycheck by depositing $15 each week in the Smithson Savings and Loan.
- To save $15 each week from my paycheck by depositing $15 each week in the Smithson Savings and Loan and earning approximately 6% interest a year.

Each step in clarifying the goal is helpful in visualizing how the end point will appear and how one will behave in reaching the ultimate goal. Changing a vague goal to a clarified, specific map of action takes time and effort.

Paul provides an example of the concerted effort needed to establish a goal showing long-range intent as well as immediate action.

CASE IN POINT

Paul took part in a goals clarification class. Although he thought the whole thing was rather silly when he began, he found the outcome to be very helpful.

Paul has enjoyed working with photography for the past four years. He has taken photos for the school paper as well as for the local weekly newspaper. He has taken photography classes, and he taught a class in basic photography to a scout troop.

When asked to state his photography goals, Paul said, "To be a good photographer." Paul's teacher said this goal was too vague and difficult to measure. Paul reluctantly thought through his goals. After much consideration, he was able to say, "My goal is to win the State Photo Contest next year."

Paul's teacher asked Paul if he could be even more specific. They discussed subgoals that would help Paul reach his desired end. Finally, Paul said, "My goal is to *win* first place in the black-and-white photo competition in the State Photo Contest next year. My subgoal is to *enter* the State Photo Contest this year."

This goal and subgoal provided Paul with a means to use his energies in careful analysis of what is required to win the contest—what the judges look for, how best to display the photos, what subjects seem to get the judges' attention. By this analysis, he was able to experiment throughout the year to perfect his work. Forming a specific goal helped Paul achieve the things that have meaning for him.

By using the Goal Chart (Figure 3-8) as a model, make your own personal goals chart. Complete the chart for several major long-term goals and short-term goals. Consider the last question seriously. Determine if you are really ready to commit yourself to striving for the goals.

Striving for Goals

A goal is well on its way to becoming accomplished if you can answer yes to the following:

1. The goal has been chosen based on your own values.
2. The goal is written, stated positively, is realistic, and personally yours.
3. The goal has been stated with subgoals and end points clarified and time periods indicated.

Figure 3-8

Goals Chart

Goal Statement: *First Refinement:* *Second Refinement:*	*Target Dates:*
Step or Subgoals to Reach Ultimate Goal:	*Target Dates for Subgoals:*
Is it worthwhile to spend my time and energy on this goal? Yes ______ *No* ______	

Several points are helpful in the actual striving for goals. These points are discussed next.

RESOURCES • There are many resources (sources of help) in achieving your goal. Unfortunately, the sources may not be obvious. You must know where and how to find them.

Let's consider the goal "to become manager and chief of the Clinton Branch of Ajax Savings and Loan within three years." Miss Michelle Jefferson, the person with this goal, works at Ajax. Miss Jefferson has consulted the director of the company (*human resource*) and has found that computer knowledge and account management were lacking in her background. She enrolled in an evening class in computer training (*educational resource*) and has worked with one of the account managers to gain advice on the account procedure process (*technical resource*). Miss Jefferson has not overlooked her own human resources. Her skills, personal qualities, and interpersonal relationships are resources that can help her reach her goal.

Becoming aware of the resources within your community can be the first step to reaching your goal. Educational resources, social service resources, counseling, and human services are available in most communities at little or no cost.

AFFIRMATION OF GOALS • Affirmation is the act of expressing a belief in the truth of a particular statement. An affirmation is one way of talking to yourself by telling yourself what you believe. Goals need to be affirmed periodically to keep us motivated and involved with the pursuit of the goal. This is especially true when the goal is long-term and seems to take forever to achieve. The goal "to become a more patient person" might benefit from affirmations, such as "I will think carefully before I respond in anger." The goal "to lose weight" might have an affirmation, such as "I will become a slimmer person." These affirmative statements can be repeated to oneself when striving for a goal that is particularly difficult. Affirmations, like the goal itself, should be positive and stated either aloud or mentally with firm conviction. A picture or photo can help the verbal affirmation. For example, cutting household costs to reach the goal of buying a new refrigerator can be made easier if a picture of the refrigerator is in sight.

The idea of affirmations may seem silly at first. Self-motivation or self-talk may appear like a game. However, think how often we give and receive affirmations in daily life. Baseball players affirm the pitcher's ability (or inability) by shouting words of encouragement on the playing field. People affirm the words of a religious leader by saying, for example, "Amen." We affirm our belief in our country with the Pledge of Allegiance. Affirmations are ways of strengthening our beliefs in particular statements.

Return to the list of goals in the previous section. Consider an affirmation of each.

REWARD • A small reward or gift to yourself when you have achieved a step toward your goal can be helpful in spurring you on to strive harder for your goals. Too often we only criticize ourselves when we don't progress fast enough. We need to counter the self-criticism with self-praise and acknowledged achievement.

A person who has lost 10 pounds when the goal was 30 pounds could reward himself or herself with a new shirt or sweater to show off a slimmer self. A person striving to earn an A in chemistry could get some self-reward after earning a good quiz grade—perhaps some extra television watching or some pleasure reading. Rewarding ourselves is not only pleasurable but also tends to urge us to strive for further gains toward the ultimate goal.

Using Figure 3-9, add a second page to the Goals Chart for your personal goals.

MAKING DECISIONS

Decisions are the outgrowth of self-concept, values, and the goals formed from these values. Goals may be set only periodically, but decisions are made many times every day. From one goal based on one particular value can come hundreds of decisions. The stronger the value and the firmer the goal, the easier will be the decision. Think of decisions as the many branches of a tree with the limbs as the goals and the trunk of the tree as the values base. The self-concept is the root system that provides all the nourishment to the entire tree.

Aspects of Decision Making

Decisions are closely related to problem solving. Decisions are usually spurred by a question such as, "How can I get a job at the steel plant?" or "What can I do to make more friends?" These are questions in which a

Figure 3-9

Goals Chart (Page 2)

Sources of Help in Reaching My Goals:
Affirmation Statement for Reaching My Goal:
Visualization of My Goal:
Rewards for Reaching My Goal or Subgoals:

decision is needed. Statements such as, "I want to get a job at the library" or "I want to make more money" are "I want" statements that show that you have a goal. Until these "I want" statements are thought of in terms of questions, you will not spur a decision.

Decisions may be long-term and require much time, deliberation, and advice from others. Some decisions are quick and produce immediate action. Little is involved from self or others.

Regardless of the type of decision, three factors will affect the decision being made. First, the maturity of the decision maker will affect the outcome. How the decision maker sees the problem will be determined by the stage of life in which the decision maker is operating. If the decision is based on the question, "What car should I buy?" the decision will likely be different for a 17-year-old purchasing a first car than for a 48-year-old who has owned and operated numerous cars. The age, maturity, and experience level of the decision maker will have an impact on the final decision.

Second, the particular situation in which the decision is taking place will be a factor in the decision making. This is called the **context** of the decision. Consider the car-buying decision. Now add the following facts to the decision-making situation:

- The decision is being made in the midst of a heavy economic inflationary period.
- The decision is a result of an automobile accident that totally demolished a former car.
- The decision maker has just won $60,000.

These facts make up the context of the decision-making situation and will be factors in the final decision.

Third, the decision maker's ability will affect the decision being made. The knowledge, skill, and number of resources the decison maker has will affect any decision. The car-buying decision will be altered if the decision maker has knowledge of car payment practices, skill in assessing components in both auto bodies and motors, comparative consumer information, and/or resources to gain this knowledge.

The various aspects of decision making need to be kept in mind as we consider the decision-making process.

The Decision-Making Process

Regardless of the time needed for the decision, the level of importance of the decision, or the range of implications involved, there is a process to use in decision making. Simple daily decisions may require less time spent on the decision-making process, but the process remains the same.

Decide! Decide!
I just cannot decide.
I think about it day and night,
No answers seem to pop in sight.
I'm working myself into a fright.
Decide! Decide!

Decide! Decide!
I just cannot decide.
I've used seven boxes of tissues.
But haven't thought through all
the issues.
All my knowledge I seem to misuse.
Decide! Decide!

DEFINE THE PROBLEM OR ISSUE • This step may sound unnecessary. But it is highly important to do some critical thinking about the real issue at hand and separate the unnecessary parts of the problem. Sometimes the issue or concern is hard to see. The disorder and confusion that often accompany a problem can block the real issue. For example, a problem statement of "How can I get more friends?" might be better stated as "How can I make myself a more friendly, outgoing person?" A problem stated as "Should I quit this job?" might be better worded, "What are the positive and negative aspects of this job?" or "What is happening on the job that makes it no longer rewarding for me?"

Identifying the real problem or decision to be made can be compared to an iceberg. The easily seen portions of the problem may not hold the real issue that we must encounter. We may have to go below the surface to discover the concern or issue involved.

REFLECT ON GOALS AND VALUES • This is necessary after you identify the real problem. This step can be very troublesome to those who have never considered their goals or the values that have motivated their goals. Aspects of the decision to be made may be in opposition to the values held. This may mean facing a value conflict. The context of the decision may require altering the goal. In essence, this step requires the decision maker to consider how the decision fits into the goals and values held. This step forces the decision to fit the individual decision maker.

SEEKING ALTERNATIVE CHOICES OR OPTIONS • All possible alternatives should be considered. Even though some options seem foolish, they may generate ideas that may be workable. This is the most creative step of the decision-making process.

Note that the *right answer* or *the* solution is not sought. It is assumed in the decision-making process that various alternatives are workable and that the decision maker must generate as many of these alternatives as possible.

WEIGHING THE POSSIBLE ALTERNATIVES • This step involves serious consideration of each choice or option generated. The consequences for the decision maker, other significant persons, and society as a whole must be considered.

The decision of whether or not to accept an evening typing job in your home as a second income will have consequences for other family members—especially if the home is small and the noise of typing bothers others. A decision of what type of house pet to buy will generate alternatives that may have consequences on apartment dwellers near you. A Great Dane and a house cat will have a different impact on self and the near society. (Friends and neighbors may receive a greater negative impact from the exercise and noise of the Great Dane than from the cat.)

Weighing alternatives provides a natural narrowing of possible solutions or options. This narrowing aids in the next step of selecting an alternative.

SELECT THE ALTERNATIVES • At this point, you decide what to do and make a plan of action. The alternative chosen may not be the same as any proposed when you sought alternative options. The final alternative may be a combination of several options or an adaptation of one of the earlier options. Refining, reshaping, and clarifying the decision is part of this step. Take time to congratulate yourself. You just made a decision!

TAKE RESPONSIBILITY FOR THE DECISION • This step requires that you fully accept responsibility for the possible outcomes. If you accept the summer lifeguard job, you also accept the fact that you may miss some of the weekend summer fun with your friends. You accept the responsibility for the lives of the small children in the pool. And you also accept the unglamorous parts of the job, such as picking up litter and emptying the trash can. Taking full responsibility for decisions can provide the opportunity to evaluate the decision and use these findings in making future decisions.

The decision-making process may be understood better if the six steps previously outlined are applied to an actual decision.

1• Define the problem:
Ann has been trying to make a decision about her post-high school education. She has been accepted in the drafting program at Simms College, a school six hours from her home. Ann has visited Simms and likes the school. Yet having never lived away from her family, Ann is hesitant to commit herself to this school. Ann has been delaying a response to the school. She knows that she must make a decision. After much thought, she defines the problem as follows: What should I do about enrolling in the drafting program at Simms College for next fall?

2• Reflect on goals and values:
Ann considers the values she has. She has high regard for education. She values being able to earn her own way. She values the

skill she has in drafting. Ann's goal is to achieve a skill that can provide for an income throughout life and will offer a good chance for promotion. She values her chance for promotion. She values her family, yet has a goal of being on her own for a while. Ann considers all of these values and goals.

3. Seek alternatives:
   With these values and goals in mind, Ann generates many possible alternatives. Some of these alternatives include the following:
   - Wait and respond later; perhaps the school will be full, and I'll not have to decide.
   - Answer yes and enroll before I change my mind.
   - Consider schools close to home, perhaps right here in town.
   - Wait and stay home for a year, then decide.

4. Weigh alternatives:
   Ann weighs each possible alternative and considers the consequences for herself and others. For example, Ann considers the option of staying at home for a year and then making a decision. She knows the consequence of this option in that her parents must support her because few jobs are available in town. Throughout this year, she would get no closer to earning her degree in drafting. This would be an obligation on her parents as well as a negative consequence to Ann since it is against her value of earning her own way. Ann considers each possible option in this manner, weighing the consequences for herself and those around her.

5. Select alternatives:
   Ann selects the alternative to respond positively to the college's acceptance. However, she is not happy with her wording of the alternative, "Answer yes and enroll before I can change my mind." She is more determined now and feels she can positively state that she will enroll in Simms College because she feels it is the best decision for her at this time.

6. Take responsibility:
   Ann takes the responsibility of enrolling at Simms College as her own decision. Though her parents and her current drafting instructor support this decision, Ann must accept any consequences, positive or negative, as her responsibility. An unhappy experience cannot be blamed on her parents or her instructor. Ann made the decision.

Decisions are part of everyday life. You will make thousands, perhaps millions of decisions throughout your lifetime. Your values and goals along with the tools of the decision-making process can lead you to the satisfaction of well-made decisions.

WRAPPING IT UP

Life involves many decisions every day. Our decisions are guided by our values and goals. *Values* are those ideas or things that we consider to be beneficial and worth striving for in life. They guide actions, judgments, and attitudes. Values determine how such resources as time, talent, energy, and money will be used. Values vary from one person, culture, and society to the next. Values are of three basic types: moral, aesthetic, and material. *Extrinsic values* serve as means to acquire other values or ends. *Intrinsic values* are those that have worth to us in their own right.

We learn values from our experiences in our *environment*. Sources of values include families, religions, peers, teachers, neighbors, community leaders, and employers. In today's world the mass media of television, radio, movies, and newspapers also have a major impact on the values we acquire. Many values change over time as a person matures. Our true values are those we voluntarily choose, those that we prize and hold dear, and live by in our actions. Knowing what your true values are is an important part of understanding your self-concept. This assists you in becoming a fully functioning person.

Goals are those ends toward which your efforts are directed. We set goals in order to gain the things or experiences that have value to us. Self-concept, values, and goals are all closely related and mutually reinforcing. Goals, too, are influenced by our families, friends, experiences, and other people in our environment. Whether they are *short-term goals* or *long-term goals*, we should set them clearly and in a positive way. Goals should also fit our individual needs and be realistic.

The decisions you make every day are rooted in your self-concept, values, and goals. Decision making is a skill that involves several steps. These steps include defining the problem or issue; reflecting on goals and values; seeking alternatives; weighing the possible alternatives; selecting an alternative; and taking responsibility for the decision. The decisions we make are also influenced by our level of maturity and the context of the decision-making situation.

Exploring Dimensions of Chapter Three

For Review

1• What is a value?
2• Why are values important?
3• List the three basic kinds of values and give two examples of each.
4• Explain the terms intrinsic value and extrinsic value.
5• List four sources of values.
6• What are the steps of the valuing process?
7• List four guidelines to help you in setting your goals.
8• What are three things you can do to help yourself in striving for goals?

9. Explain the six steps of decision making.
10. How are values, goals, and decision making related?

For Consideration

1. List three of your personal values and assess them, using the following questions as guidelines: Are they moral, aesthetic, or material values? Are they intrinsic or extrinsic values? What are the sources of the values? How would you apply the valuing process to these values?
2. Clarify or make more specific the following goals: "I want to be more responsible for my younger sisters." "I want to do better in school." "I want to be successful in a career." "I don't want to take my friends for granted."
3. List three important personal values. Now state how these values (or the means for achieving these values) may change if the following situations occurred: You move to a foreign country. You get married. You become 35 years old. You become a parent. You win $5,000. You win a four-year college scholarship.
4. Give an example to show how goals and values are related.
5. Help Terri with her problem. Explain to her the steps in the decision-making process and give her guidance in following the process. Remember, you can't decide for her. You can only give her guidance. Here is Terri's problem. Terri works at the local library. She is glad to have the job which her aunt helped her to get. However, she has learned of a better paying job that would be a challenge. She can't decide if she should try for the new job, perhaps hurt her aunt's feelings, and perhaps be less secure than in the library job, but make more money.

For Application

1. Interview an adult and ask this person to focus on an important decision made in the past. Questions should include the following: "How did the decision affect your life?" "What process did you use to make the decision?" "Who or what influenced the final decision?" "How did you feel after you finally made the decision?"
2. After considering your personal values, use your creativity to design (on paper) a bracelet or necklace of values using symbols that represent those things or ideas you value most highly. Or create a sweatshirt of values showing things and ideas you value most highly.

3• Throughout this textbook there will be many topics discussed that are based on personal values. As you and your classmates discuss various issues, it is easy to find yourself trying to instill your values in others. Keep a notebook of statements that reflect other people's attempts to force personal values on others. Discuss whether or not these people are aware of their actions.

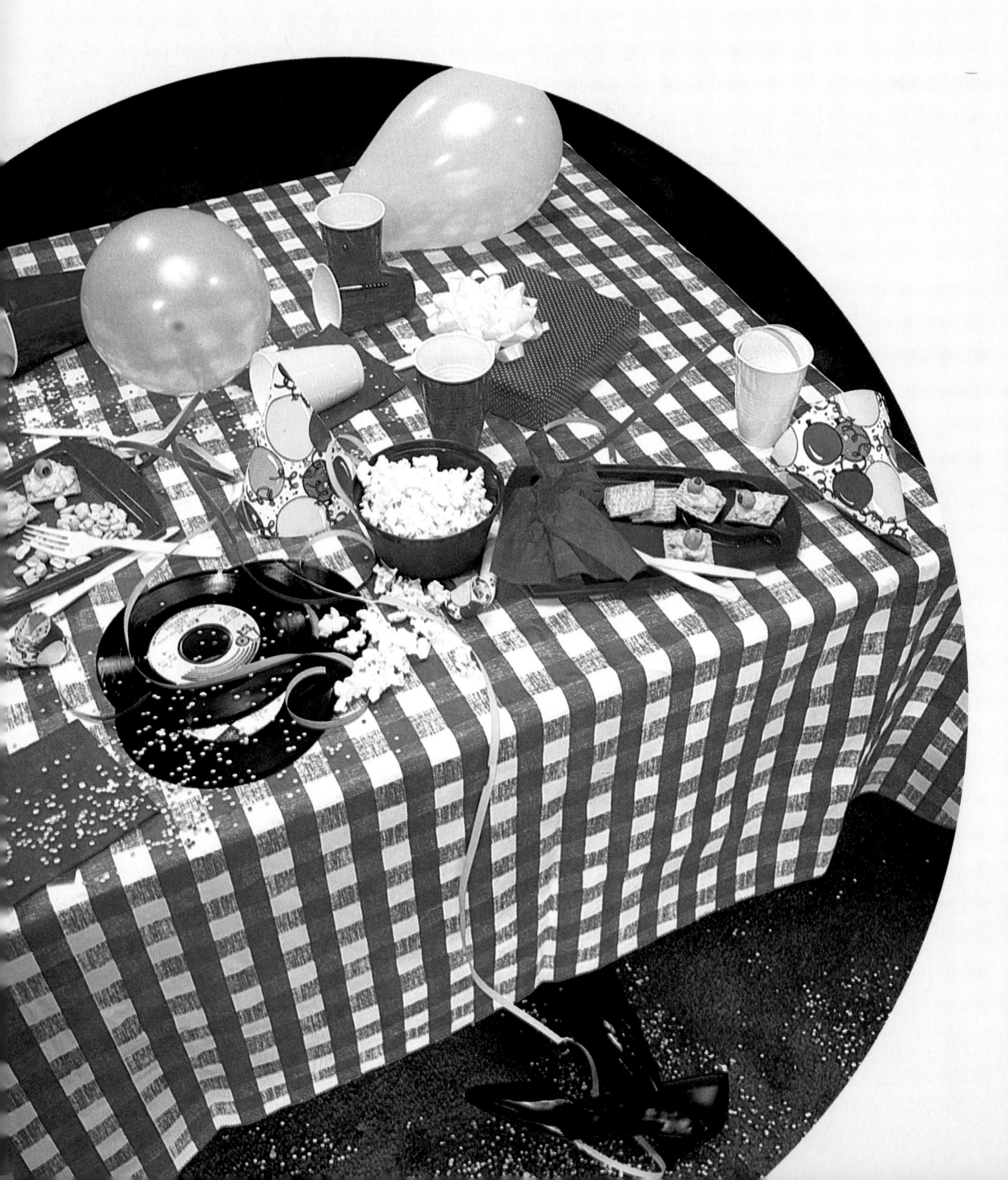

part two

Forming Interpersonal Relationships

Interpersonal relationships are important for you today and in your future life. Adult family roles and work roles require interrelating with others. Positive and meaningful relationships are more likely to occur when you know yourself and have established your own personal identity. Part One emphasized self-knowledge and identity formation. This information has set the stage for learning more about interpersonal relationship formation.

It is important to understand various kinds of relationships and the ways in which relationships grow and develop. It is equally important to understand and use effective communication. You can learn skills in both verbal and nonverbal communication as well as ways to deal with conflict in communication. Understanding persons of other cultures and subcultures is an additional pertinent aspect of forming interpersonal relationships.

Part Two includes chapters on building and strengthening relationships, communicating effectively, and understanding others. Consideration and application of these topics will help you have more rewarding and positive family and work relationships.

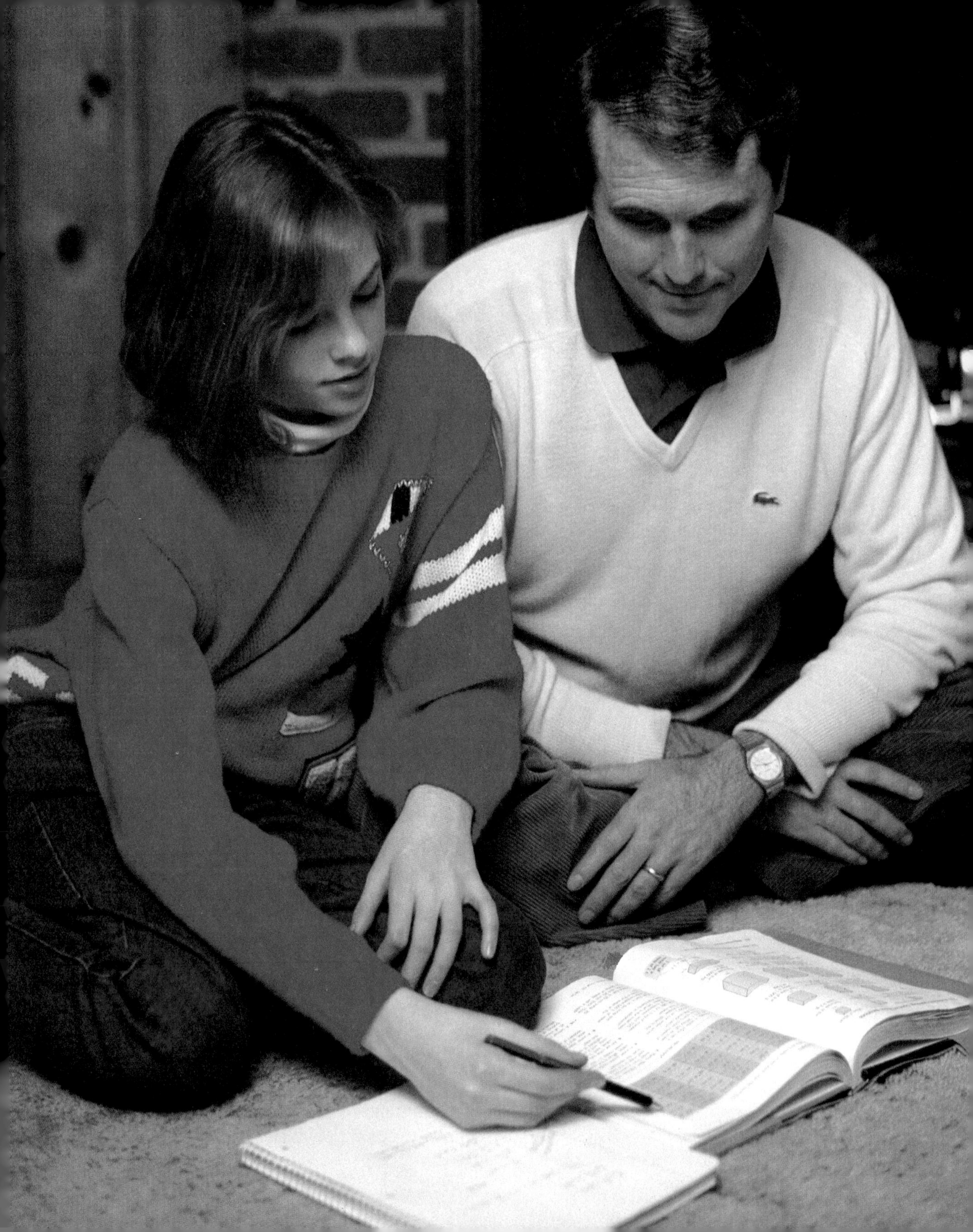

four

BUILDING AND STRENGTHENING RELATIONSHIPS

This chapter provides information that will help you to:

- Understand relationships.
- Realize the importance of various types of relationships.
- Understand the process in which a relationship develops.
- Analyze the operation of empathy, power, and reward in your personal relationships.

There once was a young girl named Kate.
With people she could not relate.
Not willing to explore,
She developed no rapport.
She felt doomed to a terrible fate.
One day when a crisis arose
Kate forgot her relationship woes.
She fostered, you see,
Mutual dependency.
Now she relates to each person she
knows.

To relate is to have a meaningful social interaction. The hundreds, perhaps thousands, of relationships you have can be positive and fulfilling or troublesome and uncomfortable.

By understanding how and why relationships develop and by considering the types of relationships that are formed throughout our lives we can develop rewarding, rich relationships that can improve life for ourselves and our society (Figure 4-1).

Figure 4-1

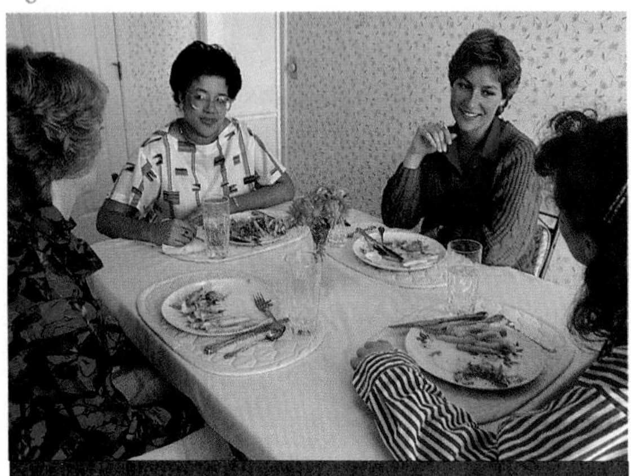

Rewarding, rich relationships can improve our lives.

UNDERSTANDING RELATIONSHIPS

Why bother to think about relationships? Obviously they can occur without planning. Actually, you might be thinking, "Who needs relationships? I function pretty well by myself."

This approach to relationships in today's society is almost like asking, "Do I have to breathe in order to live?" The compressed environment in which we live and the dependency on each other in today's world require many contacts and interactions. Consider the number of contacts you've had with people today—at home, on the bus, as you began your day, and during meals. Consider also the number of people you've interacted with today who are part of your important interpersonal relationships—a parent, a best friend, a neighbor. It soon becomes clear that even if you wanted to have no contacts or relationships, you could hardly do so.

> If a man be gracious and courteous to strangers, it shows he is a citizen of the world, and that his heart is no island cut off from other lands, but a continent that joins to them.
>
> Francis Bacon
> Essays of Praise

The important response to the question, "Who needs relationships?" is that there are immeasurable gains from building and strengthening relationships. The poet John Donne said, "No man is an island entire of itself." This means that no one can function totally alone. People need people. Henry David Thoreau wrote *Walden*, a book in which he describes his two years of living alone at Walden Pond. Thoreau writes with beauty and enthusiasm of his self-imposed solitude. His descriptions of nature and his reflections on life give the reader insight into self-searching and gaining self-reliance. Yet, throughout his book, Thoreau refers to interpersonal relationships he had in the past. These relationships sustained him and gave him peace throughout his time at Walden Pond. On completing two years of solitude, Thoreau wrote about his experiences in order to share and relate with others. Even those people who prefer large portions of solitude in their lives realize the necessity of relating to others.

In what ways might periods of solitude be beneficial in building and strengthening relationships? In what ways might relationships help solitude become more beneficial? One of the most valuable outcomes in relationships is learning to know yourself better. In Chapter 1 we found that self-concept was formed, in part, by how others react to us. Warm, responsive reactions from others show us our worth and increase our value of ourselves. Cool, negative reactions or no reactions at all from others tell us that we are of little worth and diminish our self-concept.

In Chapter 2 we learned that we must rely on others when we need help. Relationships with others can be valuable resources in times of need. You, too, can be a resource to someone else with whom you have formed a relationship. One of the values emphasized throughout this chapter, and illustrated in Figure 4-2, is that it is worthwhile for us to want to form positive relationships. Through play, children learn to form relationships, to socialize, and to enjoy the company of other human beings.

In addition to getting to know yourself better, another benefit of having positive relationships as young people is that these relationships prepare you for adult life. Learning to share, learning to get along with others and to be considerate of fellow human beings, and learning to work together for a common goal are necessary preparations for living successfully in the adult world. These learning experiences can only take place in interpersonal relationships with others.

In schools today, committee or group work often is a part of learning experiences in nearly all subjects. This is not by accident. Today's world needs individuals who are able to work together to form relationships (Figure 4-3).

Figure 4-2

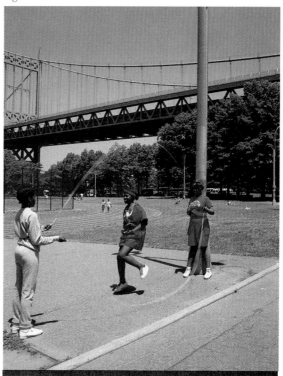

We need people for many reasons.
Audrey Gottlieb/Monkmeyer Press

A third important benefit of strong relationships is that they enrich our lives. Each new relationship has the potential for adding new experiences to our lives as well as the opportunity to share our own life experiences. Relating to others gives depth, richness, and variety to our lives. We learn of different values, feelings, tastes, and ideas that expand our lives. In essence, then, we know that all people need others. And the luckiest among us are those who can build and strengthen positive relationships.

Figure 4-3

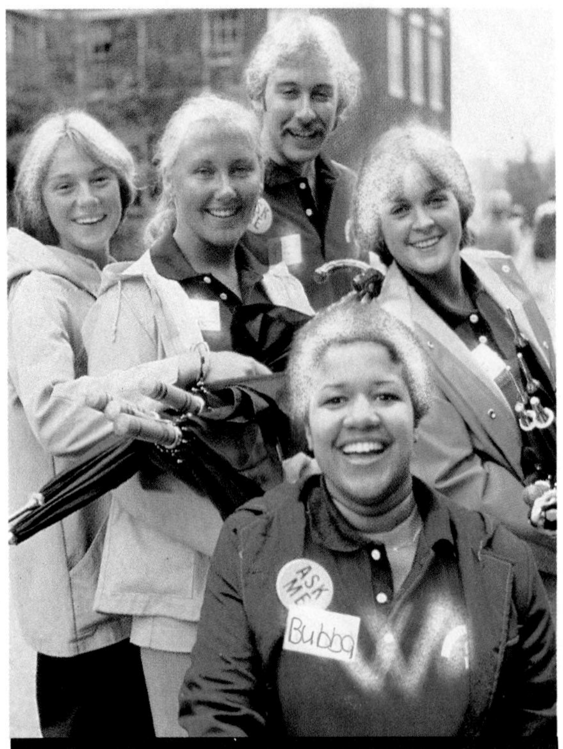

Group activities, such as serving as a college tour guide, can help young people gain relationship skills.
University of Cincinnati

GROWTH AND DEVELOPMENT OF RELATIONSHIPS

Relationships with individuals are at various levels of importance and various degrees of intimacy. You relate to the clerk in the donut shop by giving a smile, a nod, or by commenting briefly on the weather. Though you may see this person on frequent stops, you might not recognize the person in other surroundings. Yet, you still relate to each other. Quite different from this **superficial relationship** is the **intimate relationship** with a parent, best friend, steady boyfriend or girlfriend, sibling, or others you know well. Such close relationships often allow people to know each other's thoughts and feelings. Between these two types of relationships are the various relationships with teachers, physicians, employers, neighbors, relatives, and many others. Whether close and intimate, superficial, or somewhere in between, relationships can be pleasant and enjoyable or frustrating and uncomfortable. One task for people is to learn how to develop all relationships to be as positive as possible.

When two people are together there is the opportunity for a relationship to grow and develop. This growth and development may seem to happen at random. But those who have steady relationships have found that there are definite paths or processes which people follow in developing a relationship. Knowledge of some of these developmental processes can help you in forming and maintaining positive relationships.

Wheel Theory

One theory or idea that helps to show how relationships develop is the wheel theory. This idea emphasizes that all relationships develop in a basic pattern in four phases (Figure 4-4). These four phases are cyclical. The first phase, **rapport**, is the harmony or feeling of ease and comfort that is felt with another person. Rapport means that it is pleasurable being around the other person, and that we feel good just being with them. This positive feeling is necessary in order for the relationship to grow. Without rapport there is a feeling of uneasiness that will push people away from each other rather than toward each other.

Figure 4-4

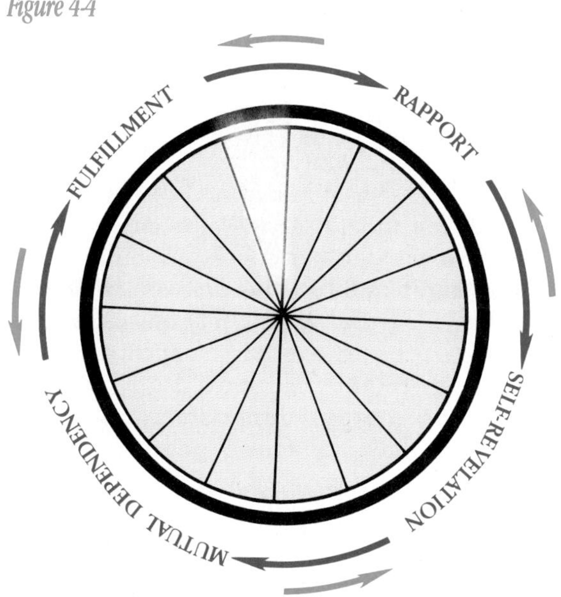

You can think of relationships, progressing through stages of rapport, self-revelation, mutual dependency, and fulfillment, as wheels rolling forward. Wheels can also roll backward, however, signifying that they, like relationships, can falter and lose ground.

Self-revelation, telling about yourself and your feelings, is the second spoke on the relationship wheel. Rapport leads to this self-revelation by fostering feelings of openness, relaxation, and sharing between the people involved. These shared ideas, experiences, and attitudes go beyond the small talk that occurs in the rapport stage. The discussion in the self-revelation stage includes more personal ideas and concerns.

The revealing of self to another person develops a **mutual dependency**. In this third spoke of the wheel, the people involved begin to rely on each other for support and encouragement. Habits and behaviors of the partners become known. Then habits and behaviors are developed to fit the partner. The dependency or reliance strengthens the relationship.

The mutual dependency leads to **need fulfillment**. The partners begin to gain confidence, assurance, respect, love, or affection. The partners feel more personally fulfilled than they did without the relationship.

Notice that this process is in a wheel formation, not a line progression. When need fulfillment is reached, the process does not end. Rather, the process continues as personal needs are fulfilled. Rapport is strengthened, thus reinforcing self-revelation, which reinforces mutual dependency, which leads to more need fulfillment. As the wheel turns, the relationship becomes stronger and stronger.

Like any wheel, however, the relationship can turn backwards and destroy itself. Self-revelation, for example, may bring out feelings and values that cause disagreements and conflicts. The wheel may move backward, and the relationship may remain at the rapport stage.

The following cases show how the relationship wheel works to strengthen and build a relationship or limit the growth of a relationship.

CASE IN POINT

Monica met Rosa by accident when she had to do a make-up session in gymnastics class. The girls shared some conversation during the class and had a snack together afterwards, where they talked about each other's strengths and weaknesses in the gymnastics routines. They made plans to meet again.

Rapport began to develop between the two girls as they discovered common interests. They began to share personal feelings and ideas related to themselves, their future plans, and life in general. This sharing was comfortable and rewarding. The knowledge shared was not abused. Ideas and concerns that were shared in confidence did not go beyond the relationship. Mutual dependency grew as the girls began to rely on each other for support. Monica knew that she could depend on Rosa to listen with feeling when she explained her difficulties with her family. Rosa could depend on Monica's words of encouragement when Rosa's schoolwork became difficult.

Needs of both Rosa and Monica were personally fulfilled by the relationship as it grew and developed. They each gained confidence and self-support from the relationship. This personal fulfillment led to increased rapport and the relationship wheel revolved again.

CASE IN POINT

Tanya and Bill met in typing class. For several weeks their conversations were limited to talk of typing and class assignments. Rapport began to develop as they talked after class and met informally during the school day. They felt at ease and comfortable with each other. They shared ideas and concerns and revealed some of their future plans. This sharing was comfortable, and the relationship grew stronger.

Mutual dependency developed as they began to rely on a nightly telephone conversation. Tanya waited for Bill each morning at her locker so they could walk to class together. Tanya listened sympathetically as Bill relayed his long-term battle with physics class. Tanya depended on Bill to listen to her struggles to get along with her sister. However, as the mutual dependency grew, Tanya began to get uncomfortable with Bill's dislike for the time she spent with her friends. Bill grew very possessive of Tanya and of the time he felt she should spend with him. When Tanya expressed her concern about their relationship to Bill, he became angry. This occurred several times. Bill and Tanya slowly began to see less of each other, and their relationship moved backward from the mutual dependency stage, although they maintained good rapport and considered each other good friends.

Their relationship will probably remain at the rapport stage unless Bill changes his possessive feelings and allows Tanya to continue her friendships, or unless Tanya allows Bill to control her personal life; thus preventing her other friendships.

It may be easier to visualize the movement of the relationship wheel as you think of close friendships and dating relationships. Yet, all relationships follow the wheel process. Employer-employee relationships, parent-child relationships, and sibling relationships progress in the same manner. You may relate with one sibling, for example, in such a way that the need-fulfillment stage is never reached. You may relate with another sibling with continuous movement around the steps of the relationship wheel while the relationship grows stronger with each revolution.

Path of Intimacy

Another tool to measure growth and development of relationships is the path of intimacy. As relationships develop and grow, they often move along a path that has three basic landmarks. Each landmark represents a level of closeness and intimacy with the other person. The first landmark on the path of intimacy is **intellectual intimacy**. When people first meet, their relationship is at this point—they share ideas and knowledge. Feelings are not yet shared, and the discussions remain on a nonpersonal basis. Conversation may center on schoolwork, a world crisis, the weather, the cost of groceries, or a movie just seen (Figure 4-5).

Figure 4-5

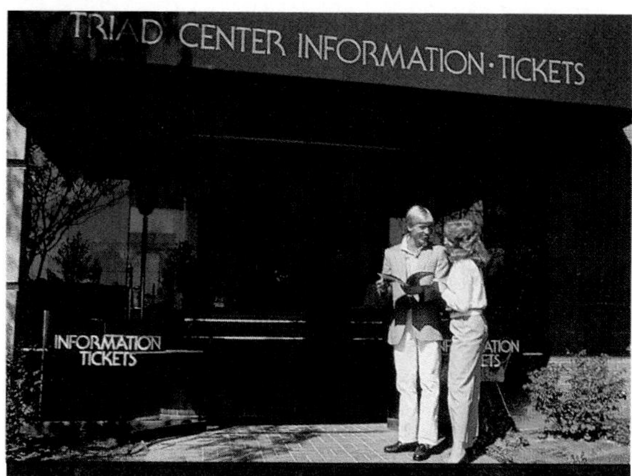

Sharing ideas or feelings about a movie creates intellectual intimacy.
Salt Lake Convention and Visitors Bureau

The second landmark is **physical intimacy**. At this stage people are comfortable touching—a pat on the back, a rough hug, a playful punch on the arm, or holding the arm or hand of another while sitting. These actions indicate a closer knowledge of the persons involved than at the intellectual stage. Relationships between family members, good friends, and dating partners are usually at the physical intimacy level.

Emotional intimacy, the third landmark on the path of intimacy, occurs when people are completely natural with each other and reveal their feelings. People operating at this landmark of the intimacy path are comfortable eliminating the masks and layers of roles they play in society. They feel free to share their most private ideas and feelings. There is a mutual trust, understanding, support, and affection. Emotional intimacy is usually found in relationships developed over time between close friends and family members (Figure 4-6).

The journey on the path of intimacy may take a long time or may be traveled swiftly. Your relationship with many people may end at the first milestone or at the second. Have you ever found after having a relationship at the intellectual level for several years that there can be a sudden movement to a close, emotional, level of relationship? For example Luis and Eric had known each other since they were babies. Because their mothers were good friends, the boys saw each other frequently and shared small talk or information about what they did at school. It was not until they were 15 that they found they had many common interests. They began sharing feelings, and their relationship quickly moved to the emotional intimacy stage. Relationships can grow and develop at different speeds. Usually time is needed in order to reach emotional intimacy.

BUILDING YOUR PERSONAL RELATIONSHIPS

Tools used to measure the growth and development of relationships have been

Figure 4-6

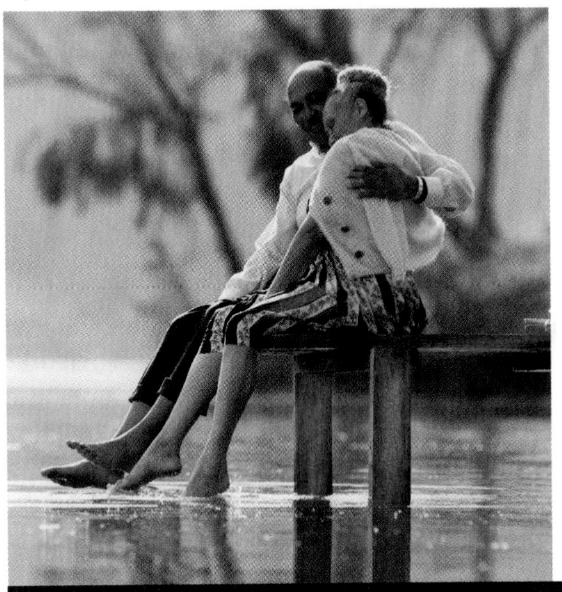

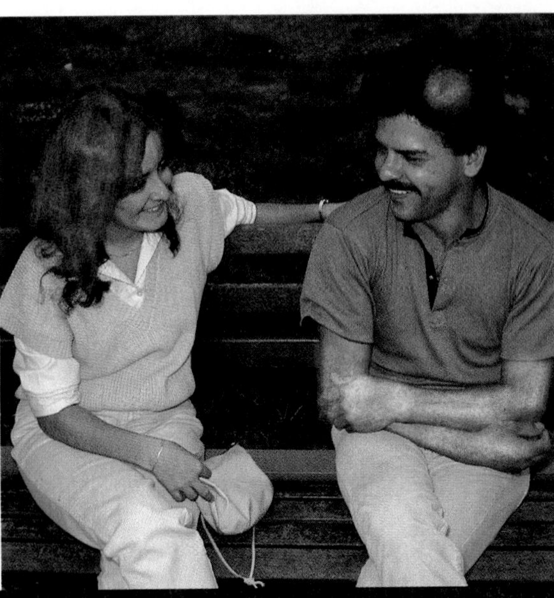

People who are comfortable touching each other and sharing their true thoughts are both physically and emotionally intimate.

Eastman Kodak Company

George C. Ferrar/Monkmeyer Press

discussed. Knowledge of how most relationships progress can make individuals more alert and aware of the growth of their own relationships. Yet, relationships do not grow and flourish by themselves. Our actions and behaviors, whether planned and purposeful or accidental, affect our relationships. Being aware of empathy, power, and rewards can build and strengthen personal relationships.

Empathy

People can more easily form and maintain relationships when they have **empathy** for others. To empathize is to mentally participate in another person's feelings or ideas. This means that you try to understand how situations appear to others while you momentarily put aside your own values and ideas. The values of others need not be accepted as your own. Rather, an attempt is made to understand the ideals, background, and experiences of others and to see the world as they see it, when you empathize.

The need for empathy in dealing with others is not a new idea. The early American saying, "Criticize no one until you walk a mile in their shoes," refers to empathy. This phrase advocates striving to understand and see things as others do. Such understanding aids in the formation and stability of relationships. Empathy is used in the following case.

CASE IN POINT

Margaret and Randy are entering the school library. Randy has six paperback books to return, each of which is a day overdue. He insists on dropping them in the return slot rather than taking them to the librarian's desk. Margaret explains that there are no late fines on paperbacks and that Randy can return the books at the desk rather than in the slot. "I know," replies Randy. "But Ms. Crotzer [the librarian] always gives me a line about responsibility to other readers and then looks at me like I just hijacked an airplane."

Margaret realizes that Randy's personal experiences might make him feel this way. Though Margaret has never found Ms. Crotzer to be disagreeable or unpleasant, she understands Randy's feelings

Several members of Randy's family have had difficulty with the law. Randy's older brother was imprisoned for shoplifting. Margaret realizes that people may react to Randy in a disapproving manner or that Randy may feel people react this way. Margaret attempts to mentally experience conflicts, attitudes, or feelings that she might have if she were in Randy's situation. She accepts Randy's decision to drop off the books without confronting Ms. Crotzer. At an appropriate time and place, she can also offer to discuss Randy's reactions related to his feelings. Over time she can emphasize the importance of individual behavior. She can highlight cases in which people have placed trust and responsibility in Randy because of *his* behavior rather than because of his family's negative behavior. By using empathy—trying to grasp the situation as it appears and feels to Randy—Margaret can strengthen their relationship.

The greater the distance from the personal problem, the easier it is to empathize. You may feel empathy for both your friend and your friend's father in their confrontation about a family matter. Yet, a similar confrontation or argument with your own father may block your ability to empathize. Sometimes it is easier to maintain our own way of thinking and not try to see others' viewpoints. It often requires maturity and effort to use empathy when we are personally involved in a situation.

Power

Power is the influence or control one partner has over the other. This power or control affects the behavior and thoughts of the partner. Power is present in all relationships, but it is more obvious in some relationships than in others.

Power can be totally one-sided with one member exerting power or dominance in all areas of the relationship. Power can also be evenly distributed within a relationship. One partner may have power in some areas, the other partner may have power in other areas, and they may share a balance of power in other aspects of the relationship.

DETERMINING POWER • It is clear that in most cases parents have power over their young children. Yet, it is also evident that in some situations a young child can manipulate a parent by use of pouting, refusing to cooperate, whining, or other means of exerting power. Though it is not always possible to determine who holds power in a particular relationship, there are certain characteristics that accompany power positions.

Age usually is related to power. Older persons typically have more power because of their age and experience. Uncomfortable situations can arise, for example, in employment relationships when a younger person is promoted to a position over an older person.

Legal positions can establish power in relationships. Parents, teachers, and police officers are examples of legitimized positions that grant power in a relationship.

Extent of education may also be a factor in power structure. Those persons with more education often hold more power. This can present some concern when younger people find themselves in a changed power structure because of their advanced education.

Money can affect the power balance in a relationship. A factor closely related to possession of money is that of wage earner or "breadwinner" status. The person who "brings home the bacon" often holds more power than the family members who only consume the "bacon" (Figure 4-7). This factor has affected women's roles in American history. Traditionally men were the sole breadwinners and therefore held major power within families. Today women's status as breadwinners has balanced power in a more equitable direction.

Personal abilities, talents, and skills give power positions in a relationship. An individual who has talents to share with others and skills to offer the relationship has a power advantage. Personal attributes such as charm, good looks, and gracious and warm behavior can also provide power in relationships.

The "**principle of least interest**" may be another factor in establishing power in relationships. The person who is less interested or cares less about continuing the relationship has more power. If a partner doesn't care if the relationship ends or flourishes, then that partner has power and can risk almost any behavior.

Figure 4-7

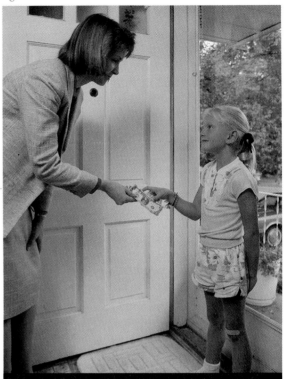

Today's mother often works outside the home. Her ability to earn money gives her economic power in the family.

CASE IN POINT

Nancy and Hans have been dating for a year. As school begins, Nancy gets involved in many activities. Though she continues to enjoy dating Hans, she has less interest in maintaining a successful relationship because of her other activities. Hans, trying harder and harder to maintain the relationship, will do whatever Nancy suggests. Nancy has established greater power because of her lessened interest in the relationship.

DEALING WITH POWER • It may seem from the above discussion that people purposely plot and slyly scheme to maintain power. This may be so in some situations, but usually people find themselves with particular levels of power without having planned it or perhaps even being aware of it. Nancy and Hans, for example, probably have little knowledge or thought about how their relationship is changing.

If power is distributed among particular areas within the relationship, the relationship moves closer to equality. There is a greater likelihood that a growing, developing relationship will be created. Powerlessness in a relationship can be degrading and humiliating. In addition, it could bring about behaviors that might otherwise be considered morally inappropriate. Excessive power by one partner can force the other partner to alter personal values and change standards of behavior. Consider the following situations in which the individuals' standards were altered because of a partner's use of power and their own desire to maintain the relationship.

CASE IN POINT

Roberto had not really been a part of Jack and Kevin's group until about six months ago. Roberto was on the edge of the group—not a real member. He wanted desperately to belong and felt a strong need to be accepted. So, to strengthen his relationship with Jack and Kevin he shoplifted several items to prove his courage to the group. He changed his own standards and values as well as broke the law in order to be a part of the group.

Carole and Patrick dated for several months. Patrick wanted a casual dating relationship with Carole. He also wanted to date several other girls. Carole was interested in a more serious and exclusive long-term relationship with Patrick. Patrick had less interest in the relationship and therefore had more power. He wanted a more intimate sexual relationship than Carole was comfortable with. Carole agreed and cooperated though going against her own moral beliefs and values in order to maintain the relationship.

We can find serious errors in judgment of all the persons involved in these cases. The powerholders misused power; the powerless persons valued their relationships beyond their own personal values and standards. Greater knowledge and understanding of power as well as personal value systems could have prevented these unfortunate situations.

Rewards and Costs

The way people handle power in relationships is by use of rewards and costs. Human behavior is often based on a system of rewards and costs. Rewards and costs are the means by which a person reinforces or strengthens the probability that a certain response or behavior will or will not occur. A simple example is that of a child who makes her bed and receives praise and smiles from her parents. The praise and smiles are her reward. The reward increases the likelihood that she will make her bed again. The parents may use the praise and smiles in order to teach or establish the habit in their child to make her bed each day. Costs may be parental disapproval, withholding an allowance, or some other form of punishment. Both rewards and costs influence human behavior.

Many people find that they have their own reward and cost system within themselves. They don't rely on many rewards or costs from others. Also, the reward and cost system is not the *only* way to bring about a change in behavior. Yet, as we attempt to build and strengthen personal relationships, it makes good sense to be aware of reward and cost systems that we follow and that we establish for others. Awareness of these conscious and unconscious rewards and costs can assist in developing sound, positive relationships that do not allow us to manipulate other people or be manipulated by others.

TYPES OF REWARDS • Rewards are known by many names. Most of the terms (reassurances, prizes, reinforcers, strokes) reflect what the reward giver does or how the person feels when receiving the reward. Regardless of what the rewards are called, they give the receiver good feelings about themselves.

Rewards can be material things—an expensive gift, a raise in pay, a box of candy, or flowers. A reward might be a task performed for another—picking up the dry cleaning, going to the grocery store, mailing a package, or washing the car.

Most rewards received in interpersonal relationships are not material. Rewards can include physical touching—a pat on the back or a squeeze of the elbow. Other rewards may be a smile, a look of praise, a nod, or a meaningful glance. Rewards are often verbal and let the receiver know how his or her action is appreciated:

- It's great to have you here; you really helped out.
- Your report was very interesting; I learned a lot.
- I would like to see you run for one of the state offices. We need people like you representing us.
- It's really fun to work with you.
- It's a pleasure to see such a well-groomed animal. It's clear that you spend time and effort caring for your pet.

Other verbal rewards may be personal compliments:

- Say, you look great today!
- Is that a new hairstyle? It looks good on you.
- You sound enthusiastic today.
- Your flowers really make my office look cheerful. It was very thoughtful of you to bring them.
- I saw you swim yesterday. It looks like you're ready for major competition.

IMPORTANCE OF REWARDS • Rewards have importance for us in two ways—as a receiver of rewards and as a sender of rewards. As a sender of rewards to others, we need to remind ourselves periodically that our partners in a relationship cannot know how we appreciate their actions or their presence unless we somehow indicate our appreciation. It is very common to overlook this simple aspect of interrelating with people. Often the closer the relationship and the greater the amount of time spent together, the less often we relay a reward. Husband-wife relationships, parent-child relationships, close friendships, dating, and work relationships where long hours are spent together often suffer from this lack of shared appreciation. Too often people forget to compliment and say thanks to the closest and most important people in their lives. This brings about commonly heard statements such as the following.

- You just take me for granted.
- You don't appreciate anything I do.
- I'm not sure if I'm doing the job correctly. You never say anything.
- I never hear a "thank you" for all that I've done.

Rewards are easily given and can do very positive things to strengthen relationships. Rewards lose their importance, however, if they're given in a meaningless fashion or purposely used to manipulate behavior of others.

As receivers of rewards, individuals can learn from the rewards given. Knowledge of personal traits and awareness of the effect of personal behavior can be gained by focusing attention on the rewards given by others. Being aware of when and why rewards are bestowed can guide individuals to behavior that is pleasing to partners. However, directing all behavior to please your partner and thereby gaining rewards can result in behavior and personality changes that are untrue to yourself.

Rewards can be beneficial or detrimental to relationships. The following guidelines signal that rewards may be playing a dangerous role in personal relationships if:

- One partner in a relationship is overly dependent on rewards from the other.
- One partner does all the performing and the other partner does all the bestowing of rewards.
- Rewards are manipulated by one or both partners in order to control behavior of partners.

COSTS • Costs are more than simply the absence of rewards. Costs are the negative results from a given action. For example, if a child purposely places chewing gum on a sofa, the child will not receive a smile and a positive reward from the parent. The child will likely have the cost of harsh words, angry looks, or punishment.

Those who control the potential costs have power. A police officer has power in controlling the cost of traffic fines. Teachers have power in controlling the cost of low grades when work is late, incomplete, or poor. Likewise, people have power in a relationship by controlling the potential loss of that relationship. Decisions about our behavior—including our behavior in relationships—involve both rewards and costs.

KINDS OF RELATIONSHIPS

Clearly not all relationships are the same. The relationship with your math teacher is different from your relationship with your parents. The way you relate to your best friend is different from the way you relate to your neighbor. Most of the relationships you have can be grouped as family relationships, friend/neighbor relationships, dating relationships, and working relationships.

Family Relationships

Relationships among family members are one of the most important types of relationships. Not only are they important for the present, but they set patterns and models for future relationships. Since family relationships are so important, they will be discussed further in Chapters 10 and 11, which emphasize interaction with family members.

PARENT-CHILD RELATIONSHIPS • The parent-child relationship begins on an unequal basis. Young children are highly dependent on parents. Parents are responsible for meeting nearly all of their child's needs. Children frequently see the parent as an all-knowing person who can correct nearly every problem and provide a safe and secure environment. At the same time, children strive to discover and experiment on their own. As the child slowly moves from dependence to independence, the parent gives guidance, care, and support.

This balanced parent-child relationship usually continues until the early adolescent years. At this time, relationships between the parents and their teens are sometimes difficult and strained because of transitional stages and development that both the teen and the parent may be experiencing. Adolescence is a time of great change. The movement from the dependence of childhood to the independence of adulthood causes strain on young people as well as the parents. Parents may warn teens to grow up and act their age and yet not allow their teens to try new, maturing experiences. Teens may feel and act like mature adults one day but return to immature, childish behavior the next day. Teenagers take giant steps toward independence; parents strive to maintain control. Body changes, peer pressure and expectations, and changes in the ways of thinking and behaving converge to make adolescence a time of transition that may sometimes be troublesome.

Lesser known than the adolescent transition period is the adult developmental transition period. Parents of many 16- and 17-year-olds are 40 years of age or older. At this point in life, like the teenager, a parent may experience bodily changes and social and cultural pressure. In today's society, gray hair and excess weight (which often accompany middle age) are biological changes that may be difficult to accept. Chances for career advancement may lessen, and adults may be faced with accepting their current career status. Women who have been out of the job market may now face reentry into that market and further education.

Parents as well as adolescents face transitional periods that are apt to bring about crises. Understanding and empathy on the part of both parents and teens can be helpful in easing conflict.

SIBLING RELATIONSHIPS • Sibling relationships, interaction with brothers and sisters, are an important part of family relationships. Sibling relationships are probably second in importance only to parent-child relationships (Figure 4-8). The degree of intimacy or closeness of the relationship is determined in large part by the ages of the siblings and the presence or absence of other children in the home or community. Usually the closer in age and the fewer other children available to interact with, the stronger the sibling relationship. Siblings often play the roles of teacher, role model, protector, playmate, companion, and mediator with parents and others. Much teaching and learning takes place among siblings throughout the life cycle.

Though many sibling relationships are close and positive, nearly all families have some sibling relationship problem. A recent study has shown that there are three basic complaints related to siblings.

1. He or she gets more things or privileges than I do.
2. My parents like him or her more than they like me.

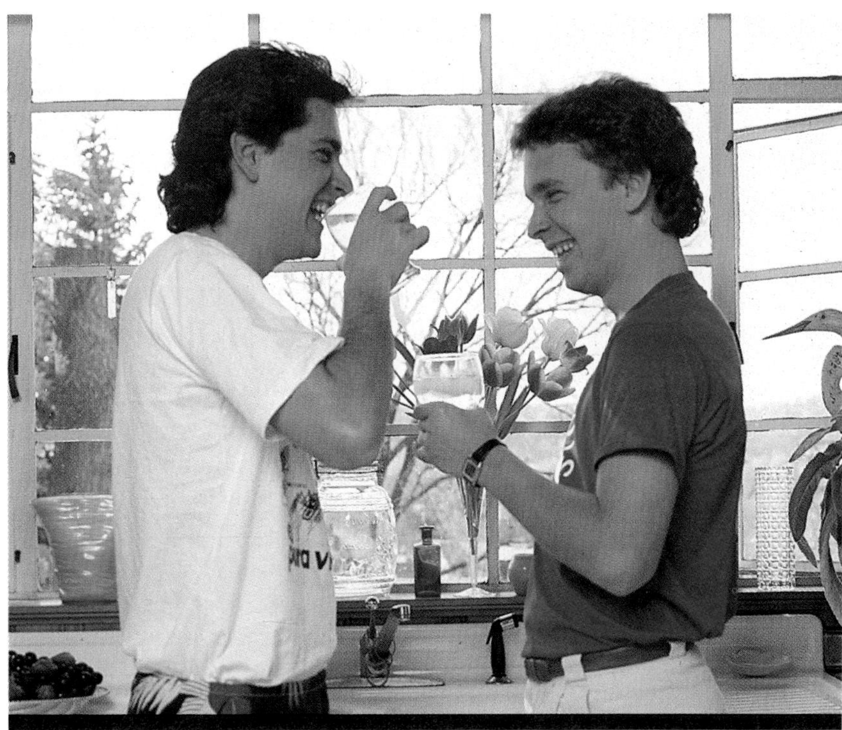

Figure 4-8
Within the family, sibling relationships are probably second in importance only to parent-child relationships. Sibling relationships include roles of confidante, friend, companion, protector, teacher, and antagonist.

3. I have to do more household chores or work than he or she does.

Most of these concerns could be met at least in part by objective family discussions and, in some cases, record keeping. A list of rotating family chores could help ease the frustration of unbalanced workloads. Lists of privileges and receipt of material goods might reflect the reality of the situation and allow the family to look at the issues objectively. However, total objectivity is impossible in families. A family is not composed of disinterested computers that can function 100 percent objectively. Consider the following situations that might affect sibling relationships.

CASE IN POINT

Connie is older and all of her clothes are purchased new. Cindy, her younger sister, gets all of her clothes secondhand from Connie.

Carlos has outstanding musical talent. He takes both violin and piano lessons from well-known and expensive teachers. Viertos has no particular musical talent and does not cost his parents the expense of lessons.

Ben just got an after-school and weekend job. Sarah, Ben's younger sister, may have to take on some of the household chores Ben used to do.

Karen loves animals and has acquired several cats, a dog, rabbits, and a bird.

Though the animals are enjoyed somewhat by the whole family, they are Karen's responsibility. Karen feels that the animal care should be counted as one of her household chores. Charles, Karen's brother, feels that animal care is an extra that should not count as one of Karen's chores.

These situations point out the inability to have full equality in many family situations. Families require give and take and a spirit of sharing that is sometimes difficult when one member feels personally short-changed. Effective communication (to be discussed in Chapter 5) is a tool to ease these feelings.

Sibling rivalry is the competition among children in a family for their parents' affections and attention. This rivalry can be controlled if parents realize individual differences and uniquenesses in their children's talents and interests and do not make unnecessary comparisons. Yet, this aspect of family life is unable to be 100 percent equal. Consider the following parents' statements:

> I know I give John more attention than I give Phil. But John seems to need so much more attention, and Phil seems so independent.

> Susan has always been like a mother to Timmy. I don't do as much for Tim like reading to him or teaching him how to do things around the house because he has Susan to help him.

> I feel badly about not doing some of the things for Anna that I did for Pete and Sandy. I was at home when they were young. But because I've gotten a job, I just can't do all the extra things. I try to make up for it in other ways.

> We had Dora when we were very young. Our budget was tight, and we just couldn't do all the things for her that we can afford to do for Linda, Andy, and David. I think we spent more time with Dora, but now we can afford more material things for the others.

It's clear that no matter how hard parents try, they cannot give equal time and attention to all their children. Unique situations and needs, changing times and places, and personality differences make no two sibling situations the same. Family members strive for understanding and empathy to meet the needs of all family members.

It is important to consider that these same siblings who may be causing you anger and frustration will likely be important people in your adult life. You will probably interrelate with and depend on your brothers and sisters throughout life. Despite the increasing mobility of individuals, sibling ties are still maintained by most people. Try to visualize yourself and your siblings in 30 years as you interact together. Consider your brother(s) or sister(s) as aunts and uncles to your children. Do you picture yourselves as having wide differences in personalities? Could these differences hinder or enhance your relationship?

Friendship and Neighbor Relationships

Friendships can promote mutual growth and development of each individual's self-concept. By sharing experiences and revealing feelings and ideas, you can learn about yourself and the world in which you live. Friendships are usually rewarding. The reward may be in what is received from the person or in what you give to the relationship.

Friendships can function at any level of the relationship wheel or intimacy path. During the middle childhood and early adolescent stage, friendships are often very intense. One or two friends are very close for a period of time and are then replaced with one or two other very close friends. Such a relationship demands that all activities be shared by the friends. Sometimes an activity or interest may be dropped because a friend has no interest in that activity. As adolescents mature, they find that there is room in their lives for many friendships at various levels of intimacy. Friendships begin to center around interests. You may have developed several friendships based on skiing or on an interest in bluegrass music (Figure 4-9). You might have one or two friends you like to spend time with, regardless of what you do together. Yet, another set of friends would be interested in

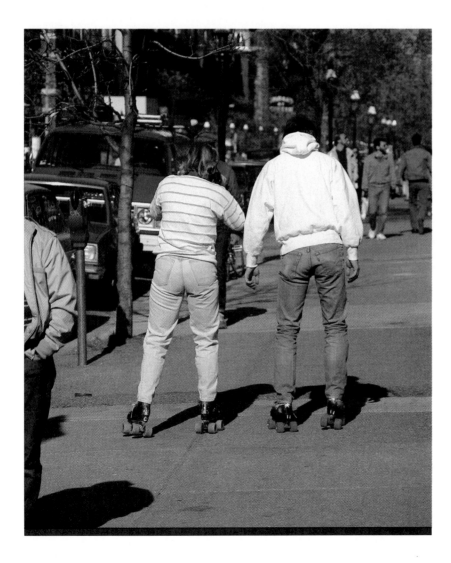

Figure 4-9
A friendship may develop based on a shared interest in skating.
Peter Glass/Monkmeyer Press

trading and discussing mystery novels. Having an array of friendships centered on a variety of shared interests is a healthy asset for entering adulthood.

Neighbors, people living in close proximity, may have friendships just like those with anyone else. Often, however, neighbor relationships are unique interactions that may occur over years without growing in intimacy. Many neighbors function at the first step in the relationship wheel and the first rung of the intimacy path. There may be rapport and intellectual or factual intimacy, but little self-revelation or physical intimacy. Knowledge of crabgrass or opinions on rent control may be shared, but relationships may not extend beyond this point. Recently this country has seen an increase in neighboring. Mutual concern for safety of people and property within communities has brought neighbors together to share neighborhood concerns. Local police have encouraged neighborhood crime watch programs that advocate getting to know your neighbors. Greater familiarity with neighbors and their daily schedules can help alert people to suspicious activities. Sharing vacation and travel plans with a neighbor who can watch your home is now very common (Figure 4-10).

Figure 4-10

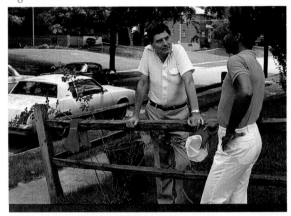

Relationships among neighbors are unique. They can vary in their degree of intimacy. For many people, there may be rapport but little self-revelation or physical intimacy.

Dating Relationships

The term dating can mean many things. To some it is a casual enjoyment of social activities. To others involved in steady dating, it is a commitment that may lead to marriage. Elementary school students talk of dating or "going together," which usually means that a certain boy and certain girl may telephone each other and discuss nothing more than homework. However people think about dating, it usually involves a form of recreation and allows the opportunity to get to know more about the opposite sex. Dating, then, is basically an enjoyable learning experience.

In years past, people dated for the purpose of choosing a wife or husband. Though dating may lead to marriage today, there are other functions of the dating relationship. Dating provides the opportunity to learn about yourself as well as about the type of person with whom you like to spend time. Dating allows you to learn what you expect in an interpersonal relationship. For example, the possessive dating partner who wants to be the only person in your life may be exciting and romantic on the movie screen, but may be boring and irritating in a daily relationship.

Earlier in this chapter the relationship wheel was discussed. Recall that the relationship can move quickly around the wheel. However, those relationships that progress at a slow, steady rate seem to grow to the greatest strength.

In general, people usually date casually before they enter a steady dating situation. This allows time to learn about one's self and expectations as well as about the partner. Too often couples enter a steady dating situation for the insurance of having a date. Though there is security in relying on someone "being there" when a date is needed, this security may prevent learning what is wanted in a dating relationship, and limit opportunities for getting to know different kinds of people.

Steady, long-term dating relationships involve responsibilities for both dating partners. Establishing limits and making these limits clear to your partner is one responsibility of dating. Knowing and expressing limits is important to any relationship, but it is especially important in dating relationships because of the close, intimate feelings that may require the need for acting on your limitations. When you set limits you establish boundaries that define and clarify personal values. Awareness of personal values is important in making decisions. Consider Fred's experience (below). Note how the limits he had established beforehand helped him make an important decision under pressure.

CASE IN POINT

Fred decided several years ago that he would not experiment with drugs. Fred's cousin had become involved with drugs. Fred saw the degrading and embarrassing behavior of his cousin who became dependent on drugs. The long-term effects of drugs on health and the extensive family problems related to drug use were clear to Fred.

Fred had been dating Ginny for several months. Fred realized that drugs were being used at a party held in Ginny's neighborhood. Ginny saw no reason to get concerned, and she teased Fred because she saw no harm in using drugs now and then. Ginny said that all the couples at these parties used drugs together and that it provided a great sharing experience. Fred's strong feelings for Ginny might have persuaded him to go against his own personal values. Fred, however, had established strong limits for himself related to drugs based on his past experience. He was aware of his own values and would not alter his convictions despite Ginny's influence.

Another dating responsibility is that of respecting limits established by the partner. This includes respect for the values and feelings of the partner. When one partner has set a limit on their own behavior whether related to sex, adherence to parents' wishes, use of drugs, driving under the influence of alcohol, or school achievement, the other partner has an obligation to respect these limits (Figure 4-11).

Responsibilities to a partner involve the dating period and after the relationship ends or changes. People who have cared for each other usually find that ending a relationship brings about a loss. Feelings of guilt, sadness, and rejection, as well as relief, are common. Recall that the *principle of least interest* indicates that the person with the least interest in the relationship has more power. This partner may also have less concern when the

Figure 4-11

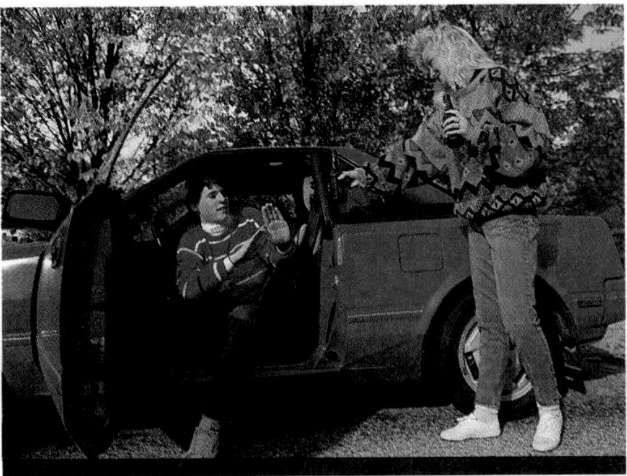

When one partner sets a limit on his or her behavior, the other partner should respect this person's values or feelings.

relationship ends. Working through the ending of a dating relationship, like participating in a dating relationship, is a learning experience.

What kind of responsibilities did Audrey have for Michael even after their dating relationship had ended?

CASE IN POINT

Audrey and Michael had dated steadily for more than a year. When they broke off their relationship, Michael was bitter. He was not anxious to be unattached. He had enjoyed steady dating, and he relied on Audrey. His bitterness and sadness could have made it easy to tell others unkind things about Audrey in order to gain sympathy and attention. However, Michael maintained his concern for Audrey by showing respect for her.

Audrey realized Michael's difficulty in ending the relationship. Because she cared about Michael, she felt obligated to slowly bring their dating relationship to an end. She made efforts to see that Michael was included in social situations in their group of friends.

Work Relationships

There are basically two kinds of work relationships: relationships between employer and employee and relationships among employees. Employer-employee relationships are generally more structured. It is clear who usually holds the power in the situation. Some jobs require a close relationship between employer-employee: other jobs do not really allow much interaction. No matter how close the relationship, it is necessary to have respect for the business, the employer, and the employee. Though knowledge and skill are usually the most important factors in getting a job, job attitude and the ability to relate well to others are necessary to keep the job.

Rewards were discussed earlier in this chapter. It is clear that the employee is rewarded by wages and perhaps special rewards for jobs done particularly well (a bonus, time off, promotion, etc.). What rewards does an employee give an employer? Remember that a reward is the means by which one reinforces or strengthens the probability that a behavior will occur.

Here are some rewards that might impress an employer.

1. Be at work a few minutes early, showing a sense of responsibility for your job.
2. Report any mistakes immediately. Try to learn from mistakes. Don't be afraid to admit it if you make a mistake.
3. Learn and abide by company rules.
4. Be respectful of superiors.

5• Give a pleasant greeting when arriving and leaving work.
6• Ask questions and be appreciative of assistance.
7• Take an interest in the job. Try to appear enthusiastic even during the less exciting parts of the job.
8• Keep your work area neat.
9• Show a willingness to perform extra duties. Go beyond the required work.
10• Don't rush to leave the moment your work time is over.

Actions such as these help to reassure the employer that good working conditions, stable wages, and other positive employment features will assure positive employee behavior. These rewards are in addition to the work carried out.

Relationships with employees can be at any stage of the relationship wheel. Persons may work together for many years and still not know each other well. Regardless of the level of the relationship, the interaction during working hours should be cooperative and respectful with the goal of accomplishing the required work. Courteous interest and concern for fellow workers is necessary for a good work relationship. Unnecessary gossip and discussion of nonwork related topics may hinder these relationships.

The work world often provides young people the first opportunity to interact closely with an older generation of people who are not relatives. This offers a good opportunity to learn respect and appreciation of life experiences as well as of job experience. Attitudes and values may differ and may present situations that result in disagreements and disharmony. The use of empathy to better understand the needs and concerns of fellow workers can be helpful in work interactions. Emphasis on the goals and objectives of the job can also assist in creating smooth employee relationships.

WRAPPING IT UP

Interpersonal relationships form the basis of your current and future life. Humans need healthy and meaningful relationships with other people in order to grow and develop in a positive manner. Some relationships are rich and rewarding, while others are troublesome and difficult.

The growth and development of an interpersonal relationship typically follows a series of stages, as depicted in the wheel theory. These stages follow the sequence of establishing rapport, self-revelation, mutual dependency, and need fulfillment. As relationships grow and develop, we move down a path of intimacy. The three steps on this path include *intellectual intimacy, physical intimacy,* and *emotional intimacy.*

In trying to build strong relationships, we must consider issues of empathy, power, and rewards and costs. *Empathy* is the ability to mentally participate in another person's feelings or ideas. In other words, empathy is the ability to place ourselves in the other person's shoes and see things as they do. Empathy is essential to understanding other people.

Power is the ability to influence or control another person in a relationship. Power is acquired from such resources as education, age, money, and legal positions. The *principal of least interest* says that the more powerful person in a relationship is the one who cares less about whether or not the relationship survives.

Rewards in relationships reinforce or strengthen the chances that a certain response or behavior of another person will or will not occur. Rewards generate good feelings and come in many forms. Rewards involve love, praise, reassurance and support, and material goods. Costs are the negative results of a given behavior. People tend to seek out and stay in relationships where the rewards outweigh the costs. In building strong interpersonal relationships, it is important to be aware of the reward and cost system which you and others follow.

Many kinds of relationships are important in our lives. Parent-child and sibling relationships within our families, friend and neighbor relationships, and dating relationships all contribute to our personal development. Relationships at work are also important. All these relationships influence your ability to be a fully functioning person and to move up the hierarchy of needs toward self-actualization.

Exploring Dimensions of Chapter Four

For Review

1• List three reasons for personal relationships.
2• List five factors that can establish power in a personal relationship and explain how these factors operate.
3• State three guidelines which signal that rewards are playing a dangerous role in personal relationships.

For Consideration

1• Select a newspaper article about international confrontations, congressional disagreement, or state issues that are currently being considered. Discuss how power is operating in these large-scale relationships. Consider how the principle of least interest is operating. Consider if reward is involved.
2• List four reasons why parents may not treat their children equally. Develop examples for each reason. Consider how these reasons may be similar to reasons why children may not treat their parents equally.
3• Develop a brief explanation to a younger sibling as to why it is important to set limits on your own behavior prior to a difficult situation. Give an example of how limits set in advance could prevent a difficult situation.

For Application

1• Create an empathy bulletin board that explains the empathetic approach. Give examples and make it clear that this approach does not require people to give up their own beliefs and values. Consider combining the bulletin boards with a skit demonstrating the use of empathy. Share the board and skit with other classes.

2• Create a short play showing how a relationship moves about the relationship wheel. Establish your own time line in relation to the movement. Consider adding music to fit the pace and style of the stages of the relationship. Remember, the wheel moves two ways.

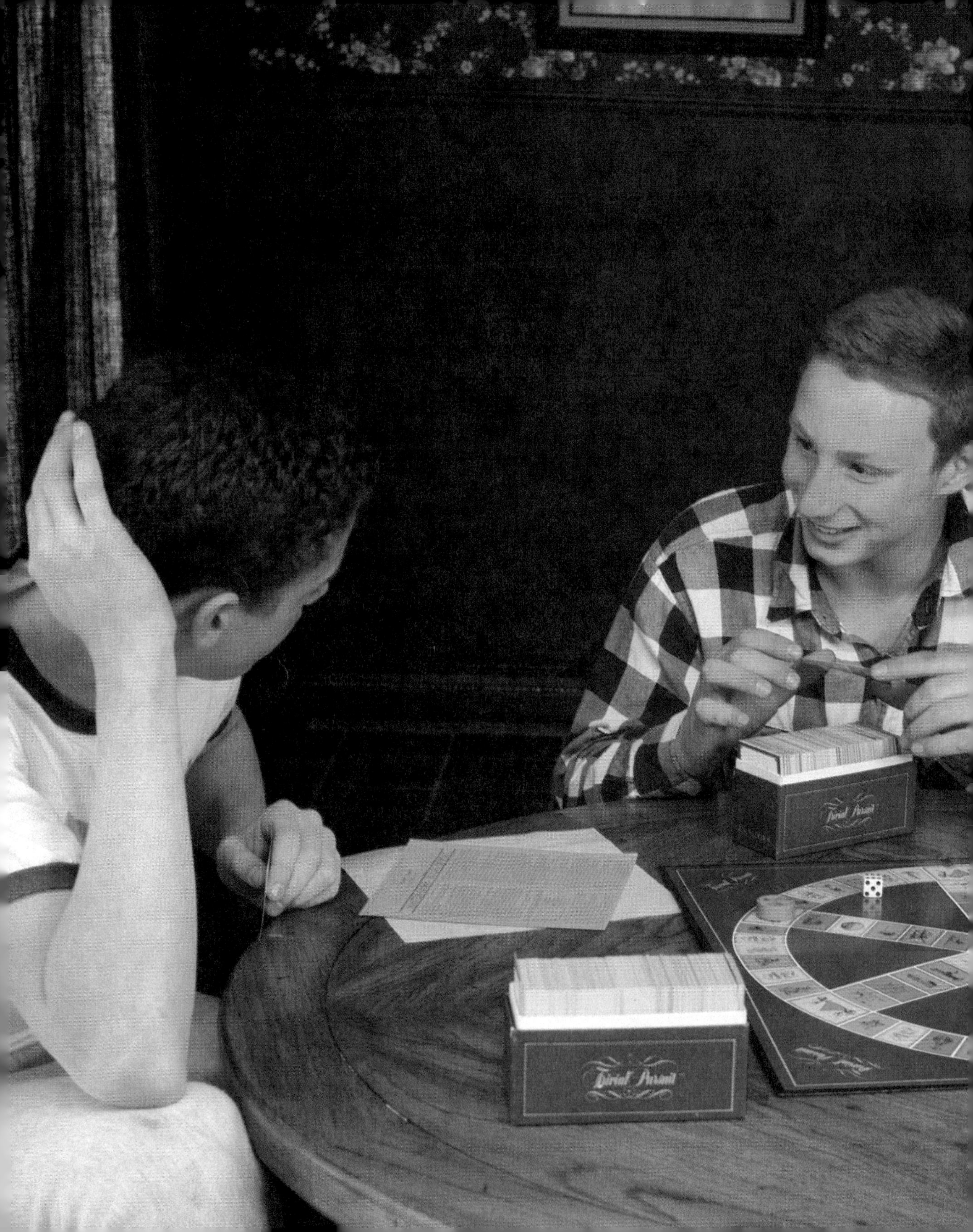
Trivial Pursuit

five

COMMUNICATING EFFECTIVELY

This chapter provides information that will help you to:

- Understand the importance of communication.
- Identify verbal and nonverbal messages.
- Analyze levels of communication.
- Apply skills in communication.
- Understand general communication dynamics.
- Apply skills in conflict resolution.

I know you believe you understand what you think I said. But, I'm not sure you realize what you heard is not what I meant.

In order to have meaningful interpersonal relationships, it is essential to have effective communication. Wondering, assuming, and guessing what others feel or think does not bring about clear and positive communication. Assumptions and guesses lead to troublesome, misleading, and frustrating conversations that may relay little of your real thoughts and feelings. Understanding the importance of communication, the dynamics operating within communication, and the skills necessary for positive communication can reduce these frustrations and concerns. This chapter focuses on building communication skills for forming positive interpersonal relationships.

Fortunately, humans have highly developed communication skills. Yet, communication can be troublesome, misleading, and frustrating in relationships.

IMPORTANCE OF COMMUNICATION

Communication involves listening and sharing information and feelings. Effective communication is necessary for satisfactory interpersonal relationships. Dating, friendships, family, and employment relationships depend on skillful communication. Communication is a vehicle or tool that helps people move around the relationship wheel and along the path of intimacy (discussed in Chapter 4).

Have you ever heard anyone say, "I just can't communicate with that person," or "We can't seem to communicate anymore"? What is really meant is that although some communication is taking place, the communication is poor or difficult between these people. These people's behaviors and/or words are saying, "You are not important enough for me to listen to," or "I'm too busy for you," or "I hear you, but you don't make any sense." One person may be sending messages that are misinterpreted. One or both people may not be listening adequately. Or, various other skills of interpersonal communication are being poorly carried out. Nevertheless, these people *are* communicating. It is impossible for us *not* to communicate.

Positive interpersonal communication brings about positive self-concepts of all those involved. As people learn to communicate positively, they learn to know themselves and others better. Thus positive, rewarding relationships are formed. The process of communication also presents some risks. As feelings and attitudes are revealed and shared, they can be used by others to inflict emotional pain. This risk, however, is usually outweighed by the benefits of positive communication.

Communication is important in all interpersonal relationships and particularly in family relationships. Specific communication concerns and skills related directly to the family will be discussed in Chapter 18. Effective communication in all relationships will be discussed in this chapter.

VERBAL/NONVERBAL COMMUNICATION

Nonverbal communication includes all the behaviors, actions, gestures, and ways of communication other than the spoken word. Primitive humans primarily used nonverbal behavior to communicate prior to the development of human languages. Even today with our highly developed verbal skills, as much as 60-70% of our communication is often nonverbal.

CASE IN POINT

The Clan of the Cave Bear by Jean M. Auel is a fictional account of the Cro-Magnon and Neanderthal races. The story provides interesting examples of various communication patterns. Messages are sent by the earlier Neanderthal people via hand motions. The more advanced Cro-Magnon girl is ridiculed for her odd ways: she laughs, cries, and has the ability to speak beyond guttural grunting sounds. Her smile is considered strange because the Neanderthals do not turn up the corners of their mouths to express their feelings.

Words often fail to relay the full meaning of what we say. Nonverbal expressions and gestures are often more effective (Figure 5-1). A wrinkled brow or frown, a wink, lowered eyes, or the slump of our shoulders often speak louder than words. In order to communicate more effectively, we need to be aware of the verbal and nonverbal messages we send and receive.

Figure 5-1

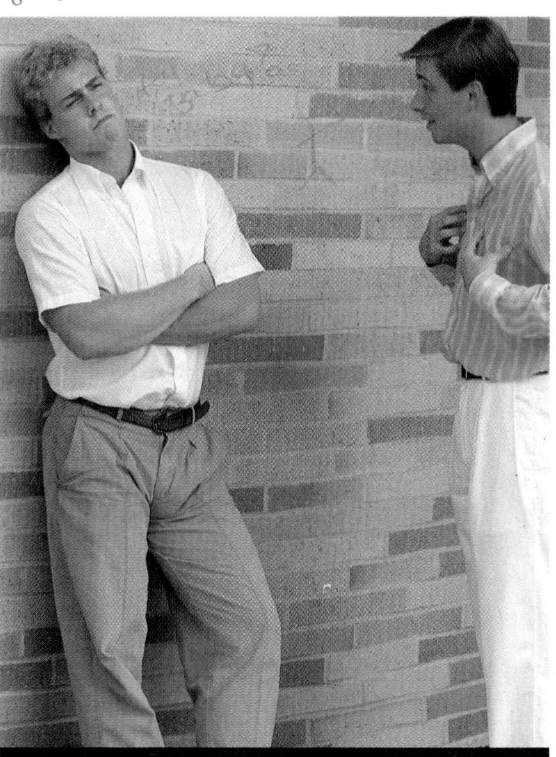

Body language such as gestures and movements are often more effective than words.

Aspects of Verbal Communication

Messages sent and received are affected by various factors of verbal communication. Consideration of these factors is helpful in making communication as clear as possible.

WORD CHOICE • Consider the following questions and the difference in messages sent:

Did your cooking create all these aromas?

Did your cooking create all these odors?

The word *aroma* is usually related to positive, pleasant, inviting smells. The word *odor* refers to negative, unpleasant smells. A specific message is being sent by the choice of either word. The choice of words must be appropriate to the meaning you wish to send. The word choice must be understood by the person receiving the message.

Slang terms such as "cool," "bad," and "heavy" have different meanings in different locations. Sometimes words are used to mean that those sending and receiving the message are of one group—group members are "in" while others are "out" of the group. Such a choice of words for use in a broad group of people with many backgrounds may cause a confused message.

Sometimes meaningless terms are chosen because the senders of the messages are not sure of what they want to say. Terms such as "like, you know," "so, okay," or "and all that stuff" are often used as fillers because the speaker cannot articulate the true meaning of the message. It is difficult, if not impossible, to always know the best choice of words. However, in order to communicate clearly, seek the most meaningful, clear, and best understood words.

SENTENCE STRUCTURE • Complex, run-on, difficult-to-follow sentences hinder communication. Likewise, incomplete sentences often leave the receiver unaware of how to respond. The following sentences communicate poorly because they send incomplete or confused messages:

> I asked her to go.
>
> I think I will ask Mary to the dance on Saturday night though she probably won't be interested because she's sort of mad about the picnic last week when Ned forgot to pick her up and didn't say the meeting had changed.

The first sentence tells us too little (who was asked, when, to go where?). The second sentence gives us too much information—much of which is irrelevant. Attention to how you organize words and relay information assists positive communication.

TONE OF VOICE • The sender's tone of voice can determine how messages are received. Low, well-modulated tones convey a calm, confident manner. High, loud, erratically spaced, grating tones relay irritation, nervousness, or frustration. Consider the following statements relayed to you by a teacher. Hear the difference in the message sent when the tone is well-modulated and pitched at a low level as compared to a high, rasping tone.

> The answers to Chapters 7 and 8 will need to be redone.
>
> I can't accept these as they are.

Consider the interpersonal messages relayed while altering your tone of voice as you repeat the following statements. In what way does tone of voice alter the message? Consider the effect of misinterpreted verbal communication on interpersonal relationships.

> This gift is too expensive.
>
> Why didn't you call me last night?
>
> Oh, I can't believe you did that.
>
> Do you know that person very well?
>
> I get very irritated when you say that.
>
> Please don't ever say that again.

Aspects of Nonverbal Communication

Aspects of nonverbal communication, such as body language, eye contact, communication space, and tactile or touching behavior are also related to verbal communication.

BODY LANGUAGE • The messages sent by our bodies are referred to as body language. We continuously send and receive messages by body language whether or not we are aware of our messages. Most people learn through experience the messages of various body actions. Drumming your fingers, for example, usually means impatience or boredom. Folding your arms can mean a defensive attitude or indicate a thoughtful position. A wink indicates a common bond of understanding. Stroking your chin usually relays a thoughtful, assessing behavior. An erect, upright body indicates interest and willingness to cooperate. A slumping, slouching position says, "I'm not interested, and I'm bored." Closing up space can mean a more comfortable relationship (Figure 5-2). Most of these behaviors become natural and automatic, yet they convey meanings with great power and strength.

EYE CONTACT • This is a particularly important aspect of body language. Direct eye contact usually shows interest in the topic discussed. If you're telling a friend about an important event and the friend looks off into space or casually leafs through a magazine, it's clear that the friend is not giving you full attention or is not listening at all. Equally frustrating is talking to people who casually look over your hair, clothes, and shoes while you speak. You have the distinct feeling that they are not completely listening nor are they very interested in your message.

You may have noticed when giving an oral report that members of your audience respond differently to you. Some people look at you directly and appear to be receiving your words. Others may be discreetly communicating to other class members. Usually you will feel more comfortable by looking at the interested person. You will likely find yourself overlooking or avoiding those who appear uninterested. You may also find different eye contact behavior among class presenters. Some speakers look directly at the members of the audience, including people in all parts of the room. Other speakers look at the ceiling, the floor, or out the window. Such eye movements on the part of the speakers affect the information sent and received just as in personal conversation.

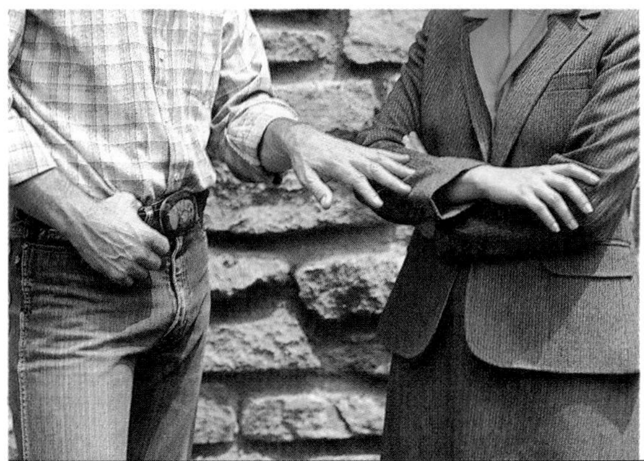

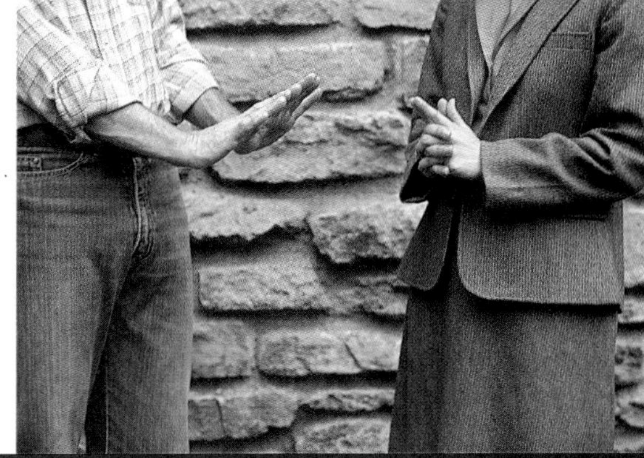

Situations can cause a change in communication space. The apparent concern and interest between the two people shown here brings them closer together.

SPACE • The distance between you and others is an important aspect of nonverbal communication. This distance varies with the closeness of the relationship. People in closer, more intimate relationships have less conversational distance between them. Studies have shown that people operate in four basic communication distances:

- Intimate distance
- Personal distance
- Social distance
- Public distance

Figure 5-3

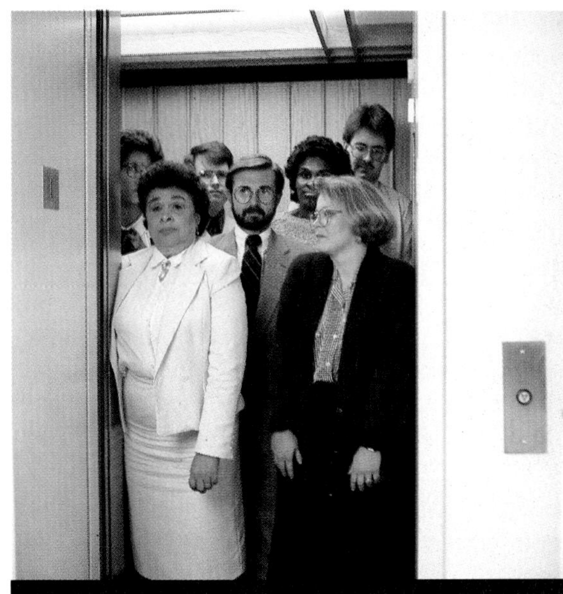

Crowded elevators can be uncomfortable when one must stand so close to strangers.

Intimate distance is usually 18 inches or less. Such distance is used in very close friendships, in kissing or hugging, in expressing an intimate thought or in sharing emotions with family members. This is not difficult to understand. You would not expect to speak loudly across a room to say, "I've really grown to like you over the past few weeks. I seem to think about you all the time. I've never felt like this about anyone else I've dated."

Some situations force a close physical distance between or among those who are not well-known to each other. Crowded buses, subways, and elevators can become uncomfortable when you must stand so close to people who are complete strangers (Figure 5-3).

Personal distance allows conversation that is private but not highly intimate. This distance of 1.7 to 3.2 feet is used when speaking with most friends and family. Conversation at home, school, or in restaurants has this personal distance.

Social distance is 3.2 to 13 feet and is the distance used by people to carry out business and daily activity. This distance is most often used in classroom situations. Employer-employee relationships and buyer-seller relationships are conducted at this distance.

Public distance of 13 or more feet is used, for example, when a school principal addresses a student body in an assembly. It is also used in plays or other public presentations. This distance is impersonal and is generally used to relay information.

The use of space in communication situations appears to be related to culture. The distances related above are found in the American culture. People from foreign cultures, particularly those from southern Europe and Latin America, communicate in closer physical space. Communication between an American and an Italian, for example, could be frustrating if neither person was aware of the differences in communication distances that are comfortable for each person. The Italian might move closer to gain a comfortable communication distance; the American might back up to gain a comfortable communication distance. Humorous but true stories relay an American backing up the length of a long corridor while a foreigner tries to catch up, each in pursuit of a comfortable communication distance.

TACTILE OR TOUCHING BEHAVIORS • People use touching in various aspects of communication. Handshaking, backslapping, roughing someone's hair, a fake punch on the shoulder, a hug, a kiss, or a soft touch on the arm are examples of communication by touch. In general, touch is used with those with whom we are closest and most intimate. In Chapter 4 it was shown that physical intimacy or touching was the second milestone on the path of intimacy. Some people have a greater need to touch and feel others when they are communicating.

Congruence

Typically, nonverbal language and spoken language are congruent. That is, the verbal and nonverbal messages agree. When Phil smiles and moves toward Annette and says, "Annette! It's really good to see you again!" the message is clear. Both Phil's verbal and nonverbal messages have expressed his good feeling about seeing Annette. When your biology teacher looks at you seriously with direct eye contact and tells you your grade won't be raised, the verbal and nonverbal messages are congruent (Figure 5-4).

Figure 5-4

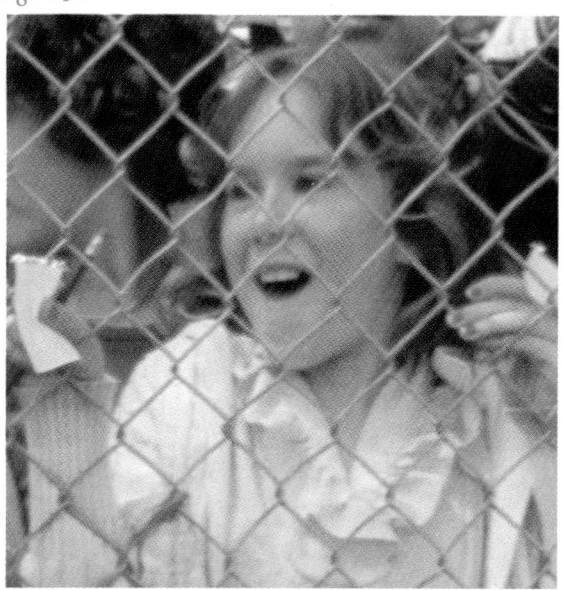

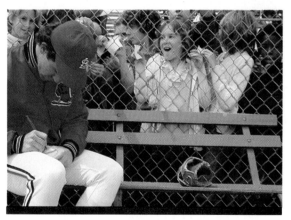

Understanding the context of a situation can help make a message clear. The photo on the bottom helps reveal the true context of the situation.

Florida Department of Commerce Division of Tourism

The communication process becomes more difficult, however, when verbal and nonverbal messages are not congruent. When words say one thing but face, gestures, and physical space chosen say something else, communication signals are hard to read. The following are examples of incongruent communication.

CASE IN POINT

Kiesha returns home after the job interview. Her steps are slow. She tosses her purse on the floor and slowly kicks off her shoes. She sits at the kitchen table with her chin resting on her hand and begins to push some spilled grains of sugar with her finger. When Kiesha's father asks about the interview, Kiesha replies, "It was great. The interview went really well."

Scott is giving a report on dangerous pesticides. He relays the information in a droning monotone and has no active or vital aspects to relay about pesticide use. Scott appears bored with the topic. As he concludes his report, Scott says that he feels this topic is very exciting and stimulating. He says that he hopes to study this area further.

These situations are confusing to the observer. Further communication would be necessary to understand the speakers' real meanings.

The verbal and nonverbal messages are so important and so interrelated that we cannot consider these factors separately. As you think about communication levels, skills, and dynamics within this chapter, realize that *both* verbal and nonverbal communication are involved throughout. Basic concepts related to messages sent, messages received, and feedback processes must be considered within the framework of verbal communication, nonverbal communication, and congruence of verbal and nonverbal communication.

LEVELS OF COMMUNICATION

Chapter 4 discussed levels of relationships. There are also levels of communication. Communication is the tool or vehicle that helps people move around the relationship wheel. As the relationship grows and becomes more intimate, the communication level changes to fit the needs of the growing relationship.

Commonplace Communication

The first level of communication provides little or no real sharing of yourself. Most communication is in the form of cliches or small talk. As you pass an acquaintance on the sidewalk you might say, "Hi, how are you?" You may not even stop or slow down, you may have no interest in how your acquaintance really is. The person may respond with, "Fine, how are you?" Yet, the person does not listen to your response. Despite what your acquaintance said, the person may have a bad headache or a severe case of poison ivy.

Such communication is commonplace and is an outgrowth of habit and custom. Have you ever passed the same people four or five times in one day, yet you've greeted each other in the same tone and words each time? This behavior remains polite and social, yet it is not even at the intellectual level of the intimacy path. Nor has the relationship reached the rapport stage on the relationship wheel. The relationship is only in the beginning stage.

Factual Report

This level also entails little sharing of self. It involves telling or explaining the facts. The following are examples:

Telling your boss that sales tags have been put on all items.

Reporting to the chemistry teacher that you will be finished with your project a day early.

Reminding your mother to call the dentist.

Telling a friend that another trombone player could be used in the pep band.

Though personal ideas may exist in these situations, they are not expressed. Facts are the important relayed ideas. This level moves close to the intellectual level on the intimacy path; it may begin to approach the rapport stage on the wheel.

Relaying Personal Ideas

Sharing begins at this third level of communication. People tell others of their judgments, ideas, and what they think should happen. The following are examples:

Relaying how you would like to see the prom decorations done.

Explaining to a teacher your ideas about forming a debate team.

Stating to your younger brother why you won't let him take your stereo on his camping trip.

This level of communication is near the self-revelation spoke on the wheel; it is not yet to the physical intimacy milestone.

Sharing Feelings

At this stage you share personal feelings and thoughts about a particular topic. The following are examples:

I'm very upset about the accident. I feel somehow we are all responsible.

It doesn't seem to me that the junior class has made a strong effort. I can't say that I feel the class has really tried.

Maybe there is something positive about the play, but I've always felt it was sort of silly and immature.

This fourth level is important and should not be confused with relaying ideas. At the idea-relaying stage, you might reveal plans to take a particular course during summer school. At the feeling-sharing stage, you might reveal worry about taking the course that may be too difficult. A personal feeling is shared at this fourth stage.

When personal feelings are shared, a risk is taken because the receiver of the message may use the information in unintended ways. For example, you may be criticized or disagreed with when you let another person know your personal feelings. Despite this risk, sharing personal feelings is worthwhile. It activates sharing by the other person or people involved and thus leads to a closer, more intimate relationship. Other examples of shared feelings include the following:

Telling how sad you feel since you stopped seeing a close friend.

Relaying how angry you feel with your brother and how you left the house crying this morning.

Sharing your good thoughts and feelings on a warm spring day.

This level of communication reaches the mutual dependency stage on the relationship wheel; it enters the emotional interaction stage on the ladder.

Maximum Communication

The highest level of communication is based on honesty and complete openness. In maximum communication the people are in accord, and their ideas and thinking are highly synchronized (Figure 5-5). Emotions and feelings of the other person are felt. Maximum communication may occur between close friends and family members. But we may have many friends and family members with whom maximum communication never occurs. The experience of complete, open, honest communication is not a permanent situation. Maximum communication is usually a brief, rare situation with satisfaction and harmony. The fact that it is brief and rare makes this situation that much more special. Usually people who experience maximum communication then return to simply sharing experiences.

Maximum communication corresponds with need fulfillment on the relationship wheel. It is at the highest level of the ladder of intimacy. The following is an example of maximum communication.

CASE IN POINT

Erin and Josh are spending the day caring for two children at the park. They have had a picnic lunch and are resting in the sun. The children have gone to the swings. Suddenly shouts from the other

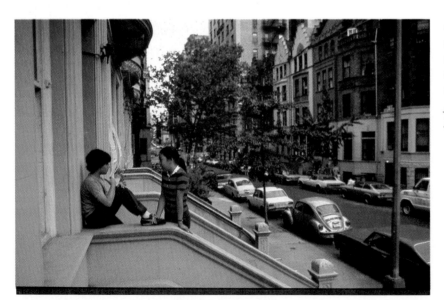

Figure 5-5
In maximum communication, emotions and feelings of the other person are felt.
Jon Lei/Stock Boston

side of the park relay that an accident has occurred. Erin and Josh quickly see that the swings are empty. Both begin running frantically across the park where a crowd has gathered. It seems like hours before they find the children, who are safely watching the police help an elderly man.

Erin and Josh hug the children and each other. It takes a few minutes before they can talk about the situation. During the few minutes of near crisis and the time afterward, Erin and Josh share few words, but their thoughts and feelings are in complete accord. Their emotions and feelings are clearly communicated.

An understanding of the basic communication level is helpful in applying communication skills. As you read and practice the skills, remember that the various levels of communication will require various degrees of the communication skills. Yet, all of the skills are applicable to all of the levels.

SKILLS IN COMMUNICATION

All communication has three components: sender, receiver, and message. The success of the communication depends on how well the sender and receiver carry out their jobs. There are specific skills to improve the sending and receiving process.

The communication process is like a volley in tennis. The server sends the messages. The opponent attempts to understand or know the type of shot so that a good return or response can be made. Just as in tennis, there are specific techniques or skills needed in order to master the sending and receiving process in the conversation game. Also as in tennis, communication skills need practice.

Consider the following communication example as the various communication skills are presented:

Anne: "Tom, I'm sorry that you and Carmen broke up. I thought you two got along really well. It was a real surprise to me when I heard about it."

Tom: "You weren't the only one who was surprised. But things just didn't work out well. We're still friends."

Anne: "That's good. I hate to see the two of you angry."

Make Intentions Clear

The sender's task is to make his or her intention of the message clear. Clarity is necessary not only in how well you speak the message, but in what intentions you relay in the message. Read the previous example in several ways with different imagined intentions of the sender. Make the sender (Anne) sound as if she is secretly happy Tom and Carmen broke up. Next, make her intentions sound genuinely sorry or a bit irritated with Tom because of the break-up. Finally, make it sound as though Anne is not really interested in the matter. Consider various nonverbal behaviors that could relay the sender's intentions. As you see, the intent of the message is affected by the way the verbal and nonverbal messages are sent. It is the sender's job to clarify intentions by being as direct as possible and by making the messages clear.

Spotlight on issues

Self-Concept and Communication

You may have heard people say, "I need to improve his self-concept," or "I'm trying to build her self-concept." In reality, no one can completely form someone else's self-concept. Each individual must build and strengthen his or her *own* feeling about self. We can, however, build an environment or establish a psychological climate to help individuals begin to feel good about themselves.

One of the best ways to establish such a climate is to communicate with people in a way that says, "You're okay," "What you do is very acceptable," "I accept you because you are a worthwhile person." In essence, we can nourish a person's concept of self with words in the same way that we can nourish a person's body with food.

You might not be nourishing the self-feelings of those you love as much as you would like. Opportunities to help your friends and family may frequently be missed. This is probably due to a lack of focused attention on the needs of others. Busy schedules and active lives may prevent us from giving attention to those we care about most.

Another reason we miss these opportunities is that we are unfamiliar with the variety of comments that are good nourishers of self-concept. In your home and school, compliments may not be too common. Praise and acceptance may be given to you in one basic pattern without much variety. "Good" and "nice job" are certainly welcomed phrases that can nourish positive feelings of self. Yet, there are many other ways to communicate to people the goodness they possess. The following phrases provide examples that affirm the worth of your parents, friends, and siblings:

Statements to Peers:

Hi, I'm glad you're here.

I'm glad to hear your opinion.

How did you ever get the scratch out of that fender? You really have a talent.

I see that differently, but I respect your feelings.

Hey, you saved enough money to buy the stereo! Good for you!

Think it through. I'm confident you'll make the best decision.

That color is good on you. You seem to have a knack for choosing nice-looking clothes.

You make a good lab assistant. You never make us feel dumb when we make a mistake.

Statements to Parents:

You're a good listener, Dad.

I bet you had a tough day. Would you like a cold drink?

I'm not sure I like your advice, but I'll give it some thought.

We're really proud of you, Mom.

I think you've given me good guidance. I can handle the pressure. Don't worry.

Hey, Dad, you fix a good batch of pancakes, and you do it with style!

I was nervous, knowing you were in the audience. But, I'm glad you came.

Can you help me with this, Mom? You have a good head for math.

Statements to Siblings:

I'm proud of you.

I can be there if you need help.

What would we do without you, Peggy?

Good luck! Win or lose, we love you.

I didn't realize that you could do that.
Sit down and tell me what happened.

I think your scores have gone up because of your hard work. You deserve the credit.

Start over. I'm not sure I heard all of your story.

These phrases are not just complimentary statements. They reflect recognition and respect. They say, "You matter," "You are a worthwhile person." By adding these and similar statements to your communication patterns, you can set the stage to improve the self-concept of those you love.

Understanding the Context

Context of the message is the situation in which the message takes place. The mood, feelings, previous experiences, physical setting, and level of physical stamina are all part of the context. Each of these factors affects the communication.

For example, you must relay messages by telephone but find it difficult to do so because of family members or friends who may be present. The context of the situation alters the message; that is, the person's presence may alter what you say. Likewise, messages may be altered because of other various contextual situations. In the previous example, if Anne had never liked Carmen and had previously told Tom that the relationship would break up, Tom would interpret Anne's comments differently. Anne's words would have a different meaning for Tom.

You cannot be aware of all the contextual situations that affect communication. You can only try to be aware of what is or has happened to others to influence the messages they send or receive.

"Where are you coming from?" or "Here is where I'm coming from," are phrases often heard within communication groups. These phrases are really attempts to explain the context of the situation. The speaker feels the need to say what she or he has experienced or which situations may have colored the statement about to be made.

I-Messages

I-messages are simple statements of fact about how you feel or think. "I really enjoy your guitar playing." "I need to have a bigger evening meal." "I never feel sure that you will pick up the mail." "It makes me feel good to find your letters in the mailbox." "I get nervous and upset when I hear the two of you argue."

Because I-messages are statements of the speaker's thoughts and feelings, they can lessen arguments and conflict. Others cannot logically argue that the speaker doesn't feel or think in a particular way. Because I-messages reflect how a particular behavior affects the speaker, the message is less threatening to the communication partner. Consider the following examples of how an I-message helps a speaker express feelings without threatening the partner:

Without I-Message:

Speaker: "Your painting is dark and spooky looking. It's sort of creepy!"

Respondent: "It is not. There's nothing creepy about it. You just don't understand good artwork."

With I-Message:

Speaker: "I get creepy feelings when I look at your painting. Is that the image you want to express?"

Respondent: "Well, no, not exactly. I hadn't thought of it as creepy. Maybe some light colors in the background would help."

Without I-Message:

Speaker: Jack Bogard is the best person for president. He's done more for the school than anyone."

Respondent: "You've got to be kidding. Jack pushes all the work off on others. He's never willing to work hard, and he's never had an original idea about anything."

With I-Message:

Speaker: "I think Jack Bogard would be a good president. From what I've seen, he seems to work hard and accomplish things. I think he's done a lot for the school."

Respondent: "Oh, I can't agree! I think he pushes too much work onto others. I can't recall one original idea he's had."

The I-messages allow individuals to disagree without threatening each other. Each person can state personal feelings and thoughts that they have because of their experiences. These thoughts and feelings do not negate or necessarily conflict with thoughts of others.

I-messages are probably most helpful in clarifying your response to the actions of others. The behavior of others often causes irritation and frustration which, in turn, may cause a quick, poorly structured response. An argument is soon generated. I-message responses help you to understand your own feelings and make yourself understood by others. Consider the possible responses to the following situation.

CASE IN POINT

As Bill enters the kitchen, he sees a note from Beth, his younger sister. The note reads, "I told Susan and Sasha that you could take us to play practice tonight at 7:00."

Though Bill has the time, he is irritated that his sister didn't ask but merely assumed he would be able to take her. This is not the first time she's done this. Instead of verbally attacking his sister and refusing to take her to the practice, he decides to use an I-message approach.

Bill: "I feel irritated that you've made arrangements for me to take you someplace without asking me. I feel like I'm being used as your personal chauffeur without being shown any consideration."

Beth: "You mean you want me to pay you for taking us?"

Bill: No. I'm saying that you make plans for my time without asking me first. I get angry when this happens. I feel like you are taking me for granted."

Beth: "Oh, well, I'm sorry. I guess I didn't think about it."

This encounter helped Bill to see why he was feeling irritation and to make himself understood by his sister. (It's easy to imagine how the discussion might have gone without I-messages.) Bill made clear statements about his feelings and about what behavior caused those feelings. Consider one more response using I-messages that increased positive communication.

Mother: "Goodbye. And don't be out too late. Drive carefully."

Sandy: "You know, mother, you say that every time I go anywhere. I feel like you think I'm going to be out until dawn driving around like a daredevil. I've never stayed out very late, and I'm a good driver. I feel irritated that you have to continually warn me as if I'm some irresponsible little kid."

Mother: "Oh, you know I always say that. It just comes out automatically. I'll try to stop. You know that I realize you're a very responsible person."

You-Messages

You-messages can threaten others and generate arguments. "You forgot to mail the letters." "You always prefer such skimpy evening meals." "You aren't reliable about getting the mail." "You fight and argue and make me nervous."

You-messages often accuse, blame, judge, and promote low self-concept. They tend to act as bait and encourage communication that achieves nothing. Consider I-messages and you-messages in the following examples and how they affect the communication outcome.

You-Messages:

Thelma: "You said we would be able to get out of your class early to get the decorations set up and then you forgot!"

Mr. Jefferson: "I didn't forget. You forgot to remind me when it was time. It's your responsibility to remind people, especially when you can't get there early in the morning."

Thelma: "You said it would be all right if I couldn't get here early."

Mr. Jefferson: "But you know better than to let the job go until the last day. I can't remember everything! You have got to take some responsibility."

I-Messages:

Thelma: "It's past time to get decorations set up. I just forgot to watch the clock."

Mr. Jefferson: "'I didn't seem to notice the time either. I think if you rush you can still get finished. Should I ask if someone else in the class is available to help?"

In the first example, the you-message example, situations were threatening to both Thelma and Mr. Jefferson. Each person fought back by adding accusation. No clear outcome is in sight. The I-messages, however, did not threaten either person in the conversation and led to the possible solution for the concern (getting others to help). I-messages are more efficient and effective.

Sending I-messages does not come about easily for most people unless they have grown up with I-message communication in their home. It may take time to learn to use I-messages easily. It also takes some self-confidence to relay how you honestly feel about certain situations. The rewards for such efforts can be close, strong, and satisfying relationships.

Listening

One of the most effective yet most difficult skills of communication is to be a good listener (Figure 5-6). Not only must you *hear* what

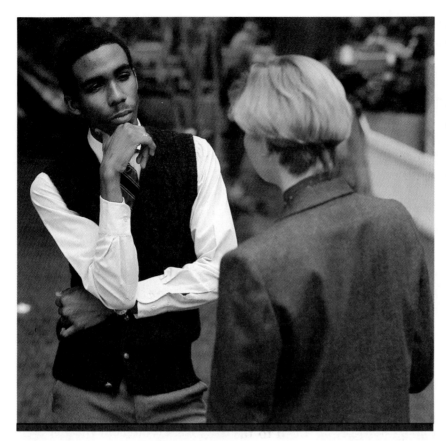

Figure 5-6
Being a good listener means observing the actions communicated by the speaker. It also means striving for the feelings and meanings conveyed by the speaker.

is said, but you must also observe the actions communicated and strive for the meaning and feeling of the words that the other person is conveying.

The biggest roadblock to good listening is that we often want to tell, share, and add our own ideas or give direction. We're sometimes so busy with ourselves that we really don't listen to the other person. A responsible listener attends to the message and attempts to tell the speaker how the message is being received or else the listener asks questions to get more clarification.

There are two basic listening techniques—active and passive listening. In **passive listening**, your responses (gestures, body language) do not relay your ideas or judgments. A passive listener may offer phrases such as "I see" or "Go on." But, the body language and eye contact can welcome the speaker to share his or her thoughts. The listener is attentive and willing to hear all the speaker offers. The listener sets up a climate for the speaker to share ideas.

Active listening involves the listener to a greater degree than passive listening. The listener is an active partner in the interaction with the goal of helping the speaker to be as clear as possible. The listener puts the message into the listener's own words and sends it back to the speaker to see if it is correct.

Marcy: "My parents said they are going to take the dog to the pound this afternoon. I'm so angry!"

Juan: "You're angry at your parents because they plan to have your dog put to sleep."

Marcy: "No, not really. I know Sparky is in pain, and the vet says she can't be helped. But I get angry when I think of how unfair it seems. She's been such a good dog, and now we have to do this."

Juan: "You feel angry because Sparky has to die. You're not really angry at your parents."

Marcy: "Yes, my parents feel just as badly as I do. I'm not really angry at them. I'm just angry and sad about the whole situation."

Juan was able to get the real message from Marcy by repeating what he thought Marcy had said. He sent messages back to Marcy for clarification. It might have been easier for Juan to hear Marcy's first statement and respond with, "I get mad at my parents, too." Marcy's real feelings would not have been shared. Active listening requires a genuine concern and interest on the part of the listener. It takes time to learn active listening. Consider how you as an active listener would respond to the following statements from a friend:

The meatloaf was a mess. I burned the rolls and the potatoes were cold.

I got such a thrill out of seeing my old friend! I was glad I went, even though I wasn't eager to go at first.

They said the report was good, but somehow they didn't act very enthusiastically.

Both active and passive listening can increase communication. Some communication situations and some people seem to work better with one or the other technique. Some people need only to have the stage set for communication (passive listening), while others need more assistance in restating and clarifying their own messages (active listening).

Feedback

Feedback is a verification or affirmation of the meaning of the message. Responsible speakers look for feedback in order to know that their message is understood. Responsible listeners give feedback to let the speaker know the message is understood. In the following brief conversation, see if you can determine the feedback statements.

Pete: "Ms. Glenn, I did a big clay sculpture in art class last term."

Ms. Glenn: "Yes, I remember the piece."

Pete: "Well, when the sculpture pieces were moved for the art show, Miss Evans wanted to borrow it."

Ms. Glenn: "Yes, I know. She asked to use it in the class play as a prop."

Pete: "She says she returned it to the art room, but it's not there now. Phil Westmont said he saw it there yesterday."

Ms. Glenn: "Let's go check it out. I can't imagine how anyone could get into the cupboards in the art room."

All of Ms. Glenn's statements are feedback to Pete's statements. Ms. Glenn could have said nothing until Pete was finished. But her statements made it clear to Pete that she was following the conversation and that she was interested and understood Pete's meaning.

Have you ever explained something on the telephone to someone who gave no feedback? Since you could not get nonverbal cues on the telephone, you had to rely on some verbal indication that the person understood. Either an "okay," "yes," or "I see" was probably needed to let you know that the person followed your explanation, that the person was "with you." Without such feedback, you probably became frustrated.

The active listening discussed earlier is one kind of feedback. Restating the person's message tells how someone understands the message and allows the sender to restate or clarify the message. Other types of feedback include statements about how you feel about the topic. You provide the opportunity for further thought and conversation on the topic. Consider the following discussion. The feedback statements allow the speaker to clarify the message.

Chad: "I'd love to go to the reception! I really would! But I just don't have the proper suit to wear."

Otis: "I didn't know that the reception was formal dress."

Chad: "No it's not. That's not what I meant. It's just that I've worn my one suit again and again. The pants are too short and the knees look worn."

Otis's feedback statements clearly help to clarify the communication.

Feedback is not limited to verbal communication. A nod, a wink of agreement, a smile, and eye contact also can show the speaker that the speaker's words are comprehended and accepted.

COMMUNICATION DYNAMICS

Several factors or dynamics operate within communication that can affect the degree of success of the exchange. Keep these factors in mind when we consider the communication process.

Limited Vocabulary of Sender or Receiver

A limited vocabulary of either the sender or receiver hinders communication. The more words you know and use freely, the better the opportunity to accurately relay your feelings. Mastery of a large, workable vocabulary provides a better chance to send and receive messages. Conversely, limited or misused vocabulary limits and even hinders communication. Consider the following examples to see how a larger vocabulary might have benefited the people involved.

Max: "I'm not sure about the job interview. She seemed to like me. She asked me if I would be dilatory. I didn't know what that meant, but I said I would surely try. Then she said she hoped I wouldn't be listless. I assured her that though I didn't have a list, I would get one."

Jack: "Well, I'm a firm believer in women's suffrage, aren't you?"

Betty: "No! As a matter of fact, I think it's the most disrespectful and degrading thing I can think of."

Jack (later to Marcia): "I couldn't believe it. Did you know that Betty doesn't think women should have the right to vote?"

Betty (later to Phil): "Can you imagine? Jack believes in abusing women. He said he believes in seeing them suffer."

Joe: "Mr. Friedman, our history teacher, really makes me mad. He wrote 'laudable work' on my paper. Every bit of that work was my own, and it was all factual!"

If you are unsure what these terms mean—"dilatory," "listless," "suffrage," "laudable"—check their definitions in a dictionary. Dictionaries are an excellent resource for expanding your vocabulary when you encounter words that are new to you.

Learned Communication

Another aspect of communication you need to be aware of is the fear and insecurity some people have related to communication. If you have grown up in an environment of nonlisteners with very little shared communication, it is likely that communication will be difficult for you. If you have grown up in an environment where there was a lot of talking but minimal communication it may be hard to break the pattern.

We need to remember that communication is learned. We are not born with highly developed communication skills. Since we know that communication can be learned, we know it can be unlearned, altered, and/or improved. Thus, one can learn to communicate more effectively.

Interpretation Inaccuracy

A third dynamic is interpretative inaccuracy. No matter how hard we strive for clarity in both sending and receiving messages, inaccuracy may exist because of background experiences.

Try visualizing a kitchen on a sunny day. Now describe the kitchen to a friend. If we could get a photo of the kitchen in the sender's mind and a photo of the kitchen in the receiver's mind, we would probably find them to be quite different. This is because of different background experiences that have occurred to each person involved.

CASE IN POINT

Ellen was only in one train station in her life. It had been a very hot, stuffy day; the train was late, and she nearly got lost. When Phyllis told Ellen of her exciting train excursion, Ellen was hardly enthusiastic. Ellen's previous experience blocked her positive feeling about train stations.

Interpretation inaccuracy may appear to be overwhelming. You must remember that the communication skills you have learned can aid you in counteracting interpretation inaccuracy. You can never know all about everyone's background. But, by being aware that background differences exist and by using communication skills, you can have effective communication.

CONFLICT AND COMMUNICATION

Conflict is a struggle between people. Conflict often occurs when one person tries to prevent or alter the behavior of another. Conflict also occurs when both parties desire a valued object that both cannot have. For example, the conflicts young children often have over who can play with a toy or who can have the bigger cookie involve struggles over limited resources. Conflict occurs periodically in

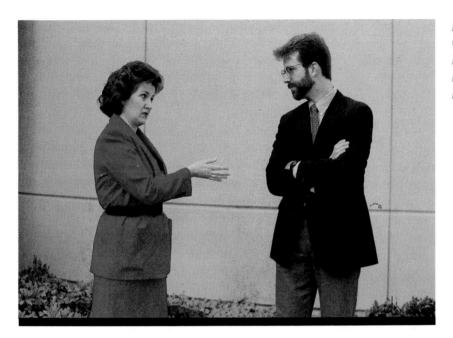

Figure 5-7
Conflict is not always bad. It can help resolve problems if constructively handled.

relationships. Since most ways to resolve conflict (and sometimes the causes of conflict) are centered around communication, let's explore conflict and conflict resolution.

There are several important points to understand about conflict before considering ways to resolve it. First, conflict is not always bad (Figure 5-7). A conflict situation can help to bring major issues into the open and can encourage action to prevent further, more serious conflict. Conflict is harmful when nothing is done to change the situation.

Second, there are negative ways to handle conflict that shut off communication. These methods are harmful and damaging to others. Physical violence is a negative, destructive way to deal with conflict. Some families use this method to deal with conflict and thereby teach this kind of conflict resolution to their children. Physical violence at the expense of self or others is never an acceptable means for dealing with conflict.

Another resolution method for dealing with conflict involves withdrawal or silence when used as a punishment. Withdrawal is removing yourself physically or mentally from the situation. Some people seem to find this the best way to deal with overwhelming feelings. It can be a method for getting your thoughts into perspective and preparing for conflict resolution, particularly for overly emotional people. In this case, temporary withdrawal can be positive. Some people retreat into silence as their method of handling conflict. Though withdrawal and silence may help prevent unpleasant confrontations, they do not allow people to work through their relationship conflicts. Withdrawal and silence without further conflict resolution are not acceptable means of dealing with conflict because they do not permit the expression or communication of people's thoughts and feelings.

Constructive Means for Conflict Resolution

There are various means to resolve conflict. Constructive means are helpful, positive ways to gain a solution to the problem while promoting a general improvement in the relationship.

FOCUSING ON THE ISSUE • This is the first step toward gaining resolution of a conflict. When angry, it is easy to make statements that are off target. These statements may be true, but they are not related to the particular issue in the conflict. When the real issue is not identified, the discussion bounces from topic to topic. The partners do not really know the central issue under discussion. The quarrel can be purposely directed at the issue or problem rather than at the people involved. The following statements help to make clear the conflict to be discussed:

> Hey, what are we arguing about anyway? I thought we were talking about our vacation, not how much work I do around the house.
>
> Let's stop all this useless talk and focus on the problem. You think I'm jealous, and I say I'm not.

The above conflicts have yet to be solved, but they have been saved from going off the issue. It requires practice and clear thinking to keep emotionally involved issues on target.

SELECTING AN APPROPRIATE TIME AND PLACE • If a conflict is to be settled, the people involved must agree to confront each other. If only one person wants to confront the issue, little can be done to find a solution. The partners need to establish a time and place when they can openly discuss the issue. Little can be accomplished when the location allows no privacy and when schedules prevent a real working through of the concern. A crowded cafeteria, a busy hallway, or a family gathering are not the surroundings necessary to resolve conflict. Statements such as the following may be necessary to establish the appropriate time and place for conflict resolution:

> We've had trouble with your curfew hours before. We need to talk about it. I'll be back at 8:30. Let's talk then.
>
> You're right. We need to work this out, but I don't want to talk with other people here. Can we sit down and discuss this tonight?

REACHING CLOSURE • Closure means that the discussion or quarrel has an end. There needs to be agreement that the issue, at least in part, has been settled. Both partners must agree on the closure. If only one partner feels the confrontation has ended, the other partner may save or hold the argument as fuel for future conflicts. Closure statements are helpful in clarifying the issue that has been resolved.

> I think it's good that we had this talk. Your opinion makes more sense to me now. Can we agree that the vacation will be split up?
>
> It seems we've got an understanding now. The money will be used only for your clothes and expenses for school activities.

It is not to be used for insurance or for gas to drive me to work. That's fine with me if you agree.

Sometimes a final solution cannot be reached. A temporary solution that further confrontation is necessary may be the best closure possible. Even this agreement should be clarified.

Well, we haven't come to a solution. It's clear we don't see eye-to-eye on this. Let's both think about it tonight and meet here tomorrow at 4:00. Maybe we can get some ideas by then.

APPLYING THE NO-LOSE METHOD • This allows conflict resolution that is acceptable to both parties. There are no winners or losers in the situation. Rather, the situation which is resolved satisfactorily by both parties is the winner. The steps to the no-lose method are similar to those of decision making.

- Define the problem or issue.
- Generate possible solutions.
- Consider possible solutions.
- Decide on the best solution.
- Implement the best way to handle the solution.
- Evaluate the solution.

People in the business and legal worlds have been successfully using the no-lose steps to negotiate conflict for some time. Specialists in parent education suggest this no-lose method to work out parent-child conflict. This method is not difficult to apply, especially if decision-making practices are familiar. However, all people involved in the situation must eliminate the idea of wanting to win at the expense of their partner. Involved parties must move from a "How can I win?" approach to a "What situation can be best for everyone involved?" approach.

Destructive Means for Conflict Resolution

Conflict is also resolved in destructive ways. Though a solution may be reached, the means for gaining the solution may cause pain to the people involved and generally weaken the relationship.

FOCUSING ON WHO IS RIGHT • This is a destructive way to reach a solution. It is a waste of time and energy to proceed in a conflict by trying to decide who is right rather than trying to reach a solution. When an argument is focused on a fact that can be proved, there is a right and a wrong answer. However, most conflict is not based on factual information. Rather, it is based on personal feelings and attitudes that are neither right nor wrong. Attempting to prove who is right can only extend the conflict.

BLOWING UP • Anger may be shown by crying, screaming, shouting, stomping feet, or otherwise visually declaring feelings. Usually those who use this means of dealing with conflict anger quickly but forgive quickly. Rarely do they hold grudges or maintain their anger. Such a method for dealing with conflict can be destructive because people sometimes say things they do not mean when they are angry. A calm discussion is preferable to exploding with hurtful, angry words. Yet, blowing up is preferable to physical abuse. It is likely that a blowup will move to positive communication more quickly than will withdrawal and silence. When one blows up, it is possible that anger can be released safely, and it is hoped that a discussion will follow.

BAGGING • This is a method of dealing with conflict by saving up irritations, hurts, and anger rather than confronting the issues as they occur. People put these saved-up frustrations in an emotional "bag" or "gunnysack" and hold them until a particular incident triggers their anger. The bag of grievances spills over in a fury of anger.

Bagging or gunnysacking is dangerous for two reasons. First, it does not allow people to deal with irritation as it happens, it permits anger to build and resentment to fester. Second, when people store up their anger and the blowup finally occurs, the fight is often very destructive. When so many issues are "saved up," it becomes difficult or impossible to focus on the most immediate or important issue.

It is safer for the communication if the blowup is aimed at the situation rather than at the person or persons involved. A situation in which a person blows up over a car not starting or a stopped-up sink is safer than a situation in which a person gets furious with a friend's, spouse's, or parent's behavior but does not release the anger immediately. The personal relationships will be damaged far less by having a few quarrels at the time the irritations take place.

USING PERSONAL ATTACKS • Perhaps the most destructive aspect of conflict occurs when people use personal attacks in their quarreling. Rather than focusing on the problem to be solved, people may belittle or ridicule their partners with harsh words. This action not only makes problem-solving difficult, it can destroy the trust that has been established in the relationship. Consider the personal attack in the following situation and the effect of the attack on the relationship.

CASE IN POINT •

Willie and his mother are having a conflict about one of Willie's friends. Willie's mother does not like some of the friend's habits. She has expressed her dislike. Willie is angered by her suggestion that his friend is sloppy and crude. Willie says, "You should talk about habits while you sit there smoking, ashes dropping to the floor." Willie knows his mother wants to stop smoking. He also knows that by mentioning the smoking he'll get to one of her weaknesses. Willie's mother counters his remark with a personal attack on Willie and his friend. The conflict becomes destructive.

There is no place for hurtful, cruel remarks in positive conflict resolution. Name calling can linger long after the confrontation and can have a harmful, permanent effect on the total relationship.

By avoiding the destructive means for conflict resolution and by using the constructive means, problems can be solved. Conflict can promote a better understanding and the total relationship can be strengthened.

WRAPPING IT UP

Effective communication is essential for building meaningful interpersonal relationships. Clear and positive communication between partners helps to forge a strong bond in the relationship. *Communication* is a skill that involves listening and sharing information and feelings. *Nonverbal communication* includes all behaviors, gestures, and ways of communicating other than the spoken word. Nonverbal expression often conveys meaning more effectively than words. Body language, eye contact, use of personal space, and touching are all forms of nonverbal communication.

Verbal communication has many components. Our ability to communicate verbally depends on the words we choose to express ourselves, sentence structure, and our tone of voice. Communication is more effective when verbal and nonverbal expressions are congruent, or consistent. Confusion and problems arise in a relationship when verbal and nonverbal messages do not agree.

Many levels of communication may exist in relationships. Commonplace communication is based on habit and custom. It is intended as a polite exchange between people without any real sharing of self. Factual reports also involve little sharing of self, but do convey information. Relaying personal information involves telling others of your judgments, ideas, and opinions. Sharing feelings involves a more personal level of communication that is somewhat more risky than the others. Maximum communication is the highest level. It involves honesty and complete openness.

Communication skills need to be learned and practiced. These include making your intentions clear; understanding the context in which the communication is taking place; using I-messages and avoiding you-messages; listening; and using appropriate feedback. Barriers to effective communication include the limited vocabularies of the sender and receiver; a poor learning environment for developing communication skills; and interpretation inaccuracy.

Conflict in relationships can be beneficial if it brings major issues into the open and encourages action to prevent further conflict. Constructive conflict management is also a skill that includes the ability to focus on the real issue. It is important that both partners participate in resolving a conflict in a way that is acceptable to each. Destructive conflict management involves focusing on who is right; blowing up; bagging (storing up) your complaints about the other; and using personal attacks. Effective communication and conflict resolution go hand-in-hand.

Exploring Dimensions of Chapter Five

For Review

1• List and give examples of four types of nonverbal communication.
2• List five levels of communication.

3• Explain the difference between active and passive listening.
4• What is the purpose of feedback?
5• List and explain four constructive means for conflict resolution.
6• List and describe four destructive means for conflict resolution.

For Consideration

1• Practice giving I-messages in small groups. Determine a topic that is most difficult for each person to handle. Create I-message statements that help deal with those topics.
2• Practice statements with a partner that help to focus on the issue in a conflict. Practice statements that help reach closure on the conflict. Practice statements to help deal with personal attacks during a conflict.
3• Write a paragraph explaining the problems caused by bagging or gunnysacking issues.
4• Discuss in small groups the kind of feedback that is helpful and the kind that is annoying. Ask teachers how they are affected by student feedback. Draw some conclusions about positive feedback, and resolve to implement certain types of feedback.
5• List people you can relate to at the various levels of communication. In general, with whom do we relay personal ideas and share feelings? With whom do we typically have commonplace communication and factual reporting?

For Application

1• Keep a log of communication. Take notes of the times you do or don't make your intentions clear. Note how and when you use feedback. Consider how knowledge of the context is important for clarity. Note how often and how well you use I-messages. After one week, review the log and set some personal goals for improving your communication. Implement your goals for a full week and evaluate your progress.
2• Create a communication book for preschoolers or elementary school children. Use pictures and simple written material to explain basic points in communicating. You may want to focus on conflict and how to resolve problems. Include only basic points; keep it simple. If possible, try out your book on a group of children. Question them to see what they learned.

3. Explore community resources that assist with problems related to physical abuse. Are resources available for children, women, men, aging people, and handicapped people who have been abused? Are resources available to help the abuser?

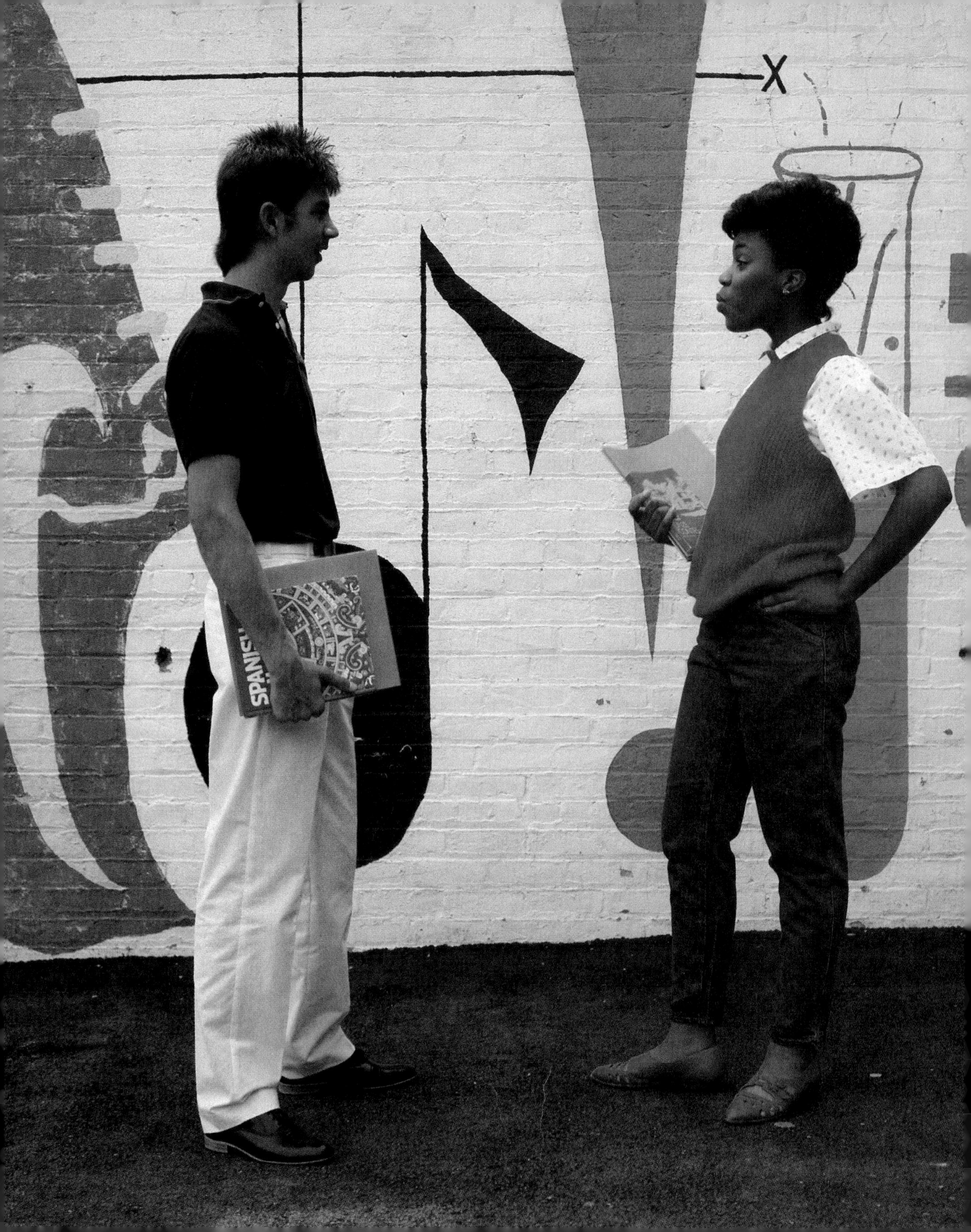

six

UNDERSTANDING OTHERS

This chapter provides information that will help you to:

- Realize the need for understanding other cultures and subcultures.
- Identify stereotypes and prejudices.
- Apply ways to break down stereotypes and prejudices.
- Consider the consequences of decisions with regard to betterment of humankind.
- Establish a personal rationale for human concerns.

Understanding and relating are key concepts in Part Two. Chapter 4 presented the importance of relating to others and building personal relationships. Chapter 5 focused on communication as a tool for building and strengthening relationships. In this chapter, the emphasis is on understanding as a tool for building strong relationships. Strong relationships require the realization and understanding of cultural differences, prejudice and stereotyping, and life in a compressed society.

UNDERSTANDING OTHER CULTURES

Culture is the social heritage of a group of people. It includes all the characteristic features, attitudes, values, traditions, customs, and rules of behavior of a particular group. Families function within cultures. Individual personalities are developed within the family and in the larger cultural sphere. A powerful conditioning is provided in culture from which young people learn the roles they will assume in adult life. In addition, children interact with other children whose families are basically of the same culture. Therefore, similar attitudes, values, and customs are observed.

Subcultures are groups within a culture which have characteristic patterns of behavior that distinguish them from others in the larger culture. Though you may exist in an American culture, you also may be part of an agrarian subculture, an oriental subculture, or an upper class urban subculture as shown in Figure 6-1. Like cultures, subcultures affect expectations, behaviors, attitudes, and overall ways of living.

Figure 6-1

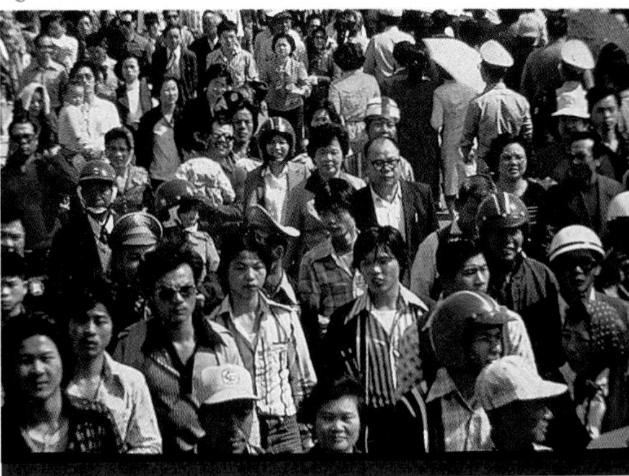

An urban subculture has distinguishing characteristics from other types of subcultures.
Taiwan Visitors Association

When people of different cultures meet, misunderstandings can occur unless attempts are made to know about the expectations, behaviors, and attitudes of the alternate culture. Consider the following situation. Will this incident hinder the relationship between these two people? How can they save their relationship?

CASE IN POINT

When Bob announced the first meeting of the Photography Club, he made a special effort to include Raul, an exchange student from Chile. Bob had seen some of Raul's photos, and he thought that the Photography Club would interest Raul and get him involved in school activities. Raul was pleased to be invited and said he would be at the meeting.

The meeting time was set for 4:00 p.m. After waiting until 4:10, Bob began the meeting. He thought that Raul had evidently decided not to attend. At 4:35, Raul entered the meeting and seemed surprised that so much had already been discussed.

Both Bob and Raul were disturbed and hurt by each other's actions. Bob felt that Raul's late arrival showed a lack of interest, concern, and respect for Bob and the club. Raul was a bit irritated that so much had been accomplished without his presence. He wondered if the club members really wanted him in the club.

Cultural differences have caused this difficult situation. Bob, a product of American culture, emphasizes being on time. Americans generally expect promptness and attention to specific appointments and schedules. Some Latin American cultures are more casual about time. Sometimes, dates and appointments are approximations—"In the afternoon," "At four or five o'clock." Raul, a product of his culture, did not think that he was late. He was surprised the meeting began without waiting for all members.

How Do You React?

While sitting in the school cafeteria, you notice the European exchange student eating her lunch. As she eats her apple, she does not stop at the core as you do. She eats core, seeds, and all. What is your response?

- Consider her poor diet and digestive system and mention it to your health teacher.
- Approach her and tell her this is dangerous and she is not supposed to eat apple cores.
- Hurry to tell your friends. It will make a good story.
- Tell her you noticed she ate the apple core. Ask if this is typical in her country.

There was a time when people needed to be concerned about only the culture in which they were born because most people remained in their own subculture. This expectation was realistic in the past. People from other cultures were considered strange, different, and were usually viewed with suspicion.

These attitudes have changed. America, which is often called the great melting pot, has grown more accepting of people from other backgrounds. Yet, some people hesitate to form relationships with those of different cultures. Realizing and accepting cultural differences are important to today's people for a number of reasons.

Today there is a much greater likelihood of having *contact with people of other cultures.* Many people will visit foreign countries during their lifetime. Increased travel to the United States, including visits of many exchange students, offers more possibilities of widening cultural horizons.

Mobility within the United States—by choice or by chance—will cause many people to live in subcultures different from their own. High levels of mobility cause relationships to be of short duration. Today we make and break relationships more quickly than in past decades.

Cultural understanding is necessary to relate to national and world issues. The front page of most newspapers can reveal actions and decisions made daily that may affect our lives. The outcomes of these decisions can be more accepted or more strongly confronted with cultural and subcultural understanding. Consider the following example.

CASE IN POINT

In the morning paper there is an article stating that the Department of Labor intends to cut benefits to many Americans considered disabled. The article implies that far too many people who are well enough to work are receiving benefits and are thereby draining the Department's budget.

In current events class, Hank is first to volunteer when the request is made for a report on a daily news article. Hank is angry and upset about the article. He criticizes the Labor Department and its decision. Sheila raises the issue of people getting undeserved benefits.

During the discussion and after class Sheila learns that Hank comes from a family of mine workers. His father, grandfather, and great-grandfather were coal miners and all had Black Lung Disease (a disease caused by habitually inhaling coal dust). Hank is deeply concerned about the need for people like those in his family to continue to receive government benefits. He feels that his family's work caused the disease and that they now deserve assistance. Hank also pointed out that people with Black Lung Disease do not look afflicted. Sometimes people have made remarks about his family members receiving aid when they appear "well."

This information helped Sheila to understand Hank's point of view. Though Sheila still contends that there are people who misuse benefits, she appreciates Hank's feelings and thoughts. The relationship between Hank and Sheila is stronger as a result.

When striving to understand those of other cultures, empathy is helpful. When we attempt to see issues as others see them, our understanding increases. We do not have to copy the ideas or philosophies of other cultures to have empathy. Empathy requires only that the situation be considered from the viewpoint of those in other cultures or subcultures. The following example shows the use of empathy in understanding other cultures.

CASE IN POINT

Deanna is a strong environmentalist. She read that the Bowhead Whale was becoming extinct in the waters surrounding Alaska, yet the whale meat was being consumed by the native villagers of Barrow, Alaska. The Alaskan state government had not made such hunting illegal. Deanna considers this inaction foolish. She cannot understand the behavior of the villagers or the government.

As she reads further about the issue, Deanna learns that the customs and traditions related to the killing of the whales are important symbols of success and strength. The Eskimos consider the skin and fat of the Bowhead Whale to be a delicacy. Traditional custom and ritual are involved in the killing of the whale. These factors do not alter Deanna's ideas about the need to preserve the Bowhead. However, she can understand the issue better by knowing the cultural background.

Two major roadblocks to understanding other cultures and subcultures are prejudice and stereotyping. Overcoming these roadblocks is a task requiring much deliberate effort.

UNDERSTANDING PREJUDICE AND STEREOTYPING

A **stereotype** is a standardized idea or mental picture of what people are or how they behave. This mental picture is often unreal and oversimplified. Examples of stereotypes include the flowing statements.

- Teenagers are reckless drivers.
- Athletes are not smart.
- Librarians are cranky and sour-faced.

Though some stereotypes may have some truth in them, they are usually oversimplified because they include *all* persons or things in a given category. Though you may know a cranky, sour-faced librarian, it is unrealistic and unfair to stereotype all librarians in this manner.

Prejudice is a preconceived judgment, attitude, or opinion. The opinion is usually without knowledge or accurate information. Prejudiced ideas and stereotypes are closely related; they are biased ideas and notions. Consider how prejudice and stereotypes function in the following situation.

CASE IN POINT

Al is from New York. He has never traveled to the southern part of the United States. His only ideas about southerners are from old reruns on television. Al's *stereotype* of *southerners* is that they are lazy, shiftless, and not too bright. This stereotype has caused Al to have a *prejudice* against southerners. Unfortunately, Al has had little opportunity to alter this prejudice since he has no contact with people from southern states who could provide Al with realistic information.

Rob has moved from Alabama to New York. When he enters Al's school, Al's prejudice prevents the two boys from forming a relationship even though their interests (tennis, math, and rock music) are similar. As the school year progresses, Rob's math scores are slightly higher than Al's and Al must work hard to defeat Rob on the tennis court. Slowly Al's prejudice begins to fade, and the boys form a strong relationship. Al begins to wonder how he could ever have been so biased and narrow-minded.

There are many kinds of stereotypes with various related prejudices. Consider the following examples. How are these stereotypes oversimplified and unfair?

Age Stereotypes:

Old people do not want change. They can't grasp new ideas.

Adolescents are the cause of most vandalism.

Geographical Stereotypes:

New Englanders are unfriendly people.

Rural people are not as up-to-date as city people. They live in old, rundown houses (Figure 6-2).

Racial Stereotypes:

Black people are very talented in music.

Jewish people are good merchants.

Occupational Stereotypes:

Doctors love to play golf.

Professors are absent-minded.

Sex Role Stereotypes:

Women are poor money managers.

Men are strong and serious.

When stereotypes become well-established and felt by large numbers of people, they can begin to control behavior. The stereotype can

Figure 6-2

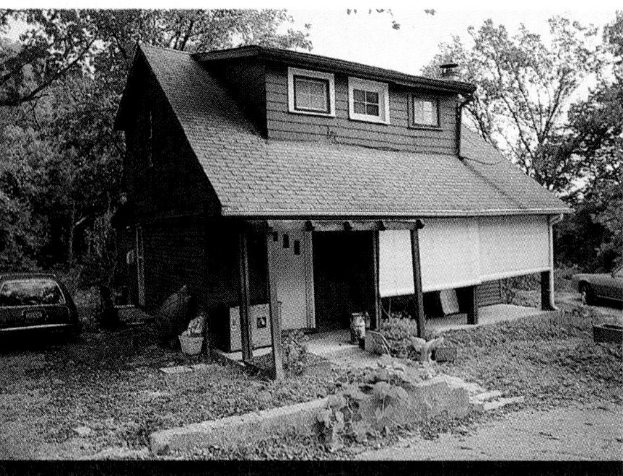

Where do you think this house is located?

prevent people from being themselves and can limit an individual's possibilities. People can lose the opportunity to relate to others as individuals. The following cases show how behavior has been controlled because of unfortunate stereotypes:

CASE IN POINT

Donna and Rose have worked in the school library for several months. They have not formed a relationship because Donna has a prejudice against people who live on Rose's side of town. Donna has stereotyped these people as poor, untidy, crude, and possibly dangerous. Rose also has prejudiced ideas about Donna. She has stereotyped Donna as rich, snobby, and unfriendly.

Helen is aware of the local prejudice against pushy or bossy girls. She's been told that girls who try to do better than boys are not considered good dates. Though Helen felt confident that she could do very well in the speech contest, she decides to withdraw her name. After all, what good would it do to win the contest if she couldn't get any dates!

Aldo emigrated from Europe when he was 12 years old. Now 17, Aldo has an accent that reminds his classmates of a popular television comedian with the same accent. The students have developed a stereotype that all people with this particular dialect are comical and full of jokes. Their expectations have led Aldo to behave comically but inappropriately at school. Aldo is having discipline problems because of these stereotypes.

Individual stereotypes and prejudices can be overcome by relating (getting to know and sharing ideas) to a person having a particular trait (Figure 6-3). Stereotypes are quickly broken when evidence is seen of inappropriate thinking. Unfortunately stereotypes and prejudiced ideas form a cycle that makes it

Figure 6-3

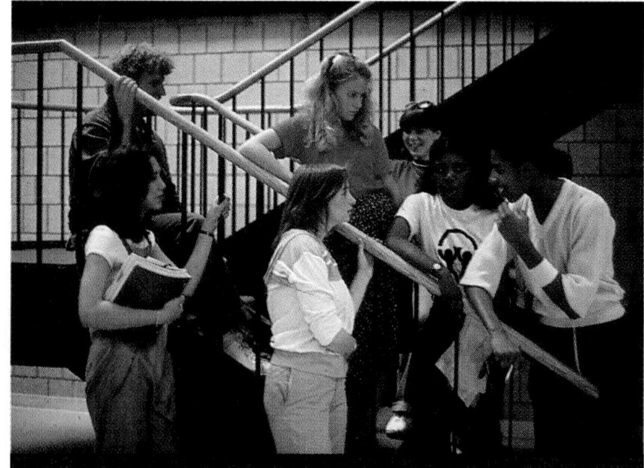

People who believe in stereotypes prevent the opportunity of establishing individual relationships with different kinds of people. Stereotypes can be overcome when we relate personally to people.

Peter Vandermark/Stock Boston

difficult to gain knowledge in order to think clearly and objectively. Teenagers may be stereotyped as destructive troublemakers, for example. Or, male ballet dancers may be thought of by some as self-centered, conceited sissies. A person who thinks this way is not likely to form a relationship with or even be near ballet dancers. Therefore, real knowledge of male ballet dancers cannot be gained. The prejudice is unfortunately maintained (Figure 6-4).

Widely accepted stereotypes can be broken by the media. Television and movies can depict people belonging to cultures or subcultures who do not portray the common stereotypes. These nonstereotyped characters can make it easier for individuals to take a first step toward establishing a relationship with the stereotyped persons. Unfortunately some media presentations reinforce stereotypes and prejudices for effect. The humor is often at the expense of the stereotyped person, or the drama highlights commonly accepted prejudiced behaviors.

Figure 6-4

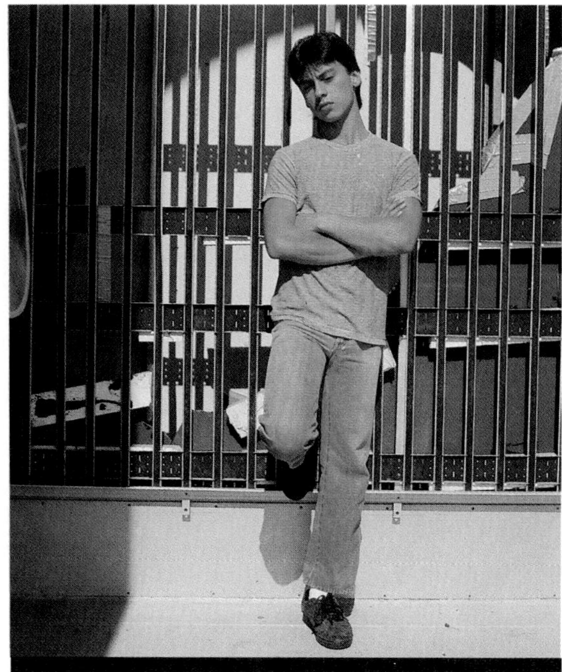

Stereotypes are quickly broken when signs of inappropriate thinking are apparent.

Spotlight on issues

Who Needs Friends?

Friendship is good for your health! It's true. People need other people. Research has shown that people who have strong supportive friends are likely to be more mentally and physically fit than those people without such supportive friends.

Humans as well as animals seem to have a biologically based attachment for others. When in danger or afraid, we seek others for protection.

Recent studies on friendship show that about two-thirds of the people surveyed have one to five friends. Women reported more close friendships than men. Trust, or the ability to keep confidences, was the leading quality people looked for in a friendship.

Friendships serve two very important functions. First, they give us a sense of who we are. Our friends serve as mirrors that reflect our *self*. Second, friendships help us enter important give-and-take relationships.

Friendships are particularly important in the adolescent years. Close friends begin to replace the family by giving positive support to build self-esteem. The school becomes a major center for social development.

Though friendship is particularly meaningful in the adolescent years, it is not uncommon for adolescents to experience loneliness. There may be a period of time when no one can provide the security, comfort, and personal attachment needed. Old friends may be preoccupied with other people or interests, and parents may not be able to fill the need. Loneliness is a universal emotion, though we may try to hide it or avoid it. As we mature, we learn to balance periods of loneliness with close friendship activity and to accept the reality of both.

CASE IN POINT

Educating people about stereotypes and prejudices is difficult because the issues and examples discussed may be interpreted as reinforcing or strengthening the stereotyped and prejudiced thinking and behavior.

An example of this is the use of Mark Twain's *Huckleberry Finn* in public schools. Many educators feel that this book can point out the injustice of racial prejudice by revealing the poor treatment of black people in the late 1800s. Some people, however, feel that this book generates more stereotyped and prejudiced thinking. It is interesting to note that there are black people and white people who favor the use of the book as well as those who are against the use of the book. How do you feel? Is it possible to teach about a topic without having people accept the topic?

Though empathy is a strong tool in increasing understanding, it is difficult to apply if little is known about the other person. It is hard to see things as others see them when the lives of others are very different from our own. Literature—short stories, novels, plays, and musical lyrics—can provide a perspective on the lives of people in other cultures.

BUILDING A RATIONALE FOR HUMAN CONCERNS

Why bother to overcome prejudice and stereotypes? Why do you need to relate to people who are different from you? You might be thinking that people from different cultures and subcultures can stay where they are, and you will manage just fine where you are.

A response to these questions includes three basic areas in which individuals must personally create a rationale or reason for having concerns for humanity. These three areas are related to altruism, living in a compressed society, and the personal gains derived from understanding others.

Altruism

Altruism is the regard for or devotion to the interests of others. Altruistic people are concerned about human good, the betterment of society, and an improved world in which all people can live.

Altruism is the opposite of self-centeredness. People who give of their own time and talent for the human good and for the betterment of society are displaying altruism. Volunteer workers of all ages attend to the needs of others for altruistic reasons. Altruistic efforts are not focused only on certain kinds of people. Rather, altruistic people see the need to understand, have concern for, and relate to all people.

Altruism is evident in communities as well as in individuals. The following are only a few examples of altruistic community action:

- Locally-sponsored schools for the handicapped
- Volunteer maintenance of school yards and parks
- Food pantries and services to help the poor
- Community sponsorship of refugees
- United community efforts to rebuild a neighbor's barn destroyed by fire
- Local fund-raising to help pay for an individual's extensive surgery or hospital care
- Blood donations for family, friends, and others in need

Give examples of such action in your community.

Altruistic ideas generally come about with maturity. Young adults begin to see themselves as human beings in a large world where all people are equal with respect to experiencing personal pain and pleasure. Young adults begin to see the need for their services to humanity and often take action to provide these services.

CASE IN POINT

Barbara does volunteer work at a refugee center. Though she can speak only a few words of the refugees' language, she shows a warmth and friendliness toward these people. As she assists them in selecting clothing, she provides the opportunity for one of their first relationships in this city. When asked why she does this work, Barbara says she feels a need to help others; she has a concern and regard for their well-being. This is an altruistic attitude. Barbara also feels she has gained from these relationships. She feels she has learned from the refugees—not only some words of another language but many things about herself and her own way of life.

Life in a Compressed Society

A second reason for overcoming stereotypes and prejudices is that we are living in a compressed society or a shrinking world. Though the actual global space may not have altered, the space per person is becoming more concentrated. In general, people live closer and interact with others in a more confined physical area than in past generations. Bertrand Russell made the following observation in an article entitled "The Science to Save Us from Science." He wrote, "Mankind has become so much one family that we cannot insure our own prosperity except by insuring that of everyone else."

There are many reasons for our society being compressed. Urban centers bring about a concentration of population for jobs and services. Rising housing costs require more compact living arrangements and sharing of public facilities and recreational centers (Figure 6-5). World trade and travel bring us closer to people and cultures different from our own.

Figure 6-5

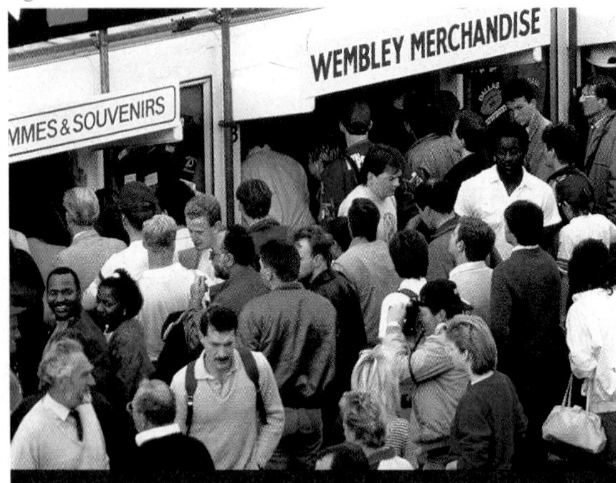

Sharing public facilities and recreational centers forces us to interact with one another in a compressed society.
Al Messerschmidt/NFL Photos

In one sense we have no choice but to strive for understanding of other cultures and subcultures if we want to live in an environment with a minimum of conflict and stress. Understanding and regard for others becomes our responsibility in a compressed society. Recognition and acceptance of this responsibility is necessary in decision making. When making a decision and considering alternatives, we must think about the consequences of our alternatives. Will these alternatives affect others? How will they affect others? If we are to live in harmony, we must consider both self and society and base our decisions on both.

How would consequences to humanity play a part in your decision making in the following situations:

- Soft drinks in throw-away cans are slightly less expensive than the same soft drinks in returnable bottles. Which will you purchase?
- Your state will vote on a mandatory seatbelt law. You do not like wearing seatbelts. Yet, you have read the statistics and realize that fewer traffic deaths occur to persons who wear seat belts. How will you vote?
- The company you work for is considering starting a small day care center for children of employees. To make this change, the size of the employee lounge will have to be cut in half. You have no children. How will you vote when employees are asked their opinion?
- You have saved some money and want to invest it. You are considering investment in a profitable, well-known corporation that manufactures roofing material. However, you learn that this company also manufac-

tures paraphernalia for illicit drug use. Will you invest in this company?

- There is a proposed change in zoning laws in your neighborhood. This change would allow a large restaurant to be built on your block. Aside from concern of lowering local property values, residents are upset about the neighborhood park near the proposed restaurant site. Small children and senior citizens who use the park may be hindered by the increased traffic the restaurant will bring. How would you decide on the issue of this zoning change?

Many factors were probably used in your decision-making efforts. Did concern for fellow humans play a major role in your final decision?

Our world has become too small for each of us to be satisfied only with doing our own thing. The following case makes this point clear:

CASE IN POINT

A ferry boat filled with people was crossing a very deep river. Midway across, one passenger began to drill a hole in the floor of the boat. "What are you doing? Stop that!" shouted the other passengers who were alarmed. "What do you care? It's none of your business!" replied the passenger. "I'm drilling the hole under my seat."

Like the passengers in the ferry boat, our world will pay the consequences of irresponsible attitudes and behaviors. Unlike the passenger with the drill, each of us must become aware of the needs and concerns for fellow humans.

Personal Gains

A third reason to strive for understanding is that the personal gains derived from relating to a diversity of people can be very rewarding. As stated in Chapter 4, we learn about ourselves when we form relationships. When we establish relationships with people of other cultures and break down stereotypes and prejudices, we begin to see ourselves and our own culture and subcultures differently. These new views are enlightening.

Opening gates and removing barriers to relationships with other people enrich our own lives. Breaking stereotypes and relating to people of other cultures and subcultures can make our society more tolerant of cultural differences (Figure 6-6).

The highest level on the hierarchy of personal needs, discussed in Chapter 2, is the self-actualizing level. Self-actualizing people are those people who strive to be the best they can be by using all talents to fulfill their

Figure 6-6

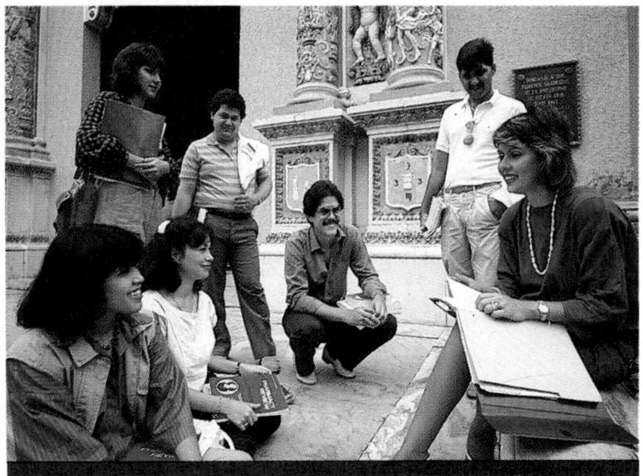

When we establish relationships with people of different cultures, we break stereotypes and remove barriers to relationships.
Michael Mauney/Walgreen Company

potential. Self-actualizing people tend to be people who have high levels of concern for others. It may be that people who are involved with something beyond themselves—something they consider worthwhile and of good to others—tend to become self-actualized.

WRAPPING IT UP

Interpersonal relationships in today's society require a sensitivity to, and an understanding of, cultural differences among people. *Culture* is the social heritage of a group of people. It includes characteristic values, attitudes, traditions, customs, and rules of behavior of the group. Culture conditions people to the roles that they will play in life, both as youth and as adults. Families serve to convey cultural attitudes and values to the individual. When individuals from different cultures interact, misunderstanding can occur if there is not mutual knowledge of each others' expectations, attitudes, and values.

The United States today is comprised of many diverse cultural groups. Mobility within the United States increases the chances that you will enter interpersonal relationships with people from different cultural backgrounds. *Stereotypes* and *prejudice* are major roadblocks to establishing positive relationships among people from different cultures. A stereotype is a standardized idea or mental picture of what people are or how they behave. Stereotypes are oversimplifications of reality. They often lead to misjudgment of the true qualities of another person. Prejudice is a preconceived judgment or opinion that is not based on fact or accurate information. Both stereotypes and prejudice impose limits on a person's ability to reach his or her potential as a human being.

Overcoming stereotypes and prejudice is important for personal growth and development. Central to the building of a rationale for human concerns is the concept of *altruism*. Altruism is a concern for human good and involves a devotion to the interests of others. Altruistic people see the need to relate positively to people of all cultural backgrounds. Altruistic people are not self-centered. Altruism plays an important role in a compressed society where many people have no choice but to live in close proximity to others from different cultures.

We stand to gain much by learning to live in harmony with many types of people. Our lives are enriched as we learn about the fascinating variety of people in the world. Self-actualizing people strive to break down stereotypes and prejudices and help both themselves and others to reach out toward realizing their full potential as human beings.

Exploring Dimensions of Chapter Six

For Review

1• Define culture and subculture.
2• Define stereotype and give two examples.
3• Define prejudice and give an example.

4. Explain how mobility can increase the need to understand other cultures and subcultures.
5. Explain how stereotypes and prejudices operate in a cycle.
6. What is meant by a compressed society or shrinking world?
7. Explain altruism and give an example.
8. What personal gains can come from relating to people of other cultures and subcultures?

For Consideration

1. Respond to the following statements from a friend: "I don't like people who are different from me. I'll be with *my* kind of people and let other people be with *their* kind."
2. Give four examples of how you are living in a more compressed society than your grandparents were.
3. Give three examples of how you have hesitated to relate to people of other cultures and subcultures. Try to explain why you hesitated.
4. Give three examples of television shows or movies that relate to stereotypes. Do they promote or help to break down stereotypes?
5. Give an example of a prejudice or a stereotype that may prevent people from being themselves.

For Application

1. Interview a person approximately your age who has emigrated from another country, who has lived in another country, or who has lived in a very distinct subculture. Ask them about examples of cultural differences and how they have adjusted to these differences.
2. Interview a grandparent or other older relative or friend. Ask about: prejudices and stereotypes that existed in their youth; how these have altered over time; new stereotypes and prejudices that have occurred; and how they would compare youth of today and of their era regarding prejudiced attitudes.
3. Using the local newspaper and other resources, list the altruistic activities that occur in your community. Do not overlook those operating in your own school, church, and immediate neighborhood. Determine how many of these activities are focused on people in the same culture and how many extend to aiding people in other cultures and subcultures. In which activities might you wish to take part?
4. Create a science fiction short story to depict life on various planets. Relay difficulties in relationship formation because of cultural differences among humans and other planetary beings.

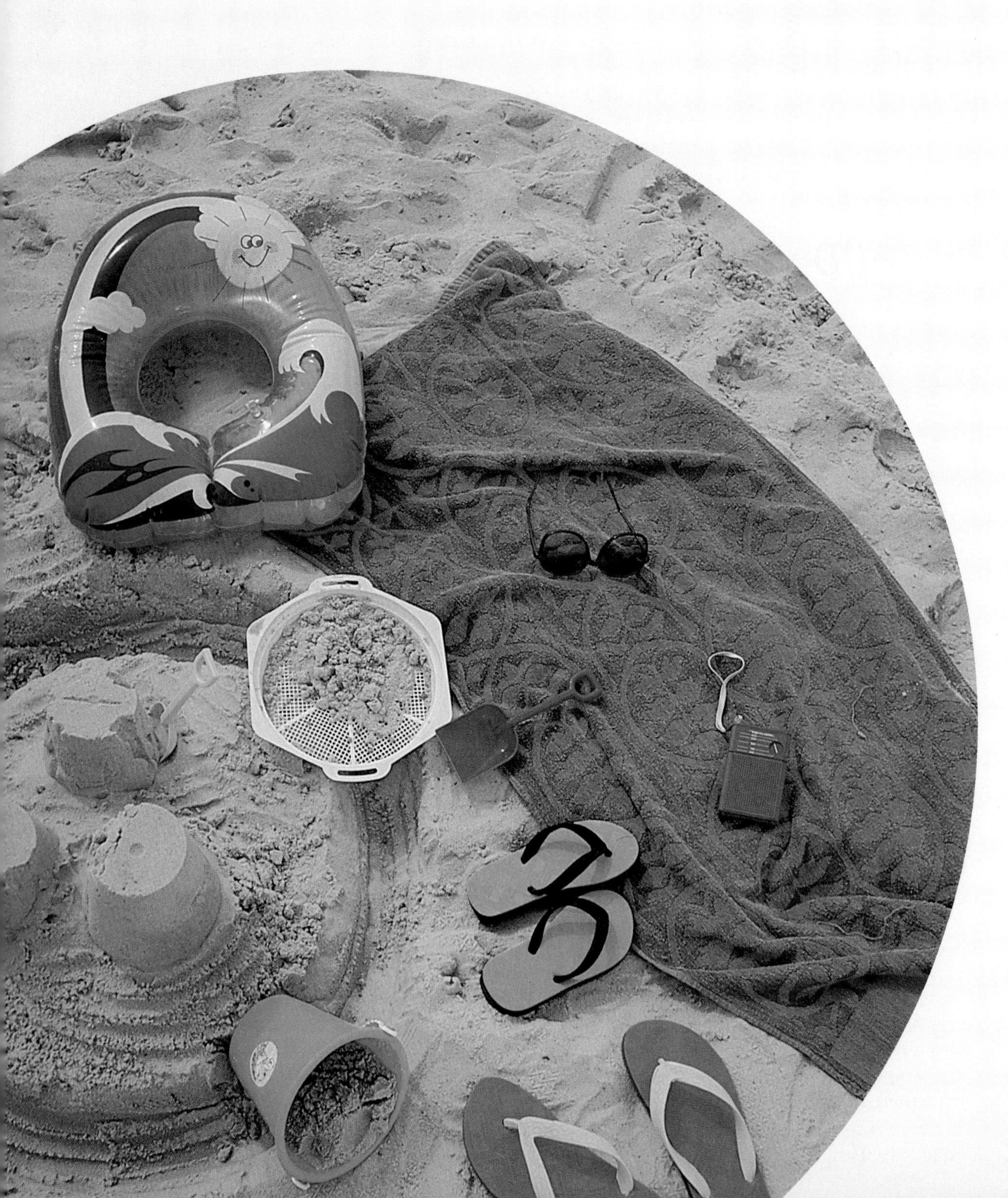

part three

Exploring Human Development

Now that we have explored the importance of interpersonal relationships in our lives, let us look more closely at human beings as individuals. Humans are complex organisms. Humans are also *dynamic* creatures who are involved in a continuous process of change. From conception until death, humans are ever growing, developing, and changing. As we grow older, our bodies change. We develop new ways of looking at and thinking about other people and the world around us. Our needs change. We develop new values and modify old ones and our expectations for ourselves and for others undergo major shifts. Because of these changes, our interpersonal relationships are greatly affected. To better understand ourselves and our relationships with others, it helps to understand the ways in which we, as human beings, develop physically, psychologically, and socially.

Part Three contains chapters on human development throughout all stages of the human life span. Chapter Seven discusses the physical growth and development of infants and children, focusing on bodily changes and changes in physical abilities. Chapter Eight discusses the mental and social development of children. Chapter Nine examines the physical and social development of adolescents and adults. While physical development slows down somewhat during adulthood, we *never* stop developing and changing as human beings.

As we explore these topics, it is important to note how all aspects of human development are interrelated. Human development does not occur in a vacuum. It is shaped and guided by the physical environment and by our contacts with other people. Therefore, you influence the development of *others* just as others influence your development.

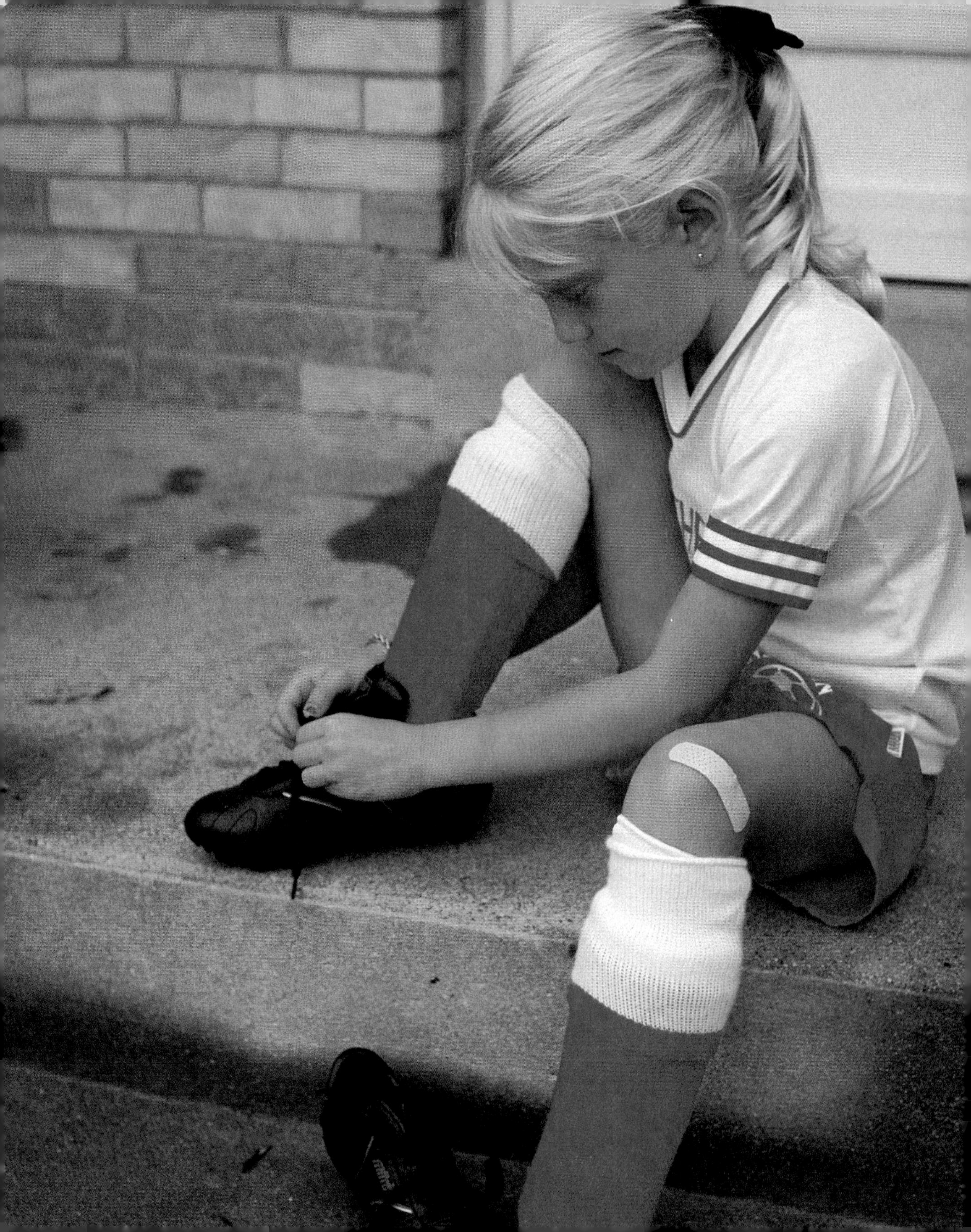

seven

THE PHYSICAL DEVELOPMENT OF CHILDREN

This chapter provides information that will help you to:

- Understand the human life span and its stages.
- Understand conception and the prenatal stage of development.
- Recognize ways of enhancing human development in the prenatal stage.
- Be aware of the physical development milestones of infancy.
- Learn ways to create a safe environment for infants and children.
- Recognize the preschool child and the school-age child stages of the human life span.

Human beings are the most intelligent, yet complex, of all creatures on earth. Although humans cannot run as fast as some animals and are not as strong or keen-sighted as others, the ability to think and to reason sets humans apart from the rest of the animal world. This ability has allowed us to develop machines to do the work that our limited strength does not allow us to do. Heavy construction equipment assists us in building large skyscrapers, highways, and bridges. Jet airplanes, automobiles, and high-speed passenger trains allow us to travel more rapidly than any other species of animal. Therefore, humans must compensate for certain limitations by employing the ability to think, to solve problems, to be creative, and to reason.

THE HUMAN LIFE SPAN

Human physical development is the manner in which one's body changes as one grows older. In studying these changes, it helps to consider the concept of the **human life span**. The human life span is comprised of a series of **stages** that exist across all years of a person's life, from the moment of conception until death. Although the division of the life span into stages is somewhat arbitrary, one usually thinks of the following stages in charting physical development:

STAGE I: Prenatal Stage
STAGE II: Infancy Stage
STAGE III: Childhood Stage
STAGE IV: Adolescent Stage
STAGE V: Adulthood Stage
STAGE VI: Aging Stage

Each of these stages can be divided into substages or phases. In this chapter, we will look at physical development in the first three stages—those relating to prenatal development, infancy, and childhood. We will also look at ways in which human physical development can be enhanced during these stages. Healthy physical development is essential to building a positive self-concept and to becoming a fully functioning person.

THE PRENATAL STAGE

The **prenatal stage** of human development begins with conception and ends with birth. This is the foundation upon which all later stages of human development are built. Although this stage for most people lasts approximately nine months, what takes place is of vital importance to later development.

Conception and the Genetic Basis of Life

The creation of human life is truly an amazing event. It involves a number of conditions that must be present between an adult female and an adult male. The female produces a number of **eggs**, or **ova**, in her reproductive organs known as **ovaries**. The male produces **sperm cells** in his reproductive organs known as **testicles**. **Fertilization** occurs when the male sperm penetrates the outer wall of the female egg (see Figure 7-1). Under normal circumstances, the fertilized egg becomes implanted in the female's **uterus** within a few days. Once this implanting occurs, conception has taken place. After becoming implanted in the uterus, the fertilized egg, or **zygote**, draws nourish-

Figure 7-1

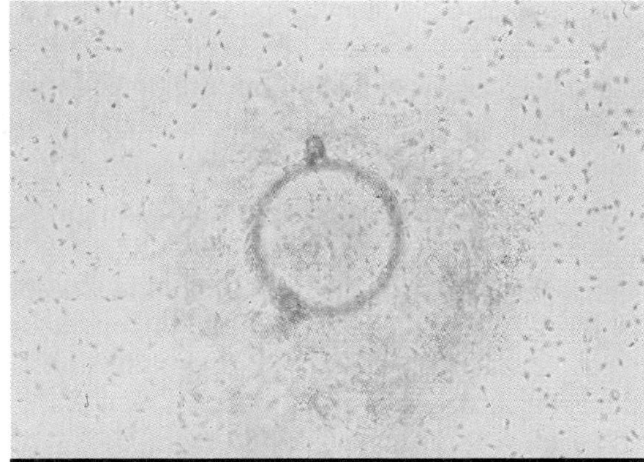

The female's egg is fertilized by the male's sperm. Only one sperm cell can fertilize the egg. After the fertilization, the egg prevents any other sperm cells from penetrating its surface.
Alexander Tsiaras/Medichrome

Figure 7-2

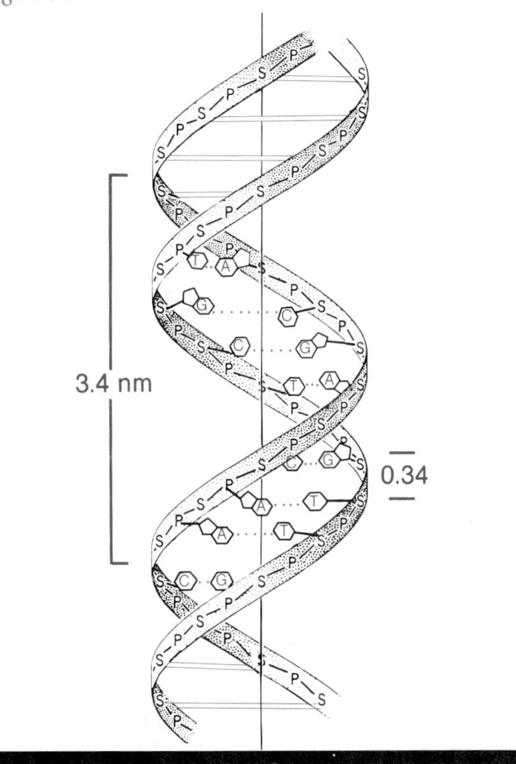

The DNA molecule is the basis for all growth of human cells.

ment from the pregnant female's bloodstream and grows during the prenatal stage of development.

The growth and development of the fertilized egg into a fully formed human being involves a remarkable process. Both the male's sperm cell and the female's egg contain **genetic material**. The most basic elements of this material are molecules known as **deoxyribonucleic acid**, or **DNA**.[1]

DNA molecules form complex strands made up of billions of atoms (see Figure 7-2). These atoms form special codes that direct the division and growth of human cells after conception. In a sense, these DNA codes are "blueprints" that guide the growth of our bodies now and in the future. Both the male's sperm cell and the female's egg contain clusters of DNA molecules known as **genes**. The genes, in turn, make up 23 **chromosomes** in both the sperm cell and the egg. When the sperm fertilizes the egg, the 23 chromosomes from each are combined into 23 pairs, for a total of 46 chromosomes, which are necessary for human cells to develop. Thus, our bodies develop out of an original combination of 23 pairs of chromosomes given to us by our mothers and fathers.

[1]The important role of DNA in human development was first discovered in 1953 by two scientists, James Watson and Francis Crick, who were awarded the Nobel Prize for their discovery.

What influence do these chromosomes have on us? They are responsible for many aspects of our physical appearance. For example, your genetic make-up, inherited from your parents, determines your hair color, eye color, height, facial characteristics, and body build. This explains the physical resemblance we are likely to have with one or both parents, our brothers and sisters, and possibly even more distant relatives such as grandparents, cousins, aunts, or uncles. Whether you are male or female is also genetically determined. To a certain extent, intelligence and other aspects of our mental functioning are genetically influenced. We also inherit **defective genes** that may be associated with certain types of diseases. Tendencies to develop certain types of cancer, heart disease, blood disorders, alcoholism, and a number of other health problems have definite genetic origins.

Once conception takes place, the fertilized egg begins to develop within the pregnant woman's uterus. The combination of genetic material inherited from the parents causes it to grow through a complex process of cell division known as **mitosis**. This growth and development are also influenced by external forces, as we shall see.

Physical Development in the Prenatal Stage

The prenatal stage of development is usually divided into three phases known as **trimesters**. Each trimester normally lasts 12 to 13 weeks. Although the normal duration of a woman's pregnancy can vary considerably, 38 weeks is the approximate time span for the prenatal stage.

THE FIRST TRIMESTER • This phase begins when the fertilized egg is implanted in the mother's uterus (see Figure 7-3). During the first several days after implantation, the egg has developed into a 32-cell organism that is only .005 of an inch long. Until it is about eight weeks old, the egg is known as an **embryo**. It draws its nourishment from the blood supply of the mother, which passes through the uterus. As cells continue to divide and growth proceeds, the embryo begins to develop a bone structure along with muscle, nerve, and blood circulation systems. The digestive and respiratory systems also begin to form in this stage, as does skin tissue. The

Figure 7-3

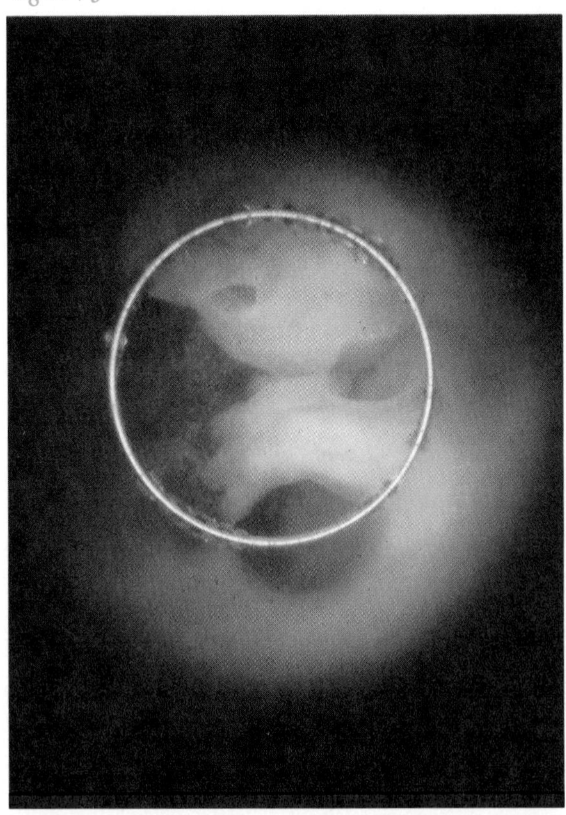

Prenatal development at approximately 8 weeks following conception.
Alexander Tsiaras/Medichrome

following schedule indicates the approximate growth times for these body parts:

Week Three:	Brain, muscles, blood vessels, and heart
Week Four and Five:	Eyes
Week Six and Seven:	Upper and lower limb buds (arms and legs), buttocks, and ears
Week Eight:	Chin, fingers, and toes

After six to eight weeks of growth, the embryo is referred to as a **fetus**. At this time, the average length of the fetus is about an inch and weighs less than 1 ounce. Just the same, the fetus has increased in mass by about 10,000 times compared with when it was a two-cell fertilized egg!

THE SECOND TRIMESTER • This phase lasts from the 13th to the 26th week following conception. Sometime between the 18th and 22nd weeks, the mother is likely to notice the fetus moving within her uterus. This is known as **quickening** and usually results from the fetus moving an arm or a leg. The fetus grows rapidly, on an average, to the levels indicated in the following schedule:

Week Fourteen:	3.5 inches long, weighing 1.6 ounces
Week Eighteen:	5.5 inches long, weighing 7 ounces
Week Twenty-two:	7.5 inches long, weighing 1 pound (16 ounces)

During the second trimester the fetus takes on a definite human appearance. The main body structures and functions are in place and operating. The fetus even shows sucking and swallowing motions. A definite heartbeat can be detected during the fourth or fifth month after conception. Leg and arm movements also grow stronger at this time. Growth continues at a remarkable pace.

THE THIRD TRIMESTER • This phase begins around the 27th week after conception and ends with the birth of the child. During this time the fetus doubles its length and weight. During the last few weeks of this stage, the fetus may gain an average of 1/2 pound per week. Major body organs continue to develop to the point that they will allow the fetus to survive, even if it is born a few weeks prematurely. There is evidence that the fetus can detect sounds outside the mother's body. The fetus also responds to touch, should the mother place her hand or push gently on her abdomen. If normal development of the fetus has taken place, a healthy full-term baby is born and the prenatal stage of human development ends.

Enhancing Human Development in the Prenatal Stage

There is much that parents can do to foster optimum development of the fetus. Although the genes we inherit have much to do with our physical development in this stage, a number of external factors also play an important role.

FACTORS HARMFUL TO DEVELOPMENT • A number of environmental factors can be harmful to the embryo or fetus and can hinder its development. Some might seriously injure or even kill the developing human in the prenatal stage. Some of these factors can be easily controlled by the parent, such as drug and alcohol use, radiation, and nourishment.

Drugs and Alcohol • Many substances commonly used today can be harmful to the unborn child. When drugs and/or alcohol are taken by the pregnant woman, they pass through the mother's uterus and enter the child's bloodstream. Medical studies show conclusively that the following substances are harmful to the unborn child:

- Cigarette smoking
- Marijuana smoking
- Heroin, cocaine, barbiturates, and other hard drugs
- Alcohol (beer, wine, hard liquor)
- Some over-the-counter and prescription drugs such as sleeping tablets, antibiotics, antihistimines, acne medication, insulin, and vitamins C, D, and K if taken in excess

The more of these substances the mother takes, the more harmful are their potential effects. Also, while any of these substances can be harmful at any time during the prenatal stage, the damage they cause is more severe during the first and second trimesters.

Two of the more common substances pregnant women use today are cigarettes and alcohol. Cigarette smoking causes babies to weigh less at birth and to be born prematurely. Alcohol can have far more harmful effects. When pregnant women consume heavy amounts of alcohol during pregnancy, the unborn child is likely to develop **fetal alcohol syndrome**. These unfortunate infants may be born with deformed faces, small heads, ear and eye problems, mental retardation, and heart defects. Such infants are also likely to be born as alcoholics. They are physically addicted to alcohol.

Household Compounds • Certain paints, pesticides, and cleaning fluids emit harmful fumes which, if inhaled by a pregnant woman, can pass to the unborn child. It is important that these be avoided or used with great caution by pregnant women.

Radiation • Pregnant women should avoid x-rays. Radiation penetrates the body and can have harmful effects on the developing fetus or embryo.

Poor Nutrition • Optimum physical development of the embryo or fetus requires sound nutritional habits of the pregnant woman. A balanced diet containing essential vitamins, minerals, and protein is essential. If the mother should be deficient in one or more nutrients, the developing fetus can be harmed. Research studies conducted during World War II found that malnutrition of pregnant women confined in concentration camps led to high rates of mental retardation among their newborns.

Disease • Certain diseases can have harmful effects on the embryo or fetus. For example, rubella (German measles) and certain sexually transmitted diseases (AIDS, syphilis, gonorrhea, herpes) can lead to a number of birth defects such as blindness, deafness, heart defects, and mental retardation.

FACTORS THAT PROMOTE DEVELOPMENT • There are certain precautions parents can take to promote the healthy physical development of their unborn children during the prenatal stage.

Regular Medical Check-Ups • It is important that a pregnant woman see a doctor or qualified medical consultant as soon as she knows or believes she is pregnant. In doing so, she will receive expert advice on how to promote the healthy physical development of her unborn child. For example, a qualified medical consultant can monitor the woman for harmful diseases, high blood pressure, poor nutritional practices, any drug or alcohol use, and any other conditions that may threaten the health of the unborn child. Without proper medical attention early in the pregnancy and throughout its duration, the risk of medical complications for both the mother and unborn child rise significantly.

Healthy Habits • Pregnant women should eat proper foods, not smoke, not drink alcohol, gain the proper amount of weight, and get adequate exercise. In this stage of the life span, the developing fetus is a helpless being. The unborn child is entirely dependent upon the mother's habits and health. The mother must assume full responsibility for this important aspect of human development that lays the foundation for all future growth.

THE INFANCY STAGE

What do you think of when you think of babies? Do you think of them as cute and cuddly or do you think of them as fussy little creatures that cry a lot? Do babies know anything about what is going on around them? At what age should they begin to walk or talk? In this section we will explore these and other questions about the physical development of humans in the infancy stage of the human life span.

Principles of Physical Development in the Infancy Stage

The **infancy stage** begins with the birth of the child and lasts until the child is 2 years of age. Newborn infants vary markedly in terms of birth weight and length. Normal birth weights range from 6 to 9 pounds, although 7.5 pounds is average.

At birth, the human infant is perhaps the most helpless and dependent of all newborns in the animal world. Infants are entirely dependent upon adult care and nurturance in order to survive or, better yet, to thrive. They require much attention to their physical needs for food, warmth, and touch. At the outset, human infants are immobile and require the assistance of others to move them about. If the physical needs of infants are neglected, they are likely to become ill or die.

Physical changes in infancy occur rapidly. Parents of young infants are often amazed at just how quickly their children grow and develop physically. However, it is important to note that the pace of child development at any stage, including infancy, varies considerably from one child to the next. For example, some infants may take their first steps at 10 months of age, while others may not walk until 14 months of age. Both ages fall within a **normal range of physical development**. When we speak of average development for infants, we will see that there is plenty of room for variation, all of which is considered to be in the normal range of development.

Research shows that infants are born with reasonably well-developed **perceptual abilities**—the senses of hearing, vision, smell, taste, and touch. These perceptual abilities allow infants to be quite adaptive to various conditions in their immediate surroundings.

For example, infants respond quickly to bright lights. Within a few days after birth they are able to follow moving objects with their eyes. They also respond to the direction from which sounds may come. The sound of the human voice is particularly interesting to infants. As is true for people of many ages, infants show a distinct preference for sweet tastes. Infants are also very sensitive to changes in temperature, particularly rapid temperature changes in the air or water. They experience pain, and they respond favorably to gentle touching, cuddling, rocking, and swaying. Infant gratification is easily recognized. Unpleasant sensations are signaled by crying and fussiness. Pleasant sensations are reflected by calm and mild behavior.

A major principle of human development is that experiences and events in one stage have a carry-over effect, shaping the person's development in later stages. In other words, stages of development build upon each other. Positive experiences in one stage, for example, increase one's chances for positive development in later stages. Likewise, problems in one stage can increase one's chances for problems in later stages.

This principle certainly applies to the prenatal and infancy stages of development. If growth in the prenatal stage is healthy and the fetus grows normally without any harmful effects from the environment, then the newborn will have an excellent chance to develop in a healthy manner and without limitations during the infancy stage.

If, on the other hand, prenatal development is harmed in some way, the infant starts out at a disadvantage. Although birth defects or handicap conditions may be genetically inherited, they also may be caused by the harmful effects of a prenatal disease or the ingestion of drugs or alcohol by the mother. In either case, these conditions of prenatal development carry over and influence later infant and child development. Depending upon the nature of the handicap, which may involve problems with sight, hearing, or limb (arm and leg) deformities, the child is often limited in physical movement, activity, or learning ability.

Physical Development Milestones

Some parents of infants and young children have a good idea of what to expect from the child in terms of **physical development milestones**. Below is a list of these milestones that infants accomplish at various ages:

- Able to roll from stomach to back
- Glances from one object to another
- Stands alone, without assistance
- Climbs stairs, both up and down
- Sits without support
- Drinks from a cup
- Recognizes his or her name
- Is toilet trained (both bowel and bladder control)
- Jumps and runs
- Takes his or her first steps alone

What do you think is the average age at which infants reach each milestone of development? The actual ages are presented in Figure 7-4.

Walking, running, jumping, climbing, and crawling involve large **motor skills**. These activities reflect **large muscle development and coordination**. These skills develop gradually during the first two to three years of life. Other types of motor activity involve **small muscle coordination**, which is the ability to pick up objects such as a rattle with the fingers. Other small muscle activities require eye-hand coordination. For example, when an infant picks up a cup to get a drink, a number of related activities are required—

Figure 7-4

Physical Development Milestones

Age in Months	Physical Ability Developed by the Infant*
1	Can hold head erect for a few seconds
3	Is able to kick legs well and glance from one object to another
5	Can lift and hold head erect, rolls from back to front
6	Can raise body onto wrists
7	Can roll from back to front, can drink from a cup
8	Can sit without being supported
9	Can turn around on the floor
10	Can stand up when held by hands or arms
11	Can pull the body up to stand by holding onto something
12	Can walk by holding onto something
13	Can stand alone without assistance, can hold cup for drinking
14	Can walk alone, recognizes own name
15	Can climb up stairs
18	Can climb onto a chair and take shoes and socks off
19	Can climb up and down stairs
20	Can jump, has established bowel control
21	Can run, has established bladder control during the day
22	Can walk up the stairs
24	Can walk up and down stairs

*These are *average* ages, with much room for normal variation.

reaching out; locating and grasping the cup; positioning the head, mouth, arms, and hands just right; raising and tilting the cup at the proper angle so that the drink goes in the mouth rather than spilling out; reversing these steps when the mouth is full to again avoid spilling; and, finally, swallowing! As infants grow older, they strengthen the motor skills they acquired as infants by playing with toys and with other children (Figure 7-5).

As Figure 7-4 shows, an infant's first motor skills involve movement and control of the head. Figure 7-4 also shows that physical development follows a progressive series of steps, from the very simple to the more complex. The old adage that "you must learn to crawl before you can walk, and walk before you can run," applies when it comes to physical development. The infant follows a learning sequence that allows him or her to continue learning more complex motor skills over time.

Figure 7-4 also shows that the infant is able to sit without support at around 8 months of age, although sitting with some support is possible around 4 months. Rolling from stomach to back occurs earlier (at about 5 months) than rolling from back to stomach

Figure 7-5

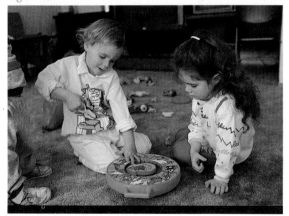

Infants and toddlers can vary in their physical appearance and development, all within a normal range.

Rick Kopstein/Monkmeyer Press

(7 months). Small motor skills required to drink successfully from a cup are usually mastered by the time the infant is 1 year old. Creeping and crawling begin at around 10 months of age, while walking with some assistance is usually accomplished by 12 months old. By 18 months, the infant can run, and by 20 months is probably able to jump.

Enhancing the Physical Development of Infants

The physical development of the infant is strongly influenced by parents and other caregivers. Infants depend on proper care if they are to develop in a normal, healthy manner—they cannot care for themselves. What parents soon discover is that they have a 24-hour job in caring for their infants. Infants are an around-the-clock responsibility.

Recall Maslow's hierarchy of needs discussed in Chapter 2 (Figure 2-1, p. 21). At the base of the hierarchy are the physical needs which are especially important for infants to satisfy. Infants have real needs for food, clothing (for warmth and comfort), shelter, nourishing liquids, sleep, and exercise. As they grow older and learn to crawl and walk, safety needs—the next step up the hierarchy—become important. We will now look more closely at each of these types of needs.

MEETING THE PHYSICAL NEEDS OF INFANTS • Proper nutrition is of major importance for infants. The growth of brain and other body cells requires that infants receive an adequate amount of nutrients in their diets, including vitamins, minerals, and proteins. Foods with high levels of salt, starches, and sugar should be avoided or kept to a minimum in the infant's diet. An excess of such elements can lead to **obesity** (being fat or overweight). Dietary needs of infants change as they grow older. The newborn infant, for example, needs only the mother's breastmilk or infant formula to acquire these essential nutrients. Only after a period of time are solid foods introduced. It is important for a parent to know when the dietary needs of the infant change.

Poor nutrition can have harmful effects on the infant's physical development. Failure to grow at a normal rate, certain diseases, or even mental retardation can result. Irreversible brain damage can occur from poor infant nutrition over a long period of time.

There are a number of books that a parent can read to get information about proper nutrition. A pediatrician is also a good source of information and should be consulted. In your community you may have professionals known as registered dieticians. These people are experts in nutrition and can provide accurate information as to what constitutes an adequate diet for infants.

In addition to proper nutrition, infants have needs for physical stimulation. Infants must be held, cuddled, touched, and talked to if they are to reach an optimum level of development. Parents or caregivers should know that infants need physical exercise to ensure proper muscle and bone development. For example, infants who are in the creeping and crawling stage should not be overly confined to playpens that restrict their ability to move freely about. Infants need space and ample opportunity to exercise arms, legs, and other parts of their bodies. At the same time, it is important to have realistic expectations of the infants' development. For example, some parents may try to encourage their infant to walk before the child is really ready. They may hold a 3-month-old infant up by the arms and force it to take steps, not knowing that this might actually be harmful. Knowing the physical development milestones helps parents understand the appropriate times that infants should be ready to do certain things.

While exercise helps large muscle development, small muscle development and hand-eye coordination can be aided by the use of colorful noise-making toys. The toys do *not* need to be expensive. Small rattles, safe objects to explore with the hands or mouth, and even kitchen gadgets, such as plastic bowls, pots, and pans, provide an interesting variety of inexpensive objects for the infant. Infants gain little from the use of expensive toys that are beyond their developmental level.

Finally, infants require an appropriate amount of rest and sleep. Each infant has his or her own patterns of sleep and rest—some need more sleep than others, while others need less. Also, infants vary in their sleep schedules. Some infants nap routinely during the day and also sleep through the night, while others follow more erratic sleep schedules. Parents soon learn that they must adjust their sleep patterns to accommodate the sleep needs and schedules of their infants.

MEETING THE SAFETY NEEDS OF INFANTS • Infants depend on their parents and other caregivers to guard their physical safety. The environment holds potential hazards for infants. Household accidents threaten the health and lives of thousands of infants each year in the United States. However, nearly all of these accidents could have been avoided had the parents or caregivers taken proper precautions to create a safe environment. Great care must be taken to assure that the environment is made as safe as possible (see Figure 7-6).

Figure 7-6

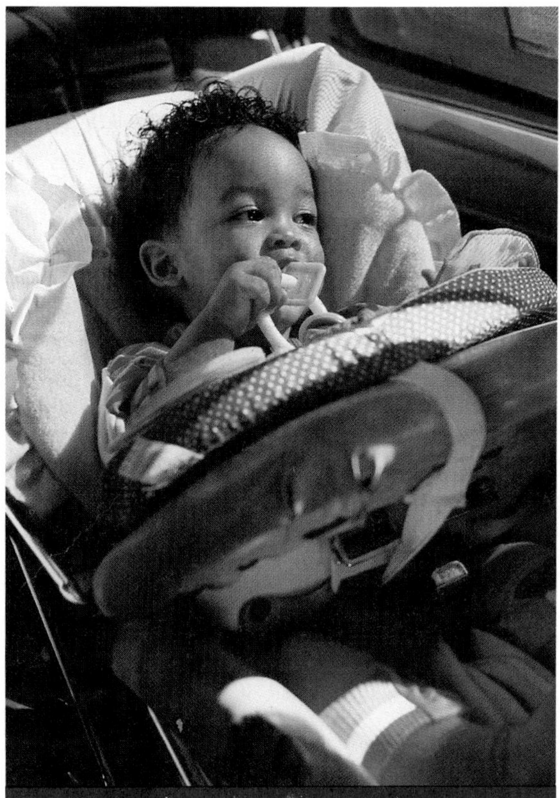

Infants must be protected from hazards in the environment.

Infants explore much of their environment with their mouths. Rattles, hands, pacifiers, and just about any object that an infant can grasp is likely to be placed in or around the mouth. The problem here is that an infant may get hold of a dangerous object. Anything that is sharp may injure the mouth. Small objects, like bottle caps, marbles, or coins, can become lodged in the infant's throat and can cause choking or even asphyxiation. The infant that is crawling or walking can also get into cupboards where poisonous substances are kept. Household cleaners, insect or rat poisons, bleach, and detergents are just some of the common household items that can seriously injure or kill infants. Many infants drown each year because they are left unattended around swimming pools, bath tubs, lakes, or other bodies of water. Others die in household fires, or suffocate in discarded household appliances (refrigerators, washers, or dryers).

Another threat to the safety of infants is unsecured automobile travel. A safe and sturdy car seat, secured with a seat belt, should be standard practice when traveling with an infant. Many states now have laws that require young children to be secured in an approved car seat and/or with seat belts. Too many infants and young children are seriously injured or killed in automobile accidents because they are not properly secured.

In providing a physically safe environment, parents and infant caregivers should follow the following basic rules for child-proofing the environment:

1. Move all sharp, small, or otherwise unsafe objects out of reach.
2. Secure all cupboards containing hazardous materials with safety latches or locks.
3. Place all poisonous substances in areas high enough that the infant cannot possibly gain access to them.
4. Cover all electrical outlets with safety caps. Move all electrical appliances to secured areas that are inaccessible to infants.
5. Block all stairways with safety gates.
6. Do not leave infants unattended for long periods of time. Know where the child is and what potential hazards might exist in the environment.
7. Never leave an infant or young child unattended in a motor vehicle. Closed vehicles heat up quickly, causing suffocation or heat stroke.

THE CHILDHOOD STAGE

The **childhood stage** begins during the third year of life. The child is now able to walk, run, and move freely about. This stage lasts until 11 or 12 years of age, when the child undergoes changes in the body that mark the beginning of adolescence.

A major feature of this stage is that the child is quickly becoming less dependent upon an adult caretaker for full-time supervision. By age 3, the child can understand simple commands and instructions and communicate with other people.

Physical development begins to slow down a bit. The average child will grow two to three inches in height per year and will gain five to seven pounds. The average height and weight of girls and boys stays about the same during this time. While boys might develop a slight edge in terms of physical strength, girls acquire better small and large muscle coordination in such activities as hopping and skipping. As was true for infant development, however, there exists a wide range of normal variation in the growth patterns of children.

CASE IN POINT

Three-year-old Monty was shorter and weighed less than the other children in his neighborhood. His mother was concerned about this, and she took Monty to the family doctor to have him examined. The doctor checked Monty's growth pattern by comparing it to national averages that are based on many years of research on children's physical development. The doctor also ran some medical tests on

Monty's pituitary gland—the gland that is responsible for growth. The doctor assured Monty's mother that there was nothing physically wrong with Monty. His genetic make-up was such that Monty was likely to remain somewhat smaller than his peers, perhaps even into adulthood. Although Monty was smaller than average, the doctor assured Monty's mother that he was still quite normal.

Physical Development of the Preschool Child

Physical development of the three- to five-year-old child continues to involve the meeting of basic physical needs for food, clothing, shelter, and safety. The major change in children this age is that they are rapidly developing the large muscle abilities to run, climb, throw, and catch. Small muscle coordination is also improving rapidly. Preschool children use crayons, scissors, and other objects necessary to be creative. They also can dress themselves. The preschool child's need for sleep during the day decreases, and the general level of activity increases significantly. Parents of preschool children are challenged just to keep up with their children's active stage of development (see Figure 7-7).

Figure 7-7

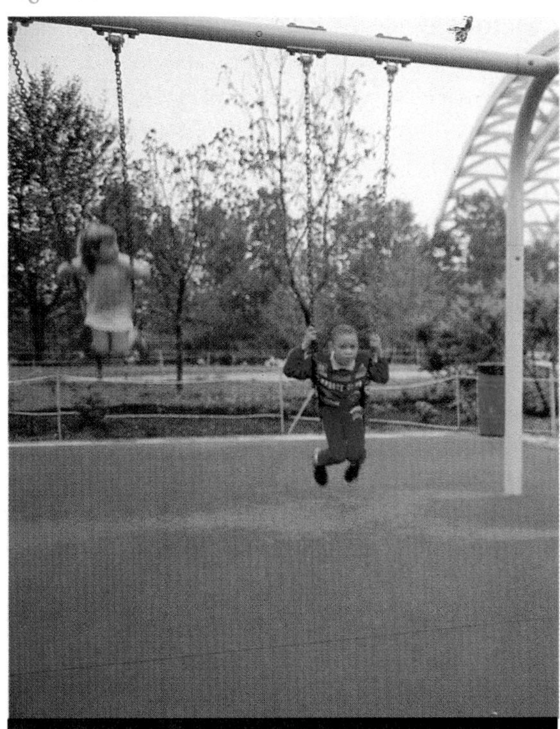

Preschool children rapidly develop physical abilities that allow them to direct and control their own activities.

Because of increased activity, the nutritional needs of the young child change as well. It is important that the child receive a properly balanced diet with appropriate amounts of protein, carbohydrates, minerals, and vitamins to ensure maximum bone, muscle, and nervous system development. Excess amounts of starches and sugar in the diet are not healthy and may contribute to obesity.

The preschool child is also developing a full set of teeth. Proper dental habits are important. These habits will carry over into later childhood and adulthood. Tooth decay is a significant threat during the preschool years, affecting nearly half of all American children by the time they are 4 years old. This is the appropriate time to introduce the child to the family dentist in order to gain proper instruction in the care of teeth. Also, early dental visits may reduce the fear and anxiety that children can experience if they have not had a timely introduction to the dental exam procedure.

Physical development of the preschool child can be enhanced by providing ample opportunities for exercise, play, and exploration of the environment. It is important to have access to swing sets, jungle gyms, and other types of playground equipment to promote large muscle development. The use of paints, crayons, and other types of drawing utensils promote the development of eye-hand coordination. Balls used to throw, catch, and kick can also increase the development of large and small muscle control as well as eye-hand coordination. Because of their rapidly growing physical activity levels and abilities, preschoolers require regular supervision and attention. The threat of injury or death due to accidents is even greater than it is for infants. Parents and other caregivers must exercise great care in supervising and controlling the activities of the preschool child in order to provide the safest possible environment.

Physical Development of the School-Age Child

Between the ages of 6 and 11, children's growth patterns maintain a fairly stable rate. Accompanying this steady growth in weight and height are rapidly developing motor abilities. The senses, particularly vision, become much sharper than they were in infancy and the preschool years as the child's body grows and matures. The child's physical development in this stage is influenced both by inherited genes and environmental conditions. Nutritional intake continues to be a major factor in the growth of muscle and bone tissue, as it is for the development of brain cells and other parts of the central nervous system. Children who were malnourished as infants or preschool children may show evidence of mental retardation or lower-than-normal growth rates during this stage. Sound nutritional habits remain an important component of the child's ability to develop in an optimum manner.

Motor skills become significantly greater during this stage. School-age children develop greater abilities to run, jump, climb, swim, catch, throw, and kick. Their physical balance and muscle coordination improve to a point where they are continually discovering new things that they are capable of doing (see Figure 7-8). The willingness of children to take risks increases because of a greater sense of confidence in getting their bodies to do what they want them to do. Thus, it is not unusual to see a school-age child with an arm or leg in a cast because of a fall from a tree or playground equipment.

Figure 7-8

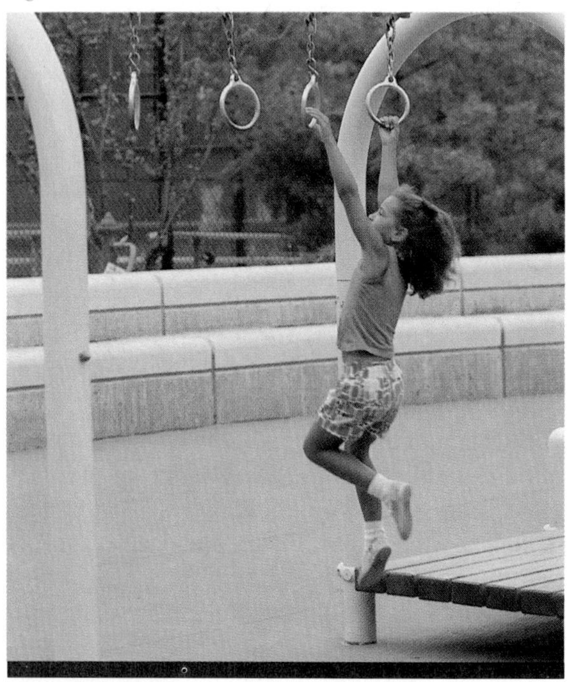

School-age children develop sharpened motor skills, such as balance and coordination, which allow them much control over their environment.

A common threat to the physical well-being of children of all ages is illness. Influenza and the common cold are nearly universal features of growing up. These can usually be handled routinely with proper care and rest. While antibiotics cannot prevent the child from contracting such illnesses as pneumonia, bronchitis, and ear infections, such drugs are useful in curing the complications that can arise from them. Chicken pox and rubella (German measles) are also relatively common among children. The development of vaccines has nearly wiped out the danger of some diseases that previously had affected many children: polio, diphtheria, tetanus, red measles, and pertussis (whooping cough), to name a few. It is important that children be fully vaccinated by the time they enter school. Pediatricians know the proper times for different immunizations. Many are given during infancy and the preschool years. Local school districts generally require that children be immunized before they enter school. Access to good medical care is an important part of promoting the healthy physical development of children. Healthy children have a better chance for optimum development.

WRAPPING IT UP

The human being is a complex organism. Our potential for living a fulfilling life and for becoming a fully functioning person is affected by the way in which our bodies develop. Physical development is closely related to social development. Our ability to form and to maintain effective interpersonal relationships depends, in large part, on our ability to grow in a positive manner.

The *human life span* can be divided into a number of *stages*: prenatal, preschool, school age, adolescence, adulthood, and aging. These stages build upon each other. How a person develops in one stage is strongly influenced by how he or she developed in prior stages. At each stage, steps can be taken to enhance the child's ability to develop in an optimum manner. Children are dependent upon others in their environment to assist them in developing toward their full potential as human beings. Parents and caregivers play a very important role.

The genetic component of physical development is important. The merging of the adult male's *sperm cell* with the adult female's *egg* combines the genes of two people into the formation of a new life. During the *prenatal stage*, cell growth and division lead to a fully formed person. The *genes* inherited from our parents comprise the blueprints for our physical development. While environmental forces also influence physical development, certain physical characteristics are primarily determined by genetic make-up: eye and hair color, height, body shape and build, and facial appearance. Normal prenatal development occurs unless something interrupts the natural growth process. Cigarette smoking, use of alcohol and drugs, poor nutrition, and certain diseases in the pregnant woman can have harmful effects on the physical development of the unborn child. Also, defective genes can cause physical abnormalities that lead to handicaps during childhood and later life. Physical development in the prenatal stage is promoted by the mother's proper health-care habits.

The *infancy stage* of human development begins with the birth of the child. Infants depend entirely upon adult caretakers for meeting their physical needs for food, water, safety, and warmth. Infants also need the physical stimulation of being touched and held by other people. Infants grow according to a sequence of physical milestones. Although average ages exist for certain milestones in physical development, there is a normal range of developmental timetables infants can follow.

To enhance infant development, parents or infant caretakers should see that the child receives a nutritious diet. In addition, infants must be given ample opportunities to move about and to develop their large and small muscle abilities. In promoting infant development, it is important that parents not expect too much too soon from the child. Proper rest and sleep are also important. An infant's sleep habits may not coincide with those of his or her parents. Therefore, parents often find themselves adjusting to their infant's sleep schedules. Infants also need a safe environment in which to grow. Great harm to the physical well-being of the infant can occur due to accidents or unsafe living conditions.

The *childhood stage* of development is divided into two substages: the preschool stage and the school-age stage. The preschool stage of development spans the ages 3 through 5. Children in this stage are developing physical skills involving *large and small muscle coordination*. Walking, running, jumping, skipping, and hopping are major physical activities for the preschooler. The preschool child is also beginning to establish skills such as drawing, writing, cutting with scissors, and other activities requiring hand-eye coordination. Preschoolers need ample opportunities to exercise their developing physical abilities. Also, sound nutrition and health care, including proper dental habits, are important for physical development in this stage.

The school-age stage of development spans the ages of 6 through 11. Children in this stage are rapidly developing relatively sophisticated motor skills. This is due to the continuing development of the central nervous system, which promotes coordination and balance. Muscle and bone growth also continue at a steady pace in this stage, so much so that the school-age child is bigger, stronger, and faster than ever before. As was true in previous stages, the school-age child depends upon adequate nutrition and sound health-care habits if physical development is to proceed in a positive manner.

Exploring Dimensions of Chapter Seven

For Review

1. What are the stages of the human life span? In what ways are these stages related to each other?
2. What influence does our environment have on our physical development in the following stages:
   a. Prenatal
   b. Infancy
   c. Childhood

3• Why is good nutrition important for the physical development of humans? What are some of the harmful effects of poor nutrition on the physical development of children?

4• How can the physical environment be made safer for children of different ages? List some of the major hazards that threaten the physical well-being of young children.

For Consideration

1• Write a paragraph explaining how a person's physical development can influence self-concept. Consider such things as physical appearance, height, weight, and body build. What will contribute to a higher level of self-esteem?

2• Consider your own personal physical development. List all the things you do to enhance your physical development. List those things you do that might hinder your development. What can you do to make your list of positive things longer? What can you do to make your list of negative things shorter?

3• Explain why some parents do an excellent job of promoting the physical development of their young children, while other parents do a poor job. What can be done to help the latter group of parents be more capable of providing optimum development of their children?

For Application

1• Seek permission to visit a maternity ward at a hospital. Observe the newborn infants and the professionals in charge of their care. Note the differences between infants in terms of their physical appearance, activity levels, size, and movements.

2• Plan a visit to a local child care facility that has preschool age children. Observe the children at play. Make notes of the different motor skills children exhibit. Also make notes of what is done at the center in terms of providing a safe environment for the children. Do you notice any conditions (equipment, practices) that might pose a hazard to the children's physical well-being?

3• Invite a registered dietician or other nutrition specialist to visit your class. Have them discuss the role of proper nutrition in physical growth. Learn what the ingredients of a sound diet are for children of different ages, as well as the function of different vitamins, minerals, and protein in the diet. What are the common elements in the food we eat that may negatively impact the physical well-being of children in some way?

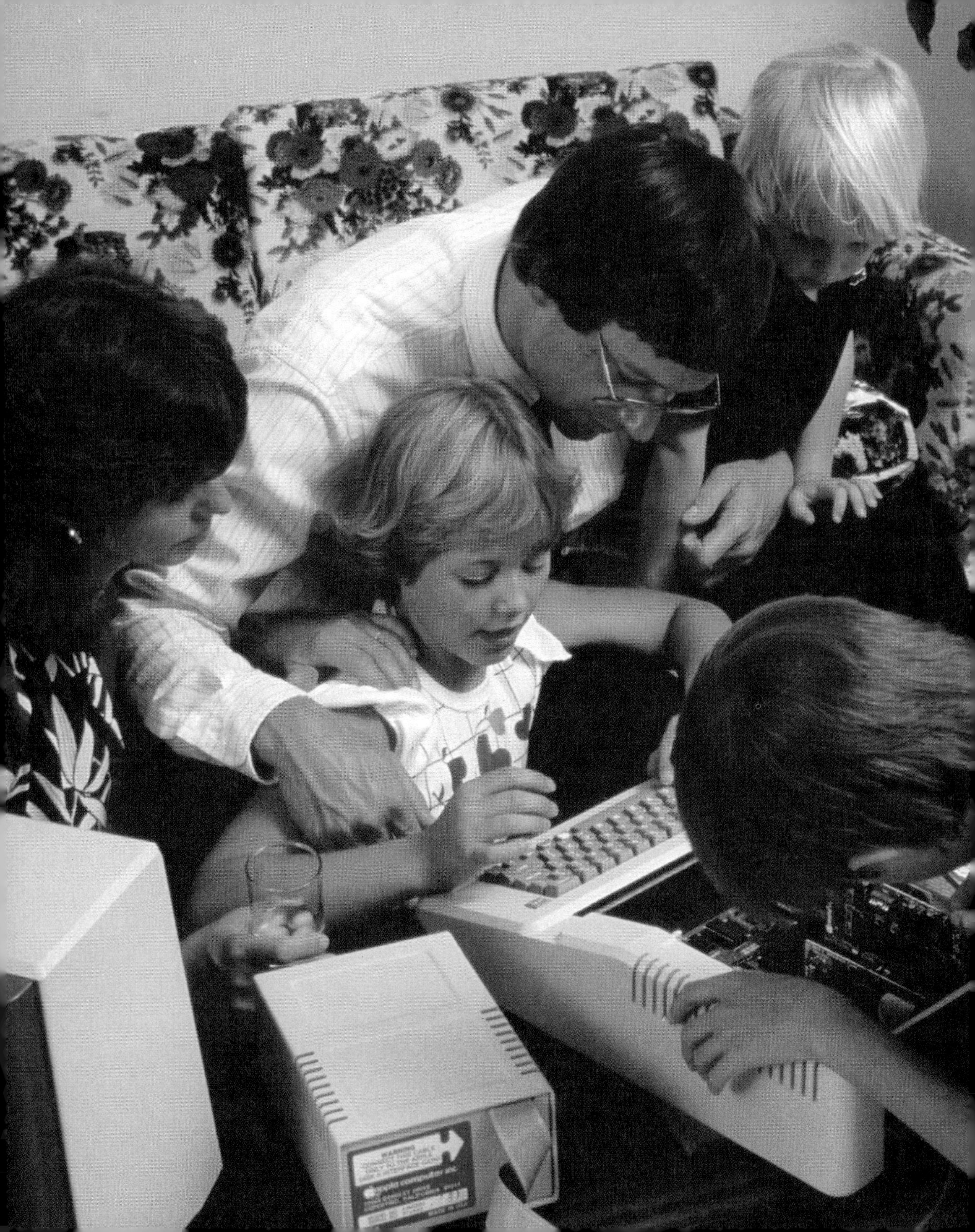
WARNING
apple computer inc.

eight

THE SOCIAL, EMOTIONAL, AND MENTAL DEVELOPMENT OF CHILDREN

This chapter provides information that will help you to:

- Understand the social, emotional, and mental development of children of different ages.
- Recognize prosocial and antisocial behavior in children.
- Become familiar with social development behaviors of infants, preschool-age children, and school-age children.
- Understand the influences of peer groups on preschoolers and school-age children.
- Recognize the different types of emotional development found in infants, preschoolers, and school-age children.
- List several types of emotions.
- Understand Piaget's theory on how children develop mentally.

The human life span involves more than just the physical growth of our bodies. The human life span also includes changes in the ways we relate to other people, in our ability to think and to solve problems, and in our expressions of feelings and emotions. Consider the following cases:

CASE IN POINT

Three-year-old Alicia is playing with a toy in her front yard. Her 3-year-old friend, Kitty, comes running over, shouting, "Let me see! Let me see!" Alicia pulls the toy back, exclaiming, "It's my toy! You can't have it!"

Nine-year-old Bonnie is proud of the new toy she received for Christmas. She calls her friend Erica on the telephone to see if Erica would like to come over to share it with her. Bonnie remembered that Erica recently shared one of her new toys, and she would like to return the favor. Also, Bonnie has more fun when she has a playmate with whom to share things.

CASE IN POINT

Four-year-old Ben is building a sand castle on the beach. When a big wave comes up and washes much of his work away, Ben immediately breaks into tears and cries for several minutes.

Ten-year-old Carmen is building a sand castle on the beach. When a big wave washes much of the castle away, Carmen throws her hands into the air and says to herself, "Well, I'd better start over, but this time I'm going to move back a few feet!"

CASE IN POINT

Five-year-old Carl is in preschool. His teacher asks Carl to watch her pour water from a cup into a tall, narrow glass. The teacher then fills the same cup with the same amount of water, and pours it into a shorter, wider glass. The teacher asks Carl, "Which glass has the most water?" Without hesitation, Carl shouts, "The tall one does!"

Ten-year-old Maria is in the fourth grade. Her teacher performs the same task with water that Carl had observed. When asked which glass contained the most water, Maria stated, "That's simple. It's the same amount in both glasses."

These cases reflect three important aspects of human development in childhood. The first case, involving the toys of Bonnie and Alicia, concerns **social development** and the acquisition of social skills. The second case, in which the sand castles of Ben and Carmen were washed away, reflects **emotional development** and the ability to control emotional expression. The third case, where Carl and Maria had to tell which glass contained the most water, concerns **mental** (or **cognitive**) **development**. Notice how children of different ages handle each situation differently. As with physical development (see Chapter 7), these other aspects of human development change over time in a particular sequence. In this chapter, we will take a closer look at the social, emotional, and mental development of children and the patterns of changes that take place as children grow older.

THE SOCIAL DEVELOPMENT OF CHILDREN

Social development means many things. Generally, social development involves the ways in which we relate to other people. Social development includes our ability to adjust to other people—learning to know their expectations and needs, what pleases or displeases them, and how to behave in acceptable ways around them. Such interpersonal skills as empathy (Chapter 4) and healthy communication (Chapter 5) are important elements of our social development.

We have already seen in Chapters 1 through 6 of this book how important healthy interpersonal relationships are in realizing our potential as individual people. As we grow through childhood, we learn how to relate to others. Parents, brothers and sisters, and friends comprise the most immediate social contacts of children. Other important social relationships, such as those with teachers, coaches, and other relatives (grandparents, cousins, aunts, uncles) also teach us how to relate to others.

Relating effectively involves the development of certain **social skills**. However, not all people acquire these skills to an equal degree. Some develop more effective social skills than others. Childhood is the stage in the human life span where we acquire our basic social skills. We learn them from our parents, siblings, friends, and others with whom we come into contact. While it is never too late to build and improve our social skills, we establish our basic pattern of relating to others in childhood. As we grow older, these patterns become habits that are more and more difficult to change in significant ways.

Prosocial and Antisocial Behavior

When we speak of social skills, we refer to the ability of the child to behave in ways designated as prosocial. **Prosocial behavior** is behavior that is oriented toward others in a positive manner. **Antisocial behavior**, on the other hand, reflects an absence of social skills. This behavior toward others is negative in its impact (see Figure 8-1). The following list contains examples of both kinds of social behavior:

Examples of Prosocial Behavior:
- Being helpful with others
- Being cooperative with others
- Comforting another person
- Encouraging another person
- Helping another
- Being sympathetic with another's misfortune
- Sharing with another person
- Giving to another person
- Taking turns

Examples of Antisocial Behavior:
- Trying to hurt another person
- Being aggressive toward others
- Being selfish or conceited
- Trying to frighten others
- Showing disrespect for another
- Teasing or ridiculing another
- Taking advantage of another for personal gain

As you read over the above list, think about the ways in which you like to be treated by others. In all likelihood, you prefer to be treated with any of the prosocial behaviors; you would prefer *not* to be treated with the

Figure 8-1

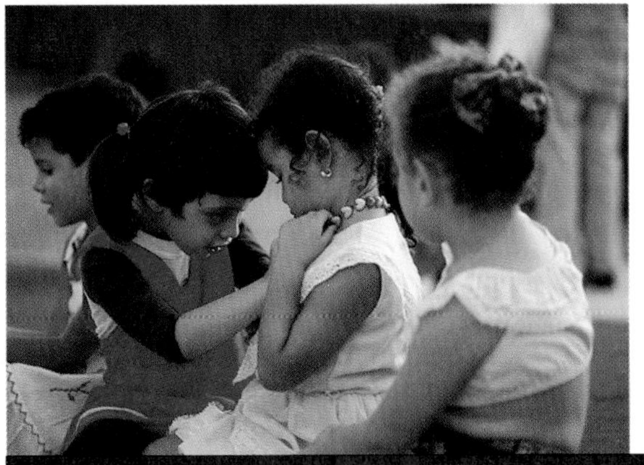

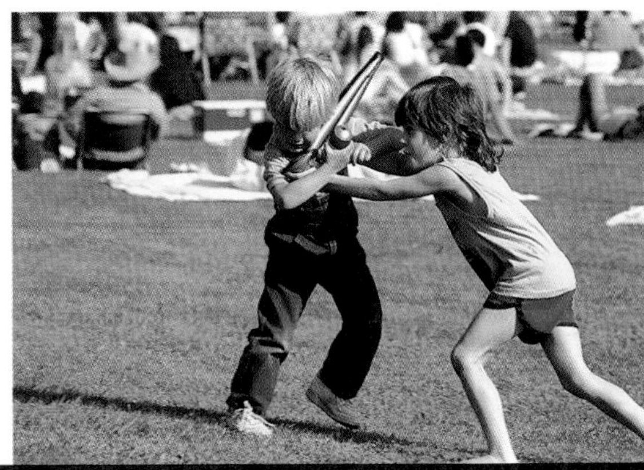

Prosocial behavior is oriented toward others in a positive way. Antisocial behavior, however, is negative in its impact on others.

Robert Torres

Peter Glass/Monkmeyer Press

antisocial ones. The *Golden Rule* of "Do unto others as you would have others do unto you" is quite valid when we consider prosocial behavior.

In the sections that follow, we will refer to **healthy social development** in children as that which shows a maximum level of prosocial behavior skills and a minimum level of antisocial behavior. Why do some children grow up as helpful, cooperative individuals who respect others, while other children grow up as "bullies" or deceitful individuals who would do anything to take advantage of others for personal gain? What are the major influences on the social development of children of different ages?

The Social Development of Infants (Ages 0–2)

Social behavior in young infants is limited to only a few simple actions. By age 4 months, infants are smiling and laughing as they interact with others. Parents and other caretakers find much enjoyment in this smiling, cooing, and "cute" behavior of young infants. Although these are not really social skills in the sense that we define them, such behaviors of infants cause others to react in loving, prosocial ways toward them.

Infants are dependent on parents and other caretakers for social involvement. Young infants merely respond and react to the social initiatives taken by their caretakers. How infants are treated by others sets the stage for the development of social skills in the preschool and school-age years.

INFANT ATTACHMENT • A major event in the social development of infants is **attachment**. Beginning at birth, warm and loving physical contact with the mother fosters a sense of security and trust in the infant's environment. Being held, gently rocked, cuddled, and talked to creates a positive feeling in infants toward people in the world around them. Like other animals, human infants need this contact to develop a strong sense of belonging. This psychological "attachment" is a healthy aspect of human social development that should take place during infancy. Further, it is not just the mother who can provide means for infant attachment. Fathers and other people in the infant's environment can give the nurturance necessary for the infant to develop a positive sense of attachment.

Spotlight on issues

Professor Harlow and His Monkeys

Imagine that you are in a scientist's laboratory equipped with several animal cages. In each cage is an infant monkey and two substitute mothers, or "surrogates," in place of the monkey's actual mother. One of the surrogate mothers has a wooden head and a wire body covered with a soft terrycloth coat. The other surrogate mother has just a wooden head and a wire body, with no terrycloth at all. Which surrogate mother do you think the infant monkey would cling to or go to for security and comfort?

This is just what psychologist Harry Harlow and his wife Margaret asked in their experiments at the University of Wisconsin Regional Primate Center laboratories. Harlow learned that infant monkeys preferred, by far, the soft contact of the terrycloth-covered surrogate mother to the cold, hard surface of the wire mother. Time after time, the infants would hug and cling to the terrycloth mother, especially when something frightened them. The infant monkeys became attached to the substitute mother who provided contact comfort, seeking comfort from the surrogate as much as they would from the warm, soft bodies of their own natural mothers.

This result is really not surprising. What did surprise Harlow, however, was the result of his next experiment. He equipped the wire mothers with feeding devices so that the infants could drink milk from them just as they would from the breasts of their natural mothers. The terrycloth mothers were not equipped with feeding devices. Which surrogate mothers would the infant monkeys now prefer: the one that provides food and nourishment but no soft contact, or the one that provides soft contact but no food? Indeed, the infant monkeys continued to prefer the terrycloth mother to the wire mother, even though the latter provided nourishment. Although the infants would go to the wire mother for feeding, they would return immediately to the cloth mother for comfort and security. Harlow concluded that, when it comes to developing mother-infant attachment, the warmth and comfort of physical contact are just as important, if not more so, than providing milk for nourishment.

Another unexpected result came from Professor Harlow's experiments. Some of his infant monkeys were raised into adulthood in isolation—that is, they had no contact with any other monkeys. The only contacts they had were the brief intrusions by the human scientists and the regular presence of the surrogate mothers. After these monkeys raised in isolation became adults, they were placed with other monkeys in the same room. What happened was astonishing, as Professor Harlow himself recounted:

> Fear is the overwhelming response in all the monkeys raised in isolation. Although the animals are physically healthy, they crouch and appear terror-stricken by their new environment. . . . They cringe when approached. . . . When the other animals become aggressive, the isolates accept their abuse without making any effort to defend themselves. . . . Their behavior is a pitiful combination of apathy and terror as they crouch at the sides of the room.[1]

Later on, after additional years in isolation, these same monkeys became aggressive themselves. They would viciously attack other monkeys, and they became totally unloving, distressed, and disturbed creatures.

So what implications does this research on monkeys have for *human* development? Can we really generalize from the studies of monkeys to humans? The answer is, "Yes," to a large extent we can generalize. Research on human infants has shown the importance of attachment to another human being. Usually this is the mother, father, or another person responsible for the care of the child. Just as Harlow's monkeys expressed a need for warm and comfortable contact, so too do human infants. Human infants deprived of this contact, or who are raised without adequate contact with other human beings, grow up with serious problems in relating to other people. These problems may involve overly shy or aggressive behavior toward others, not knowing what others expect in a relationship, or just not knowing how to act around other people. There is little doubt that human development depends upon the presence of other people and positive contacts with them.

---

[1]Harry F. Harlow and Margaret K. Harlow, "The Young Monkeys," *Readings in Developmental Psychology*, 2nd ed. (New York: Random House, 1977), pp. 154–159.

Infants who are treated in antisocial ways by parents or other caretakers soon learn to behave in antisocial ways themselves. Like the monkeys in the Harlow experiments (see *Spotlight on issues*, pp. 151–152), human infants respond negatively to being ignored, abused, or otherwise deprived of the loving attention, nurturance, and physical contact they need. Research has shown conclusively that infants who experience neglect or painful experiences grow into children (and later into adults) with serious personality disorders. They also experience problems in relating to other people in healthy ways. Such problems may include being overly hostile and aggressive, distrustful, withdrawn, or anxious and uncomfortable in relating to other people. On the other hand, infants treated with care, nurturance, and other prosocial behaviors are more likely to trust others and relate to them in a positive manner as children and adults (see Figure 8-2).

Figure 8-2

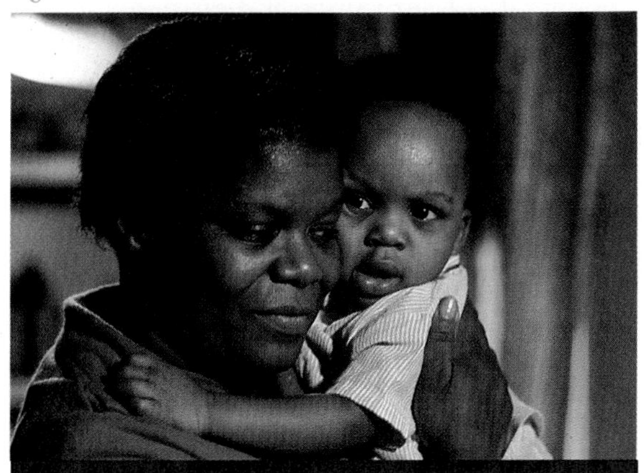

Infants who are loved, cuddled, and cared for are more likely to develop positive relationships in later stages of childhood.
USDA Photo

SOCIAL ANXIETY REACTIONS IN INFANTS • By the time infants are 8 or 9 months of age, they have established a strong bond of attachment with the mother and another nurturing caretaker, such as the father, a brother or sister, or a grandparent. They can distinguish one person from another, and are aware when the caretaker they are attached to is not around. This fact leads to two other common occurrences in the social development of infants: separation anxiety and stranger anxiety.

Separation anxiety involves crying or otherwise fussy behavior in infants when they lose sight of an attachment figure such as the parent. For example, if the mother leaves the room momentarily, the infant may cry loudly. Upon the mother's return, it may cling to the mother in order to regain the security it needs. Separation anxiety can be seen in infants up to two years of age or older. These infants seek to maintain proximity to, and contact with, the ones who have provided care and nurturance all along.

CASE IN POINT

Elena is an 8-month-old infant. Her grandmother, Mrs. Velez, was babysitting her while her mother was grocery shopping. Mrs. Velez had cared for Elena before, and never had a problem. This time, however, Elena began crying when her mother left the house. She cried for over an hour; nothing Mrs. Velez did could make Elena happy. Mrs. Velez felt badly because she thought Elena was angry with her. What Mrs. Velez did not realize is that Elena was at the age where she was experiencing separation anxiety from her mother. This is a very normal and natural occurrence in infants.

Stranger anxiety refers to the infant's negative reactions to unfamiliar people. The infant will respond to strangers in a negative way, showing an obvious fear of them and a desire to withdraw from contact with them. Thus, it is best for strangers to approach infants gradually and to do so when the infant is in the secure presence of the mother or other attachment figure. Otherwise, the infant sees the new person as a potential threat and expresses a natural fear of the unknown.

Stranger anxiety, as well as separation anxiety, are normal infant responses to uncertainty in the infant's routine environment. However, the intensity of these reactions varies from one child to the next. Some infants never display anxiety reactions. Research has shown that stranger and separation anxiety are *less* intense in infants who have been exposed to many people during the first few months of life. Anxiety reactions are also less intense among infants who have developed a secure and trusting attachment to the caretaker (usually the mother and father).

The Social Development of Preschool-Age Children (Ages 3–5)

Along with growing physical abilities (see Chapter 7), the child in the preschool-age stage of development also is quickly developing in the social realm. The potential for stranger anxiety and separation anxiety decreases after 2 to 3 years of age. This is because the child in this stage is developing **autonomy** from parents and other attachment figures. This means that the child is starting to move away from the parent caregiver toward exploring the environment on his or her own. Although the security provided by parents and other attachment figures remains very important at this age, the preschool child is developing a greater sense of independence and self-dependency. One major result of this trend is that the child takes a greater interest in other people and strives to make contact with them. In brief, the child is becoming more socially-oriented.

A major facilitator of social development at this stage is **language acquisition**. Unlike the infant, the preschool child is able to understand commands and instructions and can carry on a two-way conversation with other people. The child has an expanding vocabulary, and is even able to start talking about his or her feelings and experiences. Being able to use language opens up new doors of opportunity and learning experiences for the child which he or she finds quite rewarding.

SOCIALIZATION • An important aspect of social development in 3- to 5-year-old children is the process of socialization. **Socialization** is the learning of attitudes, values, morals, and rules for appropriate behavior in a given culture. In Chapter 3 we discussed the important role of values and attitudes in our lives; in Chapter 6 we explored how different cultures promote different values and attitudes. We begin to learn these things in this early stage of the life span. Parents are the primary teachers, but young children also learn values and rules for behavior from siblings and other relatives, friends (peer groups), preschool teachers, and in all likelihood, television viewing. Young children learn their values and attitudes by observing others who are important to them. The way a child learns to behave, whether in a prosocial or an antisocial manner, is also shaped by observations of how others around them behave.

It is in this stage that children begin to learn elementary concepts of *right* and *wrong*, *good* and *bad*. They begin to learn about such prosocial behaviors as sharing, cooperating, and respecting the rights of others. In the case of Alicia and Kitty (described at the beginning of this chapter), Alicia had not yet learned the prosocial skill of sharing. She will learn this skill if her parents, her playmates like Kitty, or an older brother or sister talk with her and help her to understand the value of sharing with others. Also, it will help if these other people in Alicia's life "model" this skill by sharing with Alicia. Alicia will have additional opportunities to learn that if she shares with others, others will share with her. It takes time and a number of different experiences for children to learn that prosocial behavior has mutual benefits for both individuals in the relationship.

An important aspect of socialization in this stage is the development of an identity as a boy or a girl. This is known as **sexual identity**. By age 3, children are aware that either they are boys or they are girls. They are able to distinguish their own sex from the opposite sex. Therefore, they begin to relate to other children based on whether the other is a boy or a girl.

Preschool-age children are encouraged to behave in ways that are appropriate for their sex, as defined by their parents and other influences in the culture that surrounds them. For example, little girls are often treated in ways defined as "feminine" in our culture. They are clothed in dresses, given dolls to play with, and may even be discouraged from rough-and-tumble play. Little boys, on the other hand, are more likely to be treated in ways that our culture defines as appropriately "masculine." They are dressed in pants, given footballs, toy guns, trucks, and baseballs, and are expected to engage in rough-and-tumble activity. Such different learning experiences provided for little boys and little girls are known as **traditional sex roles**.

Some people, however, believe that too rigid socialization of children into traditional feminine and masculine roles is harmful to personal development. Consequently, much research has focused on the consequences of how we socialize our children into sexual roles (see *Spotlight on issues*, pp. 155–158). In what ways have you learned to be traditionally

Spotlight on issues

Research on Sex Role Stereotypes

Consider the following characteristics that a person might have. Which of these characteristics do you think are usually associated with boys? Which are usually associated with girls? Are there any that are not typically associated with either sex?

aggressive	graceful
assertive	emotional
competitive	passive
dominating	dependent
rough-and-tumble	dainty
mechanical	unaggressive
unemotional	sensitive
adventurous	submissive
brave	shy
strong	flirty
mechanical	affectionate
ambitious	gossipy

Many people typically associate the characteristics listed in the left-hand column as being more common among young boys, male adolescents, and men. These characteristics are said to be traditional *masculine* characteristics. The characteristics in the right-hand column are more commonly associated with young girls, female adolescents, and women. They are traditional *feminine* characteristics. Both parents and society-in-general emphasize such sex-role traits in children from the time they are very young. Sex role stereotypes are then perpetuated through adolescence and into adulthood.

Do these distinctions generally hold true among the males and females you know (friends, parents, brothers, and sisters)? Why is this so? Are some of these characteristics more desirable than others? Which ones? What difference does it make?

You will recall from Chapter 6 that a stereotype is a standardized idea or mental picture of what people are like or how they behave. Often, this picture is oversimplified and not true in reality. We tend to see stereotyped people as having certain characteristics and behaving in certain ways even if they do not, in reality, fit that pattern.

In our society, traditional masculine and feminine characteristics are often turned into sex role stereotypes. Females may be viewed as weak, submissive, unassertive, and emotional regardless of their actual personalities. Males, on the other hand, may be seen as insensitive, unemotional, mechanically-inclined, and dominating even if they are not any of these things. This results in people not being allowed to be themselves. Sex role stereotypes limit a person's ability to become a fully functioning individual.

Sex role stereotypes might also result in discrimination. For example, an employer may hire a male over a female because the male is seen as strong and decisive while the female is seen as emotional and unassertive. This hiring decision is swayed by the employer's stereotyped beliefs about men and women and not by any objective assessment of the actual abilities of the particular man and woman applying for the job. In what other ways do you see society discriminating against either females or males on the basis of sex role stereotypes?

Apart from the limiting effects that sex role stereotypes have, actual sex role behaviors also have certain effects. Research on the sex role behavior of people has shown that children and adults who actually possess certain masculine *and* feminine characteristics have advantages over others who are exclusively masculine or feminine in their behavior patterns. For example, social and intellectual development of male and female children is enhanced when they are seen to possess the traits of being assertive and independent (traditionally masculine), as well as being sensitive to others and able to express emotions (traditionally feminine).

Among the adult population, it is commonly believed in our society that "real men" don't cry or show their emotions when upset. According to traditional role stereotypes, men are supposed to keep their feelings and problems to themselves, to "be tough," and not show weakness. Indeed, many men attempt to live up to this expectation because they have been taught to do so. On the other hand, it is more acceptable for women to show their emotions and to talk about their problems with other people. However, many medical experts and psychologists believe that this sex role pattern is responsible for the fact that men in our society are much more likely than women to suffer high blood pressure (hypertension), heart attacks, strokes, ulcers, and alcoholism. Physically speaking, holding all of your feelings and emotions inside may have harmful physical effects, in the long run.

These are just two examples of research showing that behaving in sex role stereotyped ways can limit the social, intellectual, and physical development of the individual. Why is this so? It is because some situations require a person to be assertive and strong (such as in a job interview or on a big exam in school), while other situations require sensitivity and ability to express feelings (such as in forming intimate or friendship relationships, getting along with others at work or in school). By combining certain *desirable* traits of traditionally masculine and feminine roles, a person can be more flexible in behaving appropriately across a variety of situations.

Look at yourself. Regardless of whether you are male or female, what desirable masculine sex role characteristics do you possess? What desirable feminine sex role characteristics do you possess? In what ways would you like to change your sex roles, if you could?

masculine or feminine in your own sex-role development? Can you recall any experiences as a young child that pushed you in traditionally masculine or feminine directions?

Figure 8-3

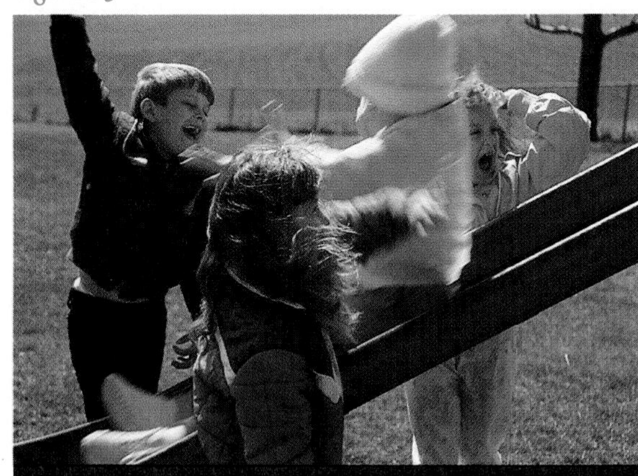

Preschool children need friends if their social development is to be healthy and positive.
Julie Habel/West Light

THE PEER GROUP • It is during the preschool years that children form their first friendships. A child's **peer group** is made up of other children who are more or less the child's own age. A person's peer group fulfills many important functions during childhood, as well as into adolescence and adulthood (see Figure 8-3). Such functions of the peer group, listed here, are important for personal development:

- Provides playmates for shared activities
- Provides a source of reinforcement, encouragement, praise, and approval
- Offers opportunities for learning prosocial skills (sharing, cooperation, helpfulness, etc.)
- Assists in language development
- Helps in the healthy separation of the child from parents and other attachment figures
- Gives a basis for comparing what one likes and what one can do with what other children the same age like or can do
- Provides opportunities for the child to be a leader as well as a follower
- Offers a sense of belonging, of being important, and of being valued by others outside the child's own family
- Helps to shape one's self-concept and build one's self-esteem

Preschool-age children need friends if social development is to be healthy. First friends are usually found in one's own neighborhood. They can also be found in child-care centers, local parks, nursery schools, or playgrounds. Young children who have no friends or who have difficulty making friends are more likely to be lonely and depressed. Without friends, childhood can be a miserable experience.

The Social Development of School-Age Children (Ages 6–12)

A major change in the child's life in this stage is entry into school. School introduces many challenges and new opportunities for children. It further separates children from parents and other attachment figures that were important in the infancy and preschool-age stages of the life span. While school is meant to educate the child in such things as reading, writing, science, and math, school is a *classroom* for social development as well. School immerses the child in the company of many other children of the same and different ages.

The School-Age Peer Group

The peer group assumes greater importance for the child in this stage. Compared with the preschool stage, friends assume greater importance in the shaping of self-concept. Whether in neighborhood play or on the school playground, children in this age range now interact more with their peers than they do with their own parents and other family members. The child becomes more dependent on friends for praise, reinforcement, and support—all of which are so very important for the positive development of self-concept. Peer groups in this stage tend strongly to be composed of children of the same sex—either all boys or all girls.

While the peer group assumes greater importance for the child in this stage, it does so in specific areas. One's friends become a more important basis for comparing one's own abilities and personal qualities—how athletic, smart, big or small, fat or thin, and attractive one is relative to peers. In this way, the peer group provides a basis for **social status**—how well-liked and important one is relative to others in the group. Peer groups also exert a strong influence on the child's behavior. School-age children are concerned about, "What will my friends think? Will they approve?" School-age children therefore try to behave in ways that will conform to their peers' expectations.

GAINING POPULARITY • Popularity with one's friends becomes a significant issue for the school-age child. Some children are more popular with peers than are others. Popular children are chosen by others to play games with, to share secrets with, to go to birthday parties, and to walk home from school with. Unpopular children are ignored, avoided, or teased. Popularity is important because of its effects on the child's sense of self-worth—one's self-esteem. Popular children feel good about themselves. They feel important and that they matter. Unpopular children believe they are not worth very much, that they don't matter, and that they have little to contribute.

What makes some children more popular than others? Research has shown that the following are characteristics of popular children in this stage:

- Healthy and attractive
- Dependable and trustworthy
- Strong self-esteem, but not conceited or boastful
- Conform to the values and attitudes of others in the peer group
- Self-confident

- Outgoing and fun to be with
- Behave in ways that make others feel good about themselves (that is, they have prosocial behavior skills)

Unpopular children, on the other hand, are more likely to have one or more of the following characteristics:

- Shy and reserved
- Reluctant to become involved in activities with others
- Physically unattractive, fat, or skinny
- Aggressive and bullying behavior toward others
- Act "babyish" in their behavior (cry and sulk a lot)
- Lack self-confidence
- Slow learners in school
- Always asking others for help and favors
- Repeatedly tattle on others and act as "goody-goodies" in front of teachers and other adults

PEER GROUPS AND SOCIAL SKILLS • Peer groups also assume a greater role for school-age children by providing an arena for competition, conflict management, and for developing effective communication skills. Competition with peers shapes the child's attitudes toward winning and losing. Competition can take place in the classroom, on the soccer or baseball field, or in striving to attain status and popularity with others in the peer group. Some children develop healthy attitudes toward competiton by learning to follow the rules of the game, not complaining every time they lose, and enjoying the competitive activity for its own sake. Other children, however, develop unhealthy attitudes toward competition. They have difficulty accepting defeat. If they can't win, they don't enjoy the activity. If they win, they brag about it and belittle the losers.

Conflict, in the form of fights and arguments, is common in the school-age peer group. It is conflict with friends that provides children with opportunities to learn the prosocial skills of negotiation, give-and-take, and sharing. By the end of this stage, children should develop a healthy attitude toward the rights and privileges of others with whom potential conflicts might take place. This is illustrated in the case of Bonnie and Erica, presented at the beginning of this chapter. By the end of the school-age years, children realize the value of sharing and cooperation with others because of the trial-and-error experiences that they have had in belonging to peer groups during this stage.

THE NEED FOR CONFORMITY • Peer groups also have more direct effects on the child's behavior. Not all of these effects are positive. In an effort to conform to the peer group's values and expectations, school-age children may engage in their first illegal or delinquent acts. These might include smoking their first cigarette, stealing or shoplifting something from a store, getting into fights, damaging property, or engaging in other anti-social acts. Conforming to the peer group is an important basis for acceptance into the group. It is also an avenue to status in the group once acceptance has been gained. Peer pressure can lead children to do things that they otherwise would not do outside of the group.

CASE IN POINT

Eleven-year-old Mark recently moved to a new neighborhood. During his first week at school, he met Paul and Ritchie. All three boys liked to play baseball and ride skateboards. Since Paul and Ritchie were already best friends, Mark felt like an outsider. Yet, he wanted to be included in anything Paul and Ritchie did together. One afternoon, Mark was invited by Paul and Ritchie to throw apples at car windows as the cars passed by on the street. Mark knew this was wrong and that it could be quite dangerous. When he told his friends that he didn't think they should do it, Paul replied, "Aw, come on Mark, we do it all the time! It's cool! You want to be our friend, don't you?" Mark was upset, but agreed to go along. These were his only friends at the time, and he wanted them to accept him.

If children receive reinforcement and approval from peers to engage in antisocial behavior, such behavior is likely to continue. Peers can also model and reinforce prosocial behavior, such as sharing, cooperation, and leadership. Which behavior—antisocial or prosocial—is stressed depends entirely on the particular values, attitudes, and moral standards that children in the peer group embrace. Thus, the peer groups that children find themselves in are very important because the influence they exert is extremely powerful.

Family and School Influences on Social Development

Much has been said about the importance of peer groups for the social development of school-age children. But what about the influence of family and school? These, too, are powerful influences on children. The influence of the peer group is limited to the degree that children maintain close ties with parents and other significant others, such as teachers.

In Chapter 12, much more will be said about the role of effective parenting in the social development of children of all ages. For now, it is important to note that most school-age children continue to maintain a strong attachment to parents and other family members throughout this stage. They do this despite their growing orientation and attachment to the peer group, which is a very normal and natural part of growing up. School-age children need to begin separating themselves from exclusive attachment to parents and the home.

The kinds of behavior that parents model for the child show up in the child's own behavior patterns. Children who observe their parents being honest, considerate toward others, and pleasant are likely to be honest, considerate, and pleasant in their own behavior toward others. Healthy social development and a positive self-concept are more likely to occur when parents treat their children with love, acceptance, and respect.

Unhealthy development and low self-esteem are related to parents who verbally or physically abuse their children. The same is true for parents who ignore or are indifferent toward their children. Under these conditions, children are more likely to seek involvement with peer groups and to move away from the painful experiences they have at home. They are also likely to develop such antisocial behavior tendencies as hostility and aggressiveness toward others. If they find peers with the same behavior tendencies, much trouble and mischief can follow. For this reason, it is important that parents strive to maintain attachment with the school-age child, while permitting the child a reasonable level of involvement with friends (see Figure 8-4).

School also influences the social development of children in this stage. The primary

Figure 8-4

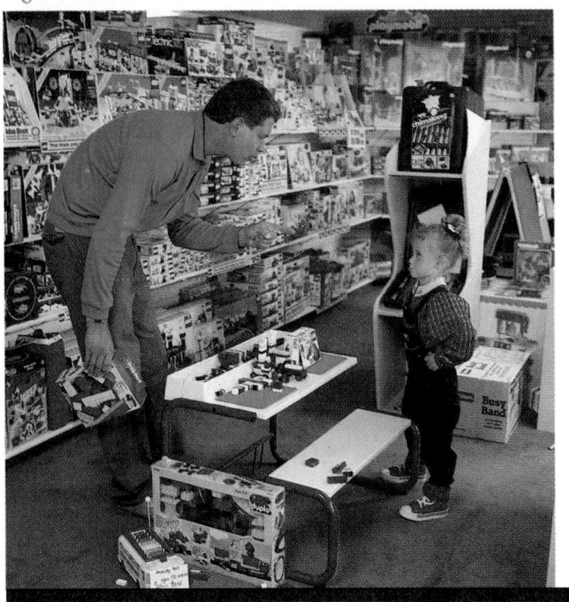

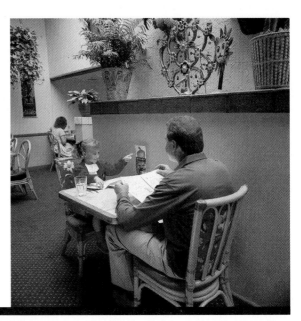

Positive interaction between school-age children and their parents offers these children the opportunity for a healthy self-esteem. Negative interactions between parents and children may encourage children to participate in antisocial behavior with peers.

person responsible for this is the school teacher and the classroom environment. Children enter school with the idea that the teacher is an all-powerful authority figure. The child's self-concept is therefore influenced by whether or not the child feels the teacher likes what the child does and who the child is. The discipline that the teacher imposes can also have a strong impact on social development. For example, if the teacher is inconsistent in enforcing rules or fails to enforce them, the child may attempt to try to "get away with anything." Discipline that is too strict or harsh may cause the child to go into a shell, avoiding friendships or involvement in socially meaningful relationships with other children. Healthy social development is more likely to occur when teachers and the school provide reasonable rules, enforce them consistently, and encourage children to develop and maintain social relationships with one another.

THE EMOTIONAL DEVELOPMENT OF CHILDREN

When someone says to you, "Don't be so emotional!" what comes to mind? Just what are emotions? What role do emotions play in our lives?

On a separate sheet of paper, write down every emotion you can think of. Beside each one, note whether it is pleasant or unpleasant. Note also whether you feel this emotion much of the time or little of the time. Now compare your response to the emotions listed in Figure

8-5. Note that there are four **core emotions** that humans experience: joy, sadness, anger, and fear. Within each of these core emotions are related emotions that we all experience at one time or another. How many of these emotions have you experienced? Most people recall only a small number of the emotions.

Emotions are simply the way our bodies and minds react to people and events around us. Think of a time you were standing in front of your class or another group to give a speech. What did you experience? You were probably experiencing the emotion of anxiety which, as Figure 8-5 shows, is related to the core emotion of fear. You may have said to yourself, "I'm really nervous!" Your mouth was dry, your heart was beating quickly, your palms were perspiring. Perhaps your voice quivered a bit as you struggled to get the first few sentences out. You may have seen someone giggling in the back of the room; that just made matters worse. This example illustrates a common emotional reaction that people experience.

Emotions involve our thoughts as well as our bodies. They arouse us to respond in a certain way. As children, we experience certain emotions very intensely: joy, happiness, anger, and frustration, for example. As we grow older, we experience a wider array of emotions. We also learn to control our emotional reactions to an extent that we could not do as children. In this section, we will look briefly at how emotional development takes place in children from the infancy stage through the school-age stage of the human life span.

Emotions in Infancy (Ages 0–2)

It is difficult to really know if young infants in the first month or two of life experience true emotions. We know that they experience *distress* when they are cold, hungry, tired, or in pain. Perhaps this reflects unhappiness.

Figure 8-5

Core Emotions and Corresponding Emotional Clusters

Joy	Sadness	Anger	Fear
Happiness	Dejection	Frustration	Wariness
Delight	Unhappiness	Jealousy	Anxiety
Contentment	Distress	Disgust	Suspicion
Satisfaction	Grief	Annoyance	Dread
Pleasure	Discouragement	Fury	Dismay
Elation	Shame	Boredom	Anguish
Pride	Guilt	Defiance	Panic

SOURCE: M. J. Kostelnik, L. C. Stein, A. P. Whiren, and A. K. Soderman, *GUIDING CHILDREN'S SOCIAL DEVELOPMENT* (Cincinnati: South-Western Publishing Co., 1988).

Over time, however, we know that infants develop emotions that are very real. By 9 months of age, infants show such emotions as joy, surprise, anger, disgust, fear, interest, and sadness. Unlike older children, the emotions of infants are not directly within their control.

The normal infant response to distress and other negative emotions is to cry. Infants cry only when something is wrong and they are in distress. Contrary to what some inexperienced parents might think, infants do not cry just to irritate the parent or to make him or her angry! Research shows that infants cry in certain ways, depending on what is the cause of their distress. One cry might reflect discomfort from hunger or cold, while other types of cries reflect anger, pain, or frustration. Parents can learn to identify the type of infant cry. This helps them to more quickly alleviate the source of the infant's unhappiness. Some people believe that crying infants should be ignored and their crying will stop. However, this is not true. Crying infants who are ignored cry louder, longer, and more frequently than those infants who are comforted when they cry. When infants cry, it is for a reason. It is always best for a parent or caregiver to try to find the source of the distress.

The most common signal of positive emotions in the infant is smiling. The smiles of newborn infants are simply reflex responses to pleasant feelings. Between 1 and 2 months of age, though, these become true *social* smiles. The infant's face will light up and smile toward familiar human faces and voices, such as those of the mother and father. Parents find these reactions to be rewarding, and parent attachment to the infant increases. By about 4 months of age, infant smiles turn into laughter when infants are gently played with or talked to by others.

Emotions in the Preschool Stage (Ages 3-5)

As the child grows older so, too, do the number of emotions that are experienced and expressed. Perhaps the most significant development, though, is in the core emotion of **fear**. Fear in infants was limited to sudden changes in the external environment, such as bright lights, loud noises, sudden or falling movements, and strange people or things. By age 3, however, the child has learned that there are, indeed, things "out there" to be afraid of. The imagination begins to have an effect, and imaginary fears are produced. While such things may not pose an actual danger to the child, the child imagines that they do.

Fear of the dark and fear of being left alone are early fears. Also, as children experience events that might have frightened them, their specific fears increase. This might include the fear of being bitten by a dog or cat, the fear of being lost, or the fear of being hurt. The child may have bad dreams, or nightmares, that inspire particular fears. To a preschool child, dreams are "real" events; they don't realize that dreams are actually their own thoughts during sleep. Children might also develop fears after watching a scary television show or hearing a scary story. Such experiences are often the root of early fears of death and of ghosts and the "bogeyman." While most people of all ages experience anxiety when thinking about death, the preschool-age child may become preoccupied with such thoughts and have more difficulty than older children and adults in controlling this fear.

Other emotions develop during this stage. For example, the emotion of **guilt** emerges as the child is now old enough to distinguish between right and wrong. Guilt is an unpleasant emotion that is quite powerful in its effects on a child's behavior. Children learn to engage in good behavior and to avoid bad behavior in order to avoid the feeling of guilt that results from doing something wrong.

The core emotion of **anger** is also heightened in this stage. Preschool children can throw genuine temper tantrums; they begin to act defiantly toward parents. It has been said that the phrase, "No!" is the most common utterance of the 2- and 3-year-old child. Excessively loud, persistent crying and fist pounding are evidence of the intensity of emotions that preschoolers can experience. They have not yet learned how to control their emotional expression of anger. They react to anger and frustration in an extreme manner. Parents often refer to this phenomenon as the "terrible twos" and "trying threes," although such tantrums are also common in older children.

Positive emotions are also growing in this stage. Expressing love and affection for others and experiencing joy and happiness are heightened. Such emotions are expressed in physical ways such as jumping up and down or firmly hugging and kissing another. The child in this stage has learned that other people also have emotions. They become concerned about how *others* are feeling; they recognize the emotional impact they have on others through their own expression of emotions. This means that the interpersonal skill of empathy (see Chapter 4) is being learned. When 4-year-old Micah smiles at his mother, he knows that it "makes her feel good inside." Likewise, when he is angered by his sister's teasing, he knows that he can make her angry by sticking his tongue out at her.

Emotions in the School-Age Stage (Ages 6–12)

A most important development in the child's emotions in this stage is that she or he gains better control over emotional expression. Rather than crying every time she or he wants something or every time something goes wrong, the school-age child expresses her or his emotional response in a more socially acceptable manner. Recall the example of Ben and Carmen at the beginning of this chapter. When Ben's sand castle washed away, he immediately cried to gain attention because he knew of no other way to express his disappointment. School-age Carmen, on the other hand, was able to rationalize what happened. She knows that crying will not help matters. If she wants a sand castle, she will have to start over in a spot that will not be threatened by the ocean's waves (see Figure 8-6).

As with the preschool child, the school-age child also has fears, although they are more realistic. These fears are more likely to be of such things as war, of being embarrassed or humiliated, or of being physically injured. School-age children fear failing a test at school, being sent to the principal's office, or "goofing up" when talking in front of the class. Being hit by a car or a threat of a nuclear attack are also possible fears. While fears of ghosts, death, and dogs usually continue into this stage, they diminish in their intensity.

Another important aspect of emotional development in this stage is learning how to

Figure 8-6

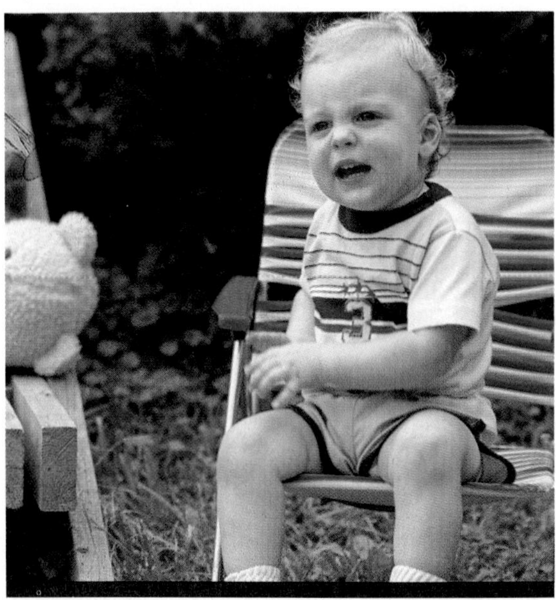

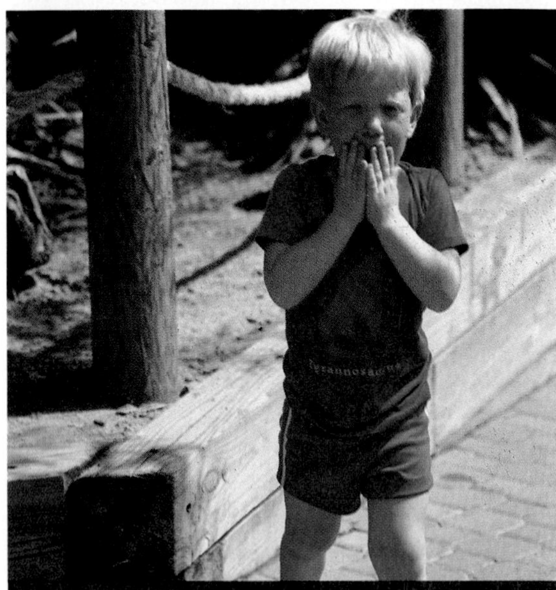

Robert Torres

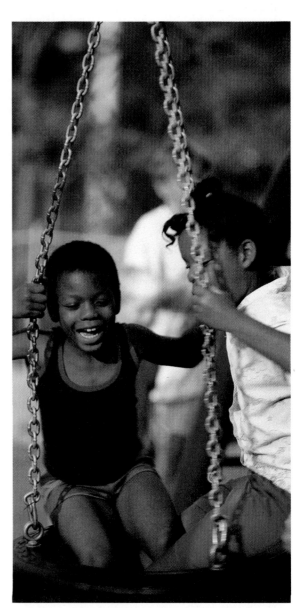

The age of the child definitely influences the type of emotional expression exhibited by the child.
Robert Torres

express emotions in ways that society considers appropriate. "Don't be a cry-baby," "You should feel sorry that you hurt him," "You shouldn't worry so much about it," are just some of the messages that society gives children of this age concerning emotional responses. School-age children learn that throwing temper tantrums and hitting other people are not considered appropriate means of expressing emotions such as anger and frustration. They learn to feel remorse when they have done something wrong, and they learn to express their remorse by apologizing to others.

Children also learn how to control and express their emotions by observing others, particularly adults. If they observe adults who openly express their emotions in certain ways, then children are likely to do the same. When 7-year-old Sondra sees her angry father pounding his fist on the table, she learns that it is appropriate to respond to anger by pounding her fist or engaging in a similar physical act. If, on the other hand, children see adults covering up their emotions and not expressing them, they, too, are likely to hide or deny their emotions. If 8-year-old Ezekial observes that his father never expresses his feelings of hurt or happiness, then Ezekial learns that such feelings are best kept inside.

In our society, differences are reflected in the way we teach boys and girls to express emotions. It is during the school-age stage that such sex differences are first emphasized. Following traditional masculine sex roles, boys are encouraged to "be tough" and not cry. Males of all ages are more likely to conceal their emotions, whether they are positive or negative. Showing emotions, especially hurt feelings or fears, is discouraged for boys in a society that holds up role models such as Rambo, He-Man, and G.I. Joe. A 12-year-old boy who cries or otherwise shows emotions may be called a "sissy." It is socially more appropriate for girls, on the other hand, to cry and to talk about their feelings. Girls, more than boys, are allowed to express feelings related to sadness, tenderness, affection, and worry.

What effect do you think this difference between the sexes in emotional expression has? Psychologists tell us that it is mentally healthy for us to be able to express our emotions. We become depressed and stressed if we are forced to hold all of our feelings inside or if we are encouraged to deny that we have feelings. When little boys are taught to deny or hold in their feelings, they grow up with an inability to reduce the stress that they feel inside. The result has shown up in the population of American adult males who have high blood pressure, heart attacks, and ulcers. It is probably a healthy sign that our society, today, permits greater expression of emotions in males, young and old alike.

THE MENTAL DEVELOPMENT OF CHILDREN

Mental development of children is closely related to their physical, social, and emotional development. Healthy development in these areas promotes healthy mental development as well.

For our purposes here, we will use the term **cognitive development** as the equivalent to mental development. **Cognitive ability** refers to the person's ability to use reason in solving problems, in being creative, and in thinking in general. Some refer to this as **overall intelligence**.

There are two basic influences on a person's cognitive development: heredity and environment. These influences are also known as the dual influence of *nature* and *nurture*. In regard to the influence of heredity, research has shown that the genes we inherit from our parents influence overall mental ability and development. This fact is well-documented by cases of gifted children and those with exceptionally high intelligent quotients (I.Q.s) that show up during the preschool years and, possibly, even in infancy. Documented cases of 2-year-olds who are reading, playing musical instruments with ease, or solving puzzles that even adults find difficult support the idea that heredity has much to do with cognitive development. These abilities show up before parents have taken any out-of-the ordinary steps to enrich the child's learning environment.

But environment also plays a major role in cognitive development. The first important environment is the home. When parents talk to their children, read to their children and encourage them to read, and provide an enriched learning environment, cognitive development of the average child is enhanced. The school is the next important influence on mental development. When schools and parents combine forces to promote learning, cognitive development increases. Environments that are deprived of communication with adults and learning opportunities appropriate for the child's age can retard the child's mental development. In this way, heredity and the environment work together to shape overall mental development of children.

The Cognitive Development of Infants

Jean Piaget, the Swiss psychologist, developed a theory about how children develop their mental abilities. According to Piaget, humans progress through four major stages of cognitive development:

- Sensorimotor (Ages 0–2)
- Preoperational (Ages 2–7)
- Concrete Operational (Ages 7–11)
- Formal Operational (Ages 11–adulthood)

Each of the first three stages will be described in the appropriate sections that follow. Formal operations will be discussed in Chapter 9.

The infant is in the **sensorimotor stage**. Just as the term implies, the infant's mental functioning is limited basically to its senses and its desire to engage in physical movement. During the first few months of life, the infant primarily responds and reacts to stimuli from the environment. It is not until later in the first year that the infant actively seeks out objects in the environment and attempts to manipulate them.

One way to test this is to study the infant's ability to determine **object permanence**. If you hold a ball in front of 3-month-old Jana, she will reach to touch it and, probably, to further explore it by putting it in her mouth. However, if the ball is removed from her sight, Jana will act as if the ball no longer exists. She seems to have forgotten it. Ten-month-old Marva, on the other hand, will search for the ball when it is hidden from view. She knows that the ball exists even though she can no longer see, touch, or taste it. For Marva, objects have *permanence* even if they can no longer be seen.

This is an important cognitive development for infants. For young Jana, objects in the environment have no separate existence from her. She is unable to distinguish other objects from her own self and senses. This is known as **egocentrism**. Older Marva, on the other hand, has learned by experience that there is a separate world, apart from herself. This is an important step in the child's understanding of how to act on and master the environment, rather than just reacting to it. Because Marva is able to see the world from a point of view other than her own, she is less egocentric than Jana.

By the time Jana and Marva are 2 years old, they will have developed a number of important cognitive abilities. They can play elementary games of hide and seek with the object, looking under blankets, chairs, and pillows when an adult hides something out of view. They have the ability to picture things in their minds, to think about what course of action is appropriate to reach a goal or get what they want. This type of activity represents the child's first attempts at problem-solving.

Jana and Marva will also develop language ability. The young infant's language is pretty much limited to crying, cooing, and babbling nonsensical syllables ("ba-ba-ba" or "na-na-na") during the first year. During the second year, these sounds begin to take the shape of actual words with meaning for the infant. Normal language development will take place if parents and others in the infant's environment talk to the infant and stimulate her or him with the proper sounds of the language. Through a process of trial-and-error, the infant will learn to imitate almost any sound in the language by 1 year of age.

The Cognitive Development of Preschool-Age Children

After infancy, the child enters the stage of cognitive development that Piaget called **preoperational**. As in infancy, children remain quite egocentric in their orientation toward the world. The 3-year-old child believes that he or she is the center of the world; that adults and other children see the world in the same way that he or she does.

Yet, the preschool child develops some important cognitive abilities that infants do not have. For example, 3-year-old Lucas is able to use **symbols** to represent such things as people and places. This allows him to engage in **symbolic play** by pretending that one object stands for another. Lucas pretends that he is a tiger in a jungle by crawling on all fours and growling. Four-year-old Marcy fastens the ends of a rope to her ears, and pretends she is Dr. Wilson listening to a patient's heartbeat with a stethoscope. These children have active imaginations that allow them to expand their mental functioning through the use of symbols in healthy ways.

Being able to use symbols also allows the child in this stage to develop an understanding of number and quantity. The preschool child can count. She or he understands that numbers stand for a particular quantity of objects, and that three cookies are more than one. Symbols increase the child's vocabulary and other aspects of language development. Preschool children are now able to understand instructions, commands, and other information communicated by others. Likewise, preschool-age children are now able to articulate their own thoughts, feelings, and desires quite effectively. They can speak in complete sentences and begin to understand proper grammar. As a 2-year-old, Martin exclaimed, "Me go swing! Me go swing!" Now, at age four, Martin states, "Mommy, please push me on the swing!" For parents, the preschool-age child is a genuine force to be reckoned with!

Preoperational children are also able to arrange objects, such as a set of sticks, according to a logical sequence. This is called **seriation**. For example, 4-year-old Bette can arrange a set of ten sticks according to their length, or a set of blocks according to their weight. She can also sort the sticks and blocks according to color, a skill known as **classification**.

There are still some skills that the average child in the preoperational stage has not yet mastered. One is the skill of **decentering**. Recall the example of 5-year-old Carl at the beginning of this chapter. Even though the tall, narrow glass and the short, wider glass had equal amounts of water, he claimed that the tall glass contained more water. When asked why, Carl held one hand above the other and said, "Because this glass is bigger!" What Carl did was centrate: focusing on one aspect of the problem to the exclusion of other relevant aspects. That is, he focused on the height of the glass, but not on the width. Other children might say the short, wide glass contains more water. They focus on the width, but not the height. Preoperational children center on one aspect of a problem, but have difficulty taking into account more than one. This leads to an incorrect solution to the problem (see Figure 8-7).

Figure 8-7

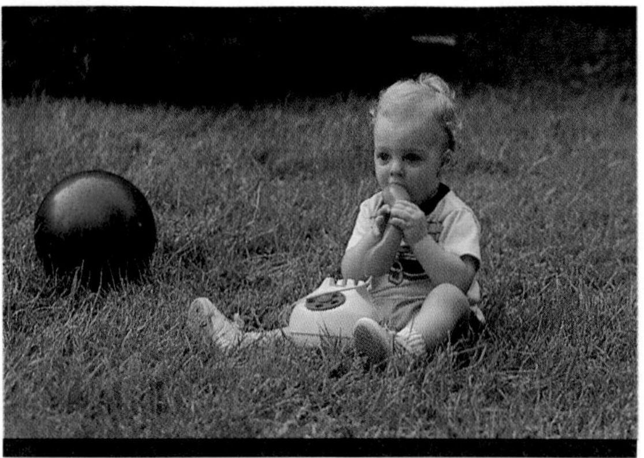

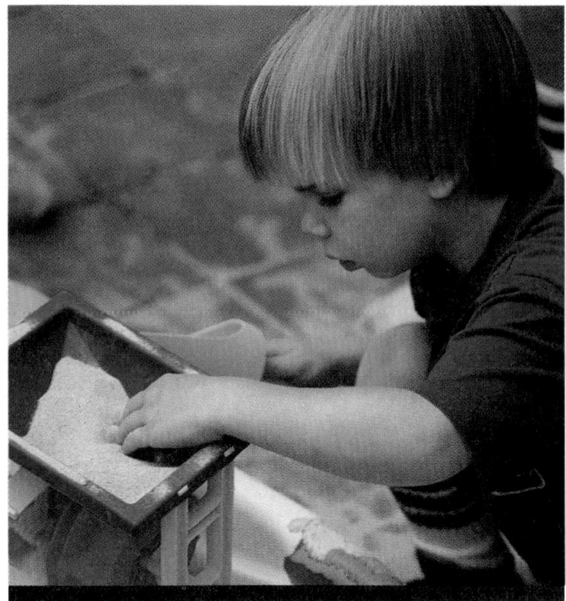

Robert Torres

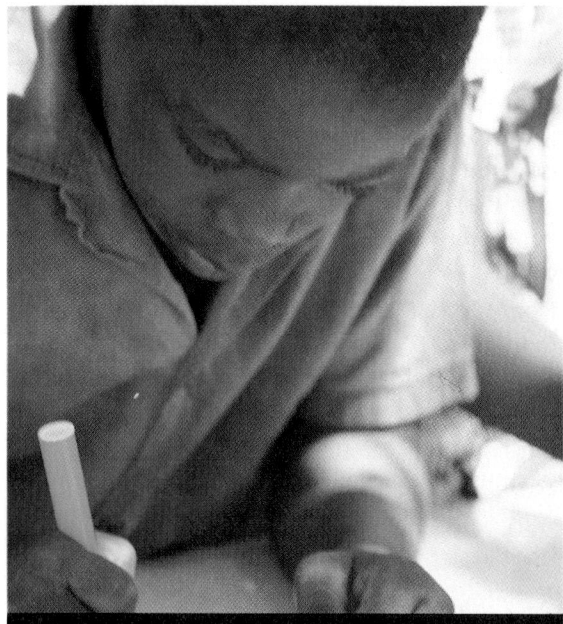

Different mental abilities are exhibited by different aged children.

Robert Torres

The Cognitive Development of School-Age Children

Between the ages of 7 and 11, children enter the stage of cognitive development known as **concrete operations**. By this time, they have mastered the skills of decentering and are able to take multiple aspects of a problem into account when trying to solve it. In the case of Maria (at the beginning of this chapter), it was obvious to her that the two glasses of water contained the same amount even though they were of different shapes and sizes. She is able to focus on the height and width of the glasses simultaneously. Unlike Carl, Maria knows that although one glass is taller, this is compensated for by the greater width of the other glass. The amount of water remains constant, regardless of the size and shape of the container.

Effective thinking and problem-solving of school-age children is assisted further by rapidly developing language, reading, and mathematical skills. Their ability to use and to manipulate abstract symbols increases dramatically as does memory and the ability to learn and retain information. School-age children use reason and logic in their thinking processes, which helps them in their learning and problem-solving activities.

School-age children also become less egocentric in their orientation toward the world. They learn that their thoughts and perceptions may not be the same as other people's. When Mookie was 4 years old, he thought that his parents and everyone else were afraid of dogs. Now that he is 10 years old, Mookie is aware that his own fear of dogs is not shared by everyone. This skill allows the school-age child to develop empathy (see Chapter 4). Mookie can put himself in the shoes of other people and is able to better predict how they might feel or behave in particular situations. This assists him in his social development as well.

Noticeable differences in the mental functioning of children begin to show up in this stage. Often these differences are not observed until children enter school and are presented with intellectual tasks. Some children are "slow learners" and have difficulty keeping up with others. School is hard for them. Some children have physical learning disabilities, such as **dyslexia**. This disability causes the child to reverse words and letters, so that normal reading is impossible. While they are just as intelligent and capable as other students, their reading difficulty causes them to fall behind and to be labeled incorrectly as "slow" or "dumb."

Other children are identified as "gifted or talented." This means that they stand out as exceptionally creative, able, and bright in whatever challenges the school offers them. However, gifted children may also have difficulty in school. This is not because the material is too difficult, but because it is too easy. Some of these children are unchallenged, bored, restless, and perhaps even rebellious.

Whether children are slow, average, or gifted in terms of mental functioning, overall mental ability is closely related to social and emotional development. Slow and gifted learners may be avoided by their peers. Slow learners may be viewed as undesirable playmates because of their poor performance in school. Gifted children may be seen as a threat to other children. Also, both types of children may become rebellious or aggressive as a result of difficulty with school work. Such behavior may turn off potential friends who view these children as not being much fun to be around.

Whatever the case, the mental development of the school-age child is a combined product of three things: (1) hereditary intelligence present from birth, (2) experiences in the home and in the way parents and others interact with child, and (3) experiences in school. In Chapter 12, we will examine some of the ways that parents can enhance the cognitive development of children along with their physical, social, and emotional development.

WRAPPING IT UP

In addition to our physical development, humans also develop along social, emotional, and cognitive lines. These areas are closely interrelated. Healthy physical development goes hand-in-hand with healthy social, emotional, and cognitive development.

Healthy social development involves the learning of *prosocial behavior* skills. Empathy, cooperation, sharing, and giving support and encouragement to others are just some examples of prosocial behavior that children begin to learn at a young age. Unhealthy social development involves the learning of such negative patterns as dishonesty, deceit, aggressiveness, and trying to take advantage of, or in some way hurt, other people.

An important aspect of social development for infants is *attachment* to parents and other caregivers. The more that infants experience pleasant, positive social relations with adults, the greater their chances of growing up to have pleasant, positive relationships with other people. They will grow up to be secure and trusting in their relations with others. Infants must be held, cuddled, talked to, and loved in order to develop socially in a healthy way. The attachment of infants to parents also leads to two types of anxiety reactions: *stranger anxiety* and *separation anxiety.* These are normal infant responses to changes and uncertainty in their usual day-to-day environment.

Preschool-age children should develop *autonomy,* or independence, from parents. While remaining attached to their caregivers, preschoolers begin to explore the environment on their own. Language development gets started, as does the learning of cultural values, attitudes, and behavior expectations, through the process of *socialization.* Preschool children develop a sense of right and wrong, good and bad, and *sexual identity* as either boy or girl. Friends, or *peer groups*, also assume importance for the social development of the child in this stage.

School-age children continue to become more peer-oriented and less parent-oriented. Popularity and conformity to the peer group become important indicators of the child's *social status* and contribute to the development of self-concept. However, peer group pressures may also lead children to engage in antisocial types of behavior. If parents, teachers, and other adults remain important role models for children in this stage, potentially negative influences of the peer group can be greatly reduced or eliminated.

Emotional development in young infants is limited primarily to responding to distress. Older infants begin to experience such *core emotions* as *anger* and *fear.* The most common signals of infant emotions are smiling to reflect pleasure and crying to reflect distress.

The range of emotions experienced and the expression of these emotions increase for preschool-age children. Childhood fears emerge in this stage as the cognitive abilities of the child to fantasize and think symbolically increase. Preschool children also develop an elementary form of the emotion of *guilt*, which is an internal check on their behaving in ways that society deems either right or wrong. In this way, emotional development is related to the development of prosocial skills. Emotional expression tends to take extreme forms in this stage: temper tantrums and persistent defiance of authority when angered or displeased; jumping excitedly and shouting when happy.

School-age children learn to better control the experience and expression of emotions. They can use reason to overcome their desires to physically respond to emotions. School-age children are less likely to strike out in anger or cry whenever something goes wrong. Emotional expression takes place in more socially acceptable ways. The nature of childhood fears in this stage changes from unrealistic to more realistic concerns. Also, society's expectations for emotional expression based on sex begin to take shape. Females, more than males, are encouraged to express a range of emotions.

A combination of one's heredity and one's learning environment contribute to *mental, or cognitive, development* in children. An enriched learning environment for children can help them to attain their full mental potential allowed by heredity. A deprived learning environment, on the other hand, places limits on what the child is able to achieve in mental functioning.

Infants in the *sensorimotor stage* of development begin life by responding and reacting to stimuli in the environment. Later, during the first year of life, they begin to act on their environment to achieve their goals and to satisfy their needs. Language development is an important part of being able to act on the environment.

The preschool-age child in the *preoperational stage* of cognitive development learns how to use symbols to increase communication effectiveness. Language development progresses to the point where the child is able to express wants and desires with adult caretakers, and to share feelings and information. Although the preschooler learns about the concepts of *number and quantity*, he or she has difficulty in solving problems that have multiple aspects.

School-age children in the *concrete operations stage* of cognitive development become adept at problem-solving by using reason and logic in their thinking. Learning to read and to write accompanies their rapidly developing language skills. By this stage of the human life span, children's mental abilities become an issue in social relationships as well. Exceptionally slow or gifted children may have difficulty forming and maintaining positive peer relationships. This further exemplifies the close connection between all aspects of human development.

Exploring Dimensions of Chapter Eight

For Review

1. What is prosocial behavior? What is antisocial behavior? What role do these types of behavior play in the child's social development?

2• What is infant attachment? How is it achieved?
3• Identify the major ways that preschool-age and school-age children differ in terms of:
   a. social development
   b. emotional development
   c. mental, or cognitive, development.
4• What are peer groups? What are their important functions for children of different ages?

For Consideration

1• Write a brief essay concerning how a person's physical, social, emotional, and mental development might be related to each other. How can development in one area enhance development in another? In what ways might failure to develop in one area lead to difficulties in another?
2• Recall your own years in the school-age stage of development (ages 6–11). List the names of as many friends as you can recall who formed your peer group. Who had the greatest influence on you? In what ways were you influenced by your peers? Which of these influences would you now say are positive? Which are negative?
3• Based on your own observations of boys and girls your own age, is there a difference in the way that each sex expresses emotions? What emotions are boys more likely to express? What emotions are girls more likely to express? What does society think about emotional expression for boys and girls? Even if the sexes do differ in emotional expression, what difference does it make?

For Application

1• Plan a visit to a recreational facility where you can observe children at play. This may be in an area where there is playground equipment, a swimming pool, or perhaps even a youth baseball or soccer game going on. Record any evidence that particular children display of: (1) prosocial behavior skills, (2) antisocial behavior, and (3) emotions. Be sure to note what they did that qualified for each of these categories. What were the immediate reactions of other children or adults to the kinds of behaviors you were recording?
2• With the help of your teacher, plan a day when parents can bring infants of different ages to class. For example, one might be 1 month old, another 6 months old, and another 11 months old. Create an area in front of the classroom where the infants can be observed. Provide an

array of safe toys (rattles, plastic cups, rings, etc.) for the infants to play with and observe. What differences between the infants do you observe in terms of motor skills? emotional expression? mental functioning? How does each parent interact with his or her child in a way that is related to the infant's age?

3• Volunteer to work at a local child care center or preschool. Learn what is done there to promote the social, emotional, and mental development of children. Maintain a written log of your experiences. What things did you particularly like? What things did you dislike? After your experience, write an essay about how your attitudes toward children have changed as a result of your volunteer contact with them.

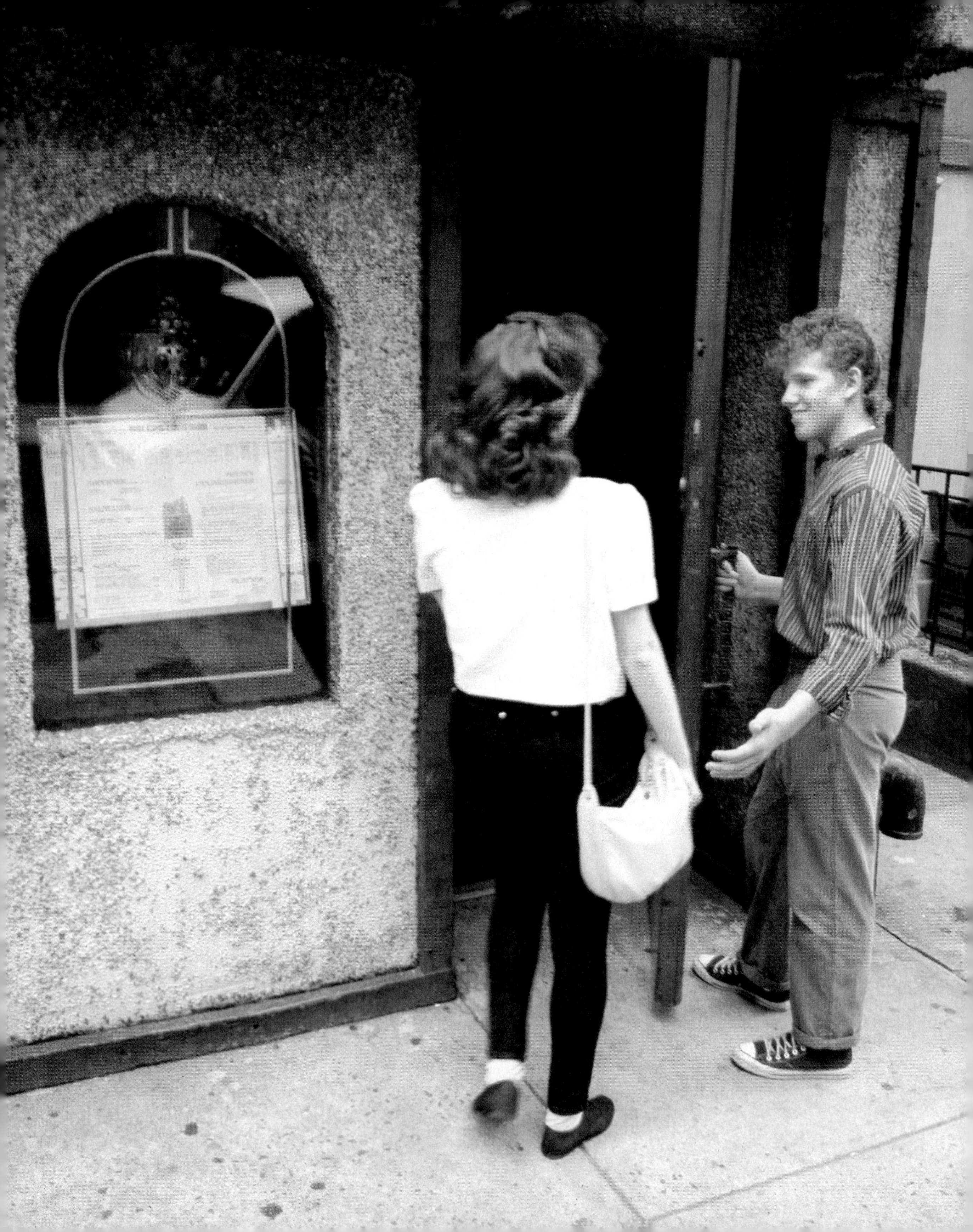

nine

DEVELOPMENT IN ADOLESCENCE AND ADULTHOOD

This chapter provides information that will help you to:

- Understand the physical, social, emotional, and mental development of adolescents.
- Recognize the strong influence of peer groups versus parents and family on adolescents.
- Understand the functions of dating in adolescence.
- Recognize some of the problem behaviors associated with adolescence.
- Familiarize yourself with physical, social, emotional, and mental development in adulthood.
- Understand the three domains of adulthood: work, marriage, and parenthood.
- Recognize signs and problems of middlescence.
- Understand the physical, social, emotional, and mental development of the aging population, and its dilemmas and assets.
- Uncover some myths about aging.
- Determine ways to meet the needs of the elderly.

In Chapters 7 and 8, we learned about the complex nature of child development. In this chapter, we will examine the remainder of the human life span as it relates to individuals in our society. The adolescent stage of development begins around the ages of 11 to 13 and continues through the teenage years. This is the stage that you, the reader of this book, are probably in. Between the ages of 18 and 20, one enters the adulthood stage. Finally, between the ages of 65 and 70, one enters the aging stage of the human life span. Each of these stages involves important physical, mental, social, and emotional changes for the individual.

ADOLESCENCE

Much of what is said about teenagers today concerns major life problems such as drug abuse, alcoholism, suicide, delinquency, running away from home, pregnancy, and rebellious behavior, to name a few. Indeed, teenagers are faced with a multitude of pressures and stresses that can result in difficult choices with negative outcomes. Just the same, the teenage years also present some exciting opportunities for learning and growth.

The unique characteristics of the adolescent stage result from the fact that teenagers, or adolescents, are in a period of transition between childhood and adulthood. Adolescents often feel as if they have one foot in each world—sometimes wanting the family security and attachment associated with childhood; other times wanting the freedom and independence of adulthood (see Figure 9-1). Many teenage problems result from society's expectations that adolescents act like adults in socially responsible ways. They should be independent thinkers who are responsible for their own actions, and are self-controlled and well-mannered. At the same time, adolescents are not supposed to enjoy many of the rights and privileges that adults are allowed—the right to vote, consume alcoholic beverages, use tobacco products, marry, and have children. This can result in confusion, uncertainty, and stress for the adolescent who is trying to answer the question, "Who am I?"

Figure 9-1

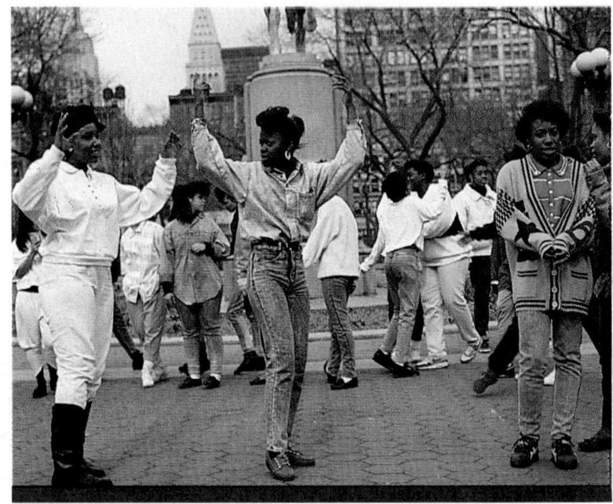

Adolescents can fulfill the need for parental and peer approval in unique ways. The parents and peers of these students, who are rehearsing a dance routine, would both approve of this activity.

Barbara R. Lewis/Monkmeyer Press

THE PHYSICAL DEVELOPMENT OF ADOLESCENTS

Adolescence begins when the person enters **pubescence**, or **puberty**. This period of time creates major physical, emotional, and social changes in the individual. Pubescence is related to the "storm and stress" that adolescents in our society go through.

The physical changes brought about by puberty are dramatic. There is a notable growth spurt in both height and weight. There is a change in the way the body is shaped and proportioned. The adolescent also attains full sexual and reproductive maturity. The male is able to produce sperm cells and the female is able to produce ova (eggs).

As with earlier stages of child development, there is much normal variation from one adolescent to the next in when puberty begins and in how much of an effect it has on the person's physical development. For some, it begins around age 11; for others, it may be delayed until 13 or 14. Girls generally begin puberty one to two years earlier than boys.

Puberty actually begins when the body starts secreting certain hormones from the pituitary gland. One hormone, commonly known as the **growth hormone**, causes changes in the body's dimensions. It causes girls to grow in height; it lengthens their arms and legs, it expands the pelvis region (widening the hips), and it adds a layer of fatty tissue under the skin. The growth hormone causes boys to increase in height; it lengthens their arms and legs, it widens shoulders, and it increases muscular strength. During this time the physical strength and endurance of the average boy surpasses that of the average girl. Adolescents in puberty grow at a rate of 3 to 4 inches per year.

Hormones secreted during puberty cause other physical changes, not all of which are welcomed by the teenager. For example, skin problems such as blemishes, pimples, and acne plague many teenagers during this time. The changing voice "squeaks" or "cracks" in a combination of childlike and adultlike tones. Some teens experience physical awkwardness, as changes in body dimensions cause them to be off-balance. For example, rapid growth in legs and feet may result in the adolescent having difficulty catching up in his or her ability to control them effectively.

Other physical changes create a more adultlike appearance for both girls and boys. The voice deepens in its tone. Growth of axillary (arm pit) hair and pubic hair in the genital region begins. For girls, **menarche**, or first **menstruation**, takes place to signal the development of the reproductive system. Also, breast development moves the adolescent girl further toward an adultlike appearance. For boys, facial hair begins to grow along with accelerated growth of the genitals (penis and scrotum). Motor skills improve along with physical strength. Because of an increase in strength and an improvement in motor skills, athletic activities become an important feature in the lives of many teenage boys and girls. Although physical development may cause some discomfort and awkwardness for adolescents, it helps the body blossom toward its fully developed adult form.

Just as with the earlier stages of child development, the adolescent can do a great deal to enhance his or her physical development. Sound nutrition and regular physical exercise are important during this stage of rapid growth. Muscle and bone growth depend upon proper diet and exercise. Personal hygiene habits should be established in such areas as dental care and the control of body orders. Preventive health care and hygiene are the keys to the successful physical development in this stage.

THE SOCIAL AND EMOTIONAL DEVELOPMENT OF ADOLESCENTS

Part One of this book discussed the importance of forming a personal identity. Indeed, this is the major social and emotional task faced by adolescents in our society. "Who am I?" "What am I worth?" and "Of what value am I to others?" are critical questions that adolescents often ask and try to answer. In doing so, the adolescent forms attitudes, goals, and values. He or she begins to get a handle on personal needs and how they might best be met. Successfully developing a personal identity contributes to the development of meaningful interpersonal relationships during adolescence and adulthood (Chapters 4–6).

Teenagers are exposed to a number of different values, attitudes, and belief systems from parents, peers, teachers, coaches, movies, and television. Many of these are conflicting influences that cause confusion: "Should I do as my parents say, or should I go along with what my friends think?" "My teacher says one thing, but my church disagrees—whom should I believe?" "If adults on television can have sex with each other, why can't teenagers?" "My boyfriend says it's ok to use drugs because 'everyone is doing it'—is that right?" The social and emotional development of adolescents is complicated by the myriad of conflicting influences, choices, and dilemmas that are experienced in our contemporary society.

Peer Group Influences on Adolescents

Compared with earlier stages of child development, the peer group becomes even more important in the social development of the adolescent. Adolescents are influenced more by peers and school activities than by parents and family. This shift is a normal aspect of adolescent development. It involves the seeking of independence and autonomy from the family. Sooner or later, the individual must leave home and establish an independent life as an adult. It is during adolescence that this process of emancipation begins. Seeking independence is important prior to the adolescent's being "launched" into a job or college after high school.

Peer groups are an important source of status and competition for the adolescent (see Figure 9-2). They help to prepare the individual for the competitive world of adulthood. Peers help satisfy the teenager's need to conform to a set of values and behaviors. Conformity assures acceptance and popularity. Acceptance by one's peers contributes to the development of social maturity, which entails a sense of competence and self-esteem. To know that friends like you and that you are capable of meeting and making new friends is an important social skill to carry into adulthood. Peer groups also provide an avenue for achievement if the teenager behaves in a way that "measures up" to peer group standards and expectations.

Figure 9-2

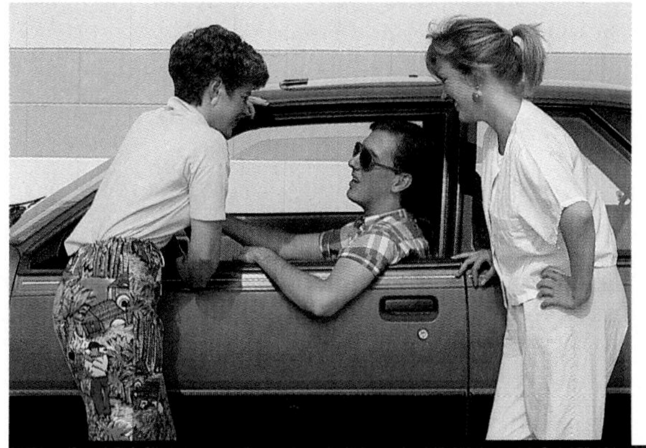

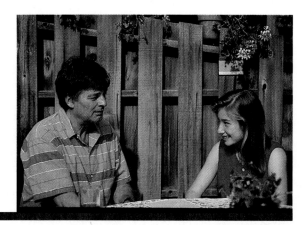

A teenager's acceptance by his or her peers and parents leads to positive development of self-esteem and competence.

Renate Hiller/Monkmeyer Press

Spotlight on issues

Sex Roles and Dating Relationships in Adolescence

Moving into the adolescent stage of the human life span introduces a new dimension into the social and emotional world of the adolescent. With puberty comes the development of one's *sexual drive*. One becomes more interested in members of the opposite sex than was true in childhood. Teenagers also develop a greater sense of what is considered to be appropriate behavior for boys and appropriate behavior for girls. In other words, sex roles become more firmly defined.

Sexual drive pushes the adolescent toward seeking more intimate relationships with members of the opposite sex, or *heterosexual relationships*. Peer groups tend to become mixed in sex composition, as both boys and girls begin to mingle in terms of recreational activities and just spending time together. When peers begin to "pair off" in couples, the adolescent is motivated to do the same. Adolescents begin to date members of the opposite sex, provided one's parents approve and the opportunity exists. For some, this begins early in the adolescent years; for others, dating begins later.

Dating is an important part of a person's experiences prior to marriage. Dating fulfills many functions, as discussed in Chapter 4. Through dating, relationships established with members of the opposite sex provide excitement for the adolescent. It also creates many new issues, such as these that follow.

QUALITIES OF A DESIRABLE DATE • What do you consider the most important qualities of a person with whom you would date? Surveys of young people show that the following qualities are most important (1 = Most Important; 9 = Less Important): (1) physical attractiveness (good looks); (2) congenial personality; (3) sense of humor; (4) intelligence; (5) good manners, considerate; (6) sincere, genuine; (7) compatible interests; (8) good with conversation; (9) fun to be with.

How many of these were on your list? It is interesting that when the same people are asked to rate qualities of a desirable *marriage partner*, being "loving and affectionate" and "honest" rate highest, while "physical attractiveness" rates lowest. What are the implications of rating the qualities of a desirable date differently from the qualities of a desirable spouse?

DATING ACTIVITIES • When you date, what do you like to do? Go to the movies, out for dinner, to a sporting event, or a party with friends? In our society, considerable freedom is granted to adolescents. Some parents, though, are more restrictive than others regarding acceptable dating activities for their adolescent children.

Male and female sex roles are also important. Is it appropriate for a girl to ask a boy out for a date, or should the boy always take the initiative? Is it acceptable for the girl to pay for the movie or the dinner, or should the boy always pay? Can a girl ask a boy to dance, or is this the boy's responsibility? Traditional sex roles dictate that males take the initiative, and females follow. Less traditional sex roles prescribe that dating activities be shared in terms of male or female initiative. What do you think?

SEXUAL INTERACTION • Controlling sexual interaction in dating relates to adolescent sex drive and sex roles. What kind of sexual behavior is appropriate for a boy and girl to engage in while dating? Should they hold hands or kiss? Should they feel and touch or pet? Should they have intercourse (go all the way)? At what point does sexual interaction between a teenage boy and girl move from the responsible to the irresponsible?

There are no simple answers to the above questions. If there were, we could solve the problem of premature sexual relations and unwanted pregnancy in our teenage population. Traditional roles in our society dictate that a male should go as far sexually as his female date will let him. However, this is not necessarily a responsible attitude. Everyone has limits as to what is considered sexually appropriate with members of the opposite sex. Your limits are dictated by your own conscience and values learned from your family, your religion, and other influences in your life (friends, siblings, and the mass media).

It is important that each person understand what sexual limits his or her conscience dictates, and not exceed them. You have the right to control your own sexual behavior on a date. *You do not have to engage in sexual behavior if you do not want to.* Beware of such lines as, "If you really loved me, you would," or, "Everybody does it." It is acceptable to say, "No!" to any sexual advance a dating partner may make. Going further than your personal values allow can lead to deception, exploitation, a premature commitment to the other person, and to deep feelings of guilt.

Any of these feelings can yield negative long-term consequences for a young person's sexuality and for his or her ability to establish healthy sexual relationships later in life. It is *your* responsibility to be aware of the consequences of any sexual interaction you undertake. Before engaging in sexual activity of any kind, ask yourself, "Am I willing to accept the consequences of my own behavior?" You, and only you, are the "boss" of your body.

STAGES OF DATING • Would your answers to the above questions be different if you were "going steady" with the person, rather than just casually dating? How about if you were engaged to the person?

In our society we go through different stages of seriousness in relationships with members of the opposite sex. We usually begin by casually dating a number of different partners; that is, we "play the field." This allows the young person exposure to a number of different personalities. After dating a number of individuals, young people often begin to narrow the field of potential partners before selecting an eventual marriage partner. Others may come to believe that marriage is not for them.

When partners feel a special bond of affection with each other, "more steady" relationships are established. In steady relationships, partners do not date others. Some people go steady too soon, before they have had a chance to "play the field" and date a number of others. Others go steady simply to engage in sexually intimate behavior. They may feel that they are "in love," and that advanced levels of sexual intimacy are therefore appropriate.

What do you think? At what point is steady dating appropriate? At what point are various types of sexual interaction acceptable?

Parents and Teens—A Generation Gap?

What about the so-called "generation gap" between adolescents and parents? If teens are becoming peer-oriented and possibly exposed to such negative influences as drugs or alcohol, isn't there a high degree of conflict between adolescents and their parents? Is this conflict between adolescents and parents normal? Or is parent-adolescent conflict abnormal and something to worry about?

Research offers an answer to this question. Adolescents expect more *power* relative to their parents in making decisions about themselves on a daily basis. Hairstyle and length of hair, curfew on school nights, choosing a boyfriend or girlfriend, and the kind of music to play and how loudly it can be played in the house are examples of some of these concerns. Wanting more of a say in personal and family matters is a *normal* expectation of the teenager who is moving toward adulthood and feeling a need to conform to the expectations of the peer group. Naturally, conflicts can arise if the adolescent wants more of a say than parents are willing to give.

Many adolescents have heard parents make exclamations like the following:

"Be home by midnight!"

"You can't date that person—I won't allow it!"

"You cannot go to that party!"

"Turn down that radio!"

However, it is interesting that the conflict actually may not be over any of these issues, *per se*. Rather, the *real* issue may be the adolescent's need to establish independence and autonomy contrasted with the parents' difficulty in "letting go" of the child who has been dependent upon them for so many years.

Such issues as hair length, style of clothing, and musical preference are clearly related to the teen's involvement with his or her peer group. Parents may feel threatened by their teenager's increasing involvement with the peer group and their child's need to conform.

Parents often resist the idea that their "child" is growing up. Out of love and affection for their teenager, parents may not want to think about the day their child will become an adult and leave home. It is not easy for parents to relinquish the influence that they have had over the childhood years. Parents may also mistakenly believe that the teen's search for independence is a sign that the parents are no longer loved, needed, or wanted by the teen. Conflict arises, then, when the teenager's need for more power is met by the parents' fear of losing power, love, and, ultimately, their "child" to the world of adulthood.

Such conflicts can take on major proportions for both parties. Adolescents and parents can become alienated from each other if conflicts are not successfully resolved. Such emotions as anger and frustration can make matters worse if they are not handled well. Parents and their teens may say to themselves, "I just don't understand her," or "He just doesn't understand me." Parents may believe that their teenager's friends are leading him or her astray with their unacceptable ways of behaving. Adolescents may say that their parents are "old-fashioned," "square," or "not with it."

Despite such conflicts, research also shows that parents retain a good deal of influence over teens in several major ways. For example, parents are a stronger influence than peers when it comes to the adolescent's major life values, religious beliefs, and plans for college or an occupation. Parents and adolescents agree far more than they disagree on these more basic "core" issues in life. In a sense, it is more important for parents and teens to agree on these issues, than the relatively trivial matters such as hair length and clothing style. Thus, while a "generation gap" may exist, the gap is much narrower than many people believe.

Problem Behavior in Adolescence

Unfortunately, not all influences of peer groups are positive for the social development of adolescents. Furthermore, adult society can also provide models of behavior that have negative influences on teens. Because of these negative influences, adolescents can engage in behavior that, for onc reason or another, gets them in trouble. These behaviors may be antisocial, illegal, immoral, or simply dangerous to the physical and psychological well-being of the adolescent (see Figure 9-3). Each of the following problem behaviors should be of great concern to adolescents, parents, and society in general.

ALCOHOL AND DRUG USE • Why do teenagers use drugs and alcohol? A major reason is that such substances are usually available to anyone who is able to pay for them. One's friends may exert pressure by saying, "Come on, everyone's doing it." Adolescents also see drugs and alcohol used in adult society, perhaps by parents or older siblings. In an effort to act in a grown-up manner, teenagers may copy the behavior of adults they observe engaging in alcohol or drug use. Drugs and alcohol may also be used as a psychological "crutch" for adolescents who have difficulty with the task of establishing a personal identity (see *Spotlight on issues*, Chapter 2, pp. 30–31). They cannot handle the stress involved in all of the changes going on with adolescence, and they turn to these substances for help.

One problem with this is that substance use is habit-forming. There is no cut-and-dry

Figure 9-3

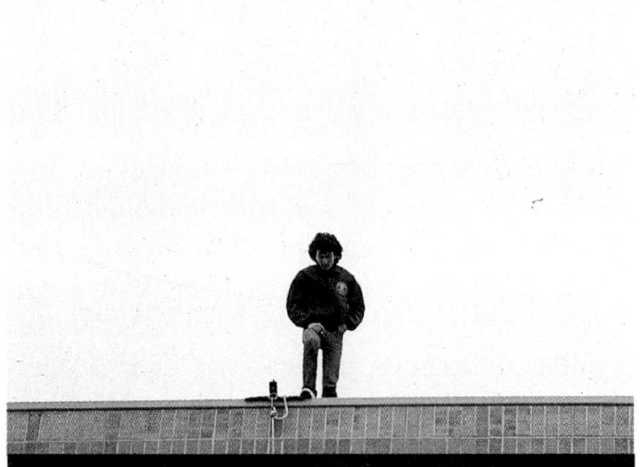

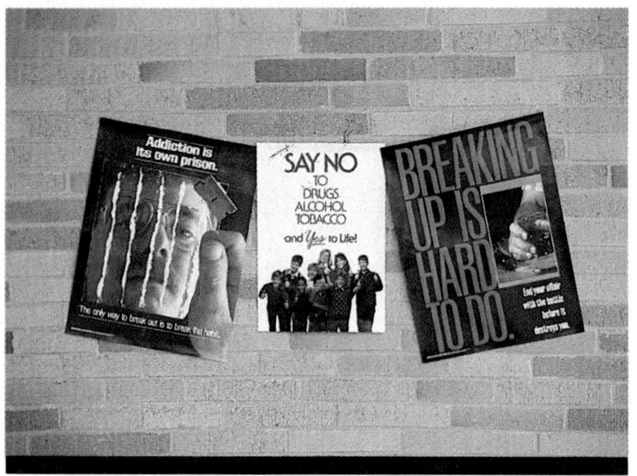
Addiction is
its own prison.
SAY NO
TO
DRUGS
ALCOHOL
TOBACCO
and Yes to Life!
BREAKING
UP IS
HARD
TO DO.

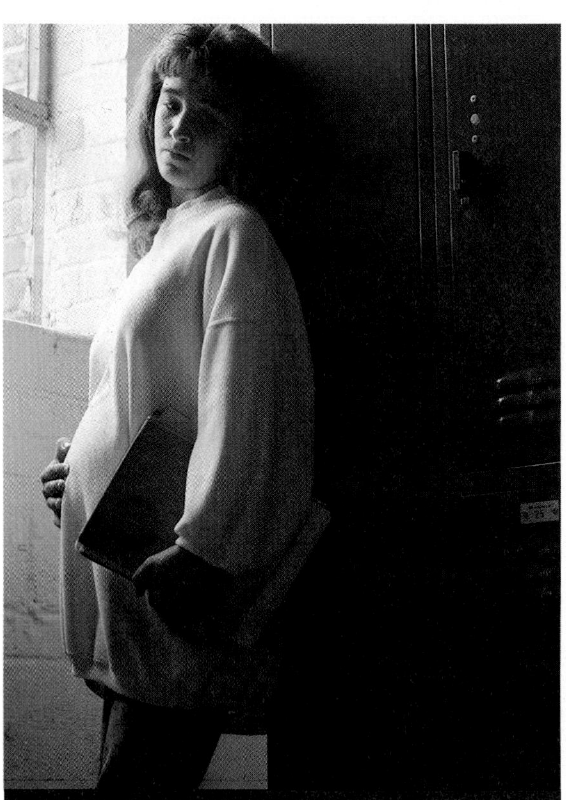

Some behaviors associated with adolescence are antisocial, illegal, immoral, and dangerous.
Jim Erickson/The Stock Market

distinction between what might be considered *normal use* and *abuse* of drugs and alcohol. The typical adolescent is not mature enough to control substance use, or to stop it when it becomes too much. Many adults, in fact, have similar difficulties, as evidenced by the high rate of drug addiction and alcoholism in our society today. These substances give the person a false sense of security and of being "in control." The person with a drug or alcohol habit has trouble functioning when they are not "high," and they become far less than a fully functioning person.

Use of drugs and alcohol by teens is illegal. Getting caught can create problems with the police and juvenile courts. Selling and/or using drugs can give the adolescent an arrest record, which can create problems later on when he or she applies for a job, or some other desirable activity. Adolescent substance use can also create major conflicts with parents. Often these conflicts are destructive and involve much resentment and anger on both sides.

Furthermore, both drugs and alcohol have physically dangerous side effects. The more they are used, the more dangerous they become. Heroin, cocaine, "crack," and barbiturates ("downers") can cause death. Of course, any drug can cause death if used by someone who is driving a car under the influence of a mind-altering substance. The automobile driver not only risks his or her own life, but also the lives of innocent others when driving under the influence of drugs or alcohol.

The best advice for any teenager is to say "NO!" to the pressure to use these dangerous substances. When substance use becomes an important avenue to status and popularity in one's peer group, it is best to search for other friends who don't expect such behavior. You, too, might be able to influence your friends who use drugs or alcohol by encouraging them to find alternative ways of enjoying life. A substance-free adolescent is healthier in the long run.

ADOLESCENT SEX AND PREGNANCY • Why is it that more than 1,000,000 unmarried teenage girls in the United States become pregnant each year? This is among the highest rates of adolescent pregnancy of all countries in the world. What impact does adolescent pregnancy have on the lives of the teenager mother or father?

As noted earlier, the adolescent matures sexually and develops the physical ability to reproduce. More teens today are deciding to experiment with sexually intimate behavior than ever before. The result has been a marked increase in the number of adolescents experiencing unwanted pregnancies.

As with drug and alcohol use, teens who engage in sexual intercourse are influenced by peer group attitudes and behavior. Adolescents are easily influenced by friends who claim that sex is "fun," "OK to do," and that "everybody's doing it."

Adolescents also observe permissive attitudes toward human sexuality in adult society. Whether it is portrayed in television shows, in the movies, in commercials for toothpaste or perfume, or in sexually suggestive books and magazines, teenagers today are given the message by *adult society* that you should be "sexy," "seductive," and sexually involved. Consider, too, the titles and lyrics of popular songs which also carry strong sexual messages.

When the pressure of peers and the stamp of approval by adult society are combined, many teenagers really see no compelling reason to wait to engage in full sexual relations.

While society may appear to be granting legitimacy to sexual involvement for teens, it certainly does not approve of teenage pregnancy. Yet, an unwanted teenage pregnancy is a definite risk of adolescent sexual activity. Adolescent sexual activity also has other potential negative consequences. Sadly, few teens give adequate thought to the following matters before they become sexually involved:

- Exploitation of one person by the other (being "used" for sex)
- Going against one's moral beliefs, religious values, or sense of what is "right or wrong"
- Becoming sexually involved with someone you really don't love
- Losing the respect of friends, parents, and other family members who believe that sexual intercourse in adolescence is wrong

- Contracting a sexually transmitted disease from an infected sex partner (see Chapter 13, pp. 308–311)
- Feeling guilty due to any of the above concerns

Clearly, teenage sexual activity has consequences. What happens when teenagers have babies? What are the consequences of adolescent pregnancy? The following list provides some examples of why pregnancy has negative consequences for the social development of teenage mothers and fathers:

- Medical complications in delivering the baby, due to the girl not yet being physically mature enough for childbirth
- Medical complications in the baby (premature, low birth weight, mental deficiency, injuries at birth)
- Stress, depression, and a feeling of helplessness in one's life (teen parents are more likely to attempt suicide)
- Low self-esteem and the perception of one's self as a failure or a "bad" person
- Greater-than-average chance of dropping out of school; not reaching educational goals after high school (college, trade school)
- Lower-paying jobs and a greater chance for unemployment
- Greater chance for abusing the child due to frustration, immaturity, and a sacrifice of educational and career goals
- High probability of marital problems and divorce for teenage parents who marry
- Children of adolescents perform poorly in school, achieve less education, receive lower incomes, and are more likely to be adolescent parents themselves.

Pregnancy and parenthood during your teenage years are threats to becoming a fully functioning person. It places limits on one's future. Rather than writing one's own "life script," the teenage parent has much of it written for him or her.

ADOLESCENT SUICIDE • A most tragic situation in our society today is that of adolescents who take their own lives. There is no greater sign of just how stressful adolescence can be for some teens. For one reason or another, some teenagers are less able to cope with and manage the pressure that they are under. Why do you think this is so?

During the past several years, the number of teenagers who commit suicide has increased. More than 5,000 young people in the 15- to 24-year-old range take their own lives each year. Next to accidents, suicide is the second leading cause of death among teenagers in our society.

Adolescents may commit suicide for a number of reasons. Some feel isolated from friends. They may not have established a meaningful tie with a peer group. Poor grades or other problems in school may create unbearable pressure. Others have boyfriend or girlfriend problems. They are unable to cope satisfactorily with the emotion of love. Still others may be unhappy with the conflict they are having with their parents. Or, they may be depressed if their parents should get a divorce. They may feel unwanted or unloved at home, if they are made the "scapegoat" for their family's unresolved problems. Being rejected by parents or friends is difficult for adolescents to handle emotionally. They have been hurt, and their desire to "hurt back" becomes stronger than their desire to live.

Any of these circumstances can lead to severe mental depression. Depressed adolescents feel alienated; they see life as not worth living. They see themselves as failures, worthless, or unlovable. They may blame themselves for their parents' marital or financial problems, experiencing an overwhelming sense of guilt. They see no future for themselves and come to believe that they cannot go on. They feel "trapped." The only way to escape the trap is to kill themselves.

What can be done to prevent this tragic event from happening? Depressed adolescents can be helped by counseling and support from friends and family. The key to suicide prevention lies mainly with the troubled teenager's friends and family. The ability to observe and recognize the signs of danger by friends and family is of critical importance. Troubled adolescents usually give some indication that something is wrong. The following warning signs should be observed:

- A shift in the adolescent's mood, from generally being happy-go-lucky to brooding, sulking, or just not talking
- Excessive drug or alcohol consumption that happens more than once in a while
- Stray comments such as, "Life is such a drag," "Some days I'd just like to kill myself," "Where I'm going, it won't make any difference," or, "I just don't know if it's all worth it" (These may not be idle threats.)
- A relatively sudden and unexpected withdrawal from social activities with friends
- An apparent loss of weight, appetite, or sleep
- Unusually risky behavior, such as reckless driving or careless stunts
- Change in school work or school attendance
- Making "final arrangements," such as giving away favorite personal possessions.

There may be other signs that tell you the person is just not the same or just not right. They may be acting "out of character," or they just "aren't themselves lately."

What should you do if you think a friend of yours is depressed to the point of being in trouble, and is not able to manage her or his emotional state? One thing that you can do is to talk with him or her and see if there is something wrong. Be supportive, nonjudgmental, and compassionate. Find out if there is anything you can do to help. The opportunity to share problems and feelings, and knowing that someone is there to listen, can be helpful. If you believe that the friend is indeed in trouble and needs help, contact a teacher or school counselor to discuss the situation. Many communities offer suicide prevention counseling and telephone "hot lines." Your family doctor can also give you good advice as to what services are available in your community for providing help to troubled teens. Take any threats or warning signs seriously—laughing or making fun of a person's serious threat to commit suicide may increase their feelings of desperation. Never dare a person to carry out a suicide threat. Taking some positive action is far better than ignoring or making light of a potentially life-threatening situation. The needless waste of human life and potential can and should be avoided whenever possible.

The Joys of Adolescence

Despite all of the change, stress, and potential problems that complicate the life of the average adolescent today, many adults look back on these years and exclaim, "Those were the greatest years of my life!" Most parents and their adolescent children enjoy each other's company. They enjoy a number of fun activities together. Parents wind up taking great pride in watching their children make the transition to adulthood.

Teenagers today have many desirable characteristics. They are idealistic and concerned about the future. They have a great deal of energy and a zest for life. They are courageous and willing to take risks—to experiment and try on various social roles "for size," discarding those that just don't fit. Adolescents are striving for independence; they can be relied on to handle responsibility. They are open, honest, and loyal to family and friends. While many adolescents have an active sense of humor, they are also serious deep-thinkers. Their positive attitude toward life is unsurpassed by any stage in the human life span.

THE MENTAL DEVELOPMENT OF ADOLESCENTS

Recall from Chapter 8 that the mental development of children proceeded through three stages: the sensorimotor, the preoperational, and the concrete operational. As children enter adolescence, they move into the stage known as **formal operations**. Adolescents develop higher level thinking skills and problem-solving abilities. They are able to use abstract concepts effectively, which explains why teenagers are able to handle the more complex language, math, and science tasks presented in junior high and high school.

School is an important element in the mental development of adolescents. By the time they are in high school, teenagers are developing literacy skills in reading and writing that will carry them into adulthood. School is the training ground which prepares the adolescent for entry into the world of work or college. The better able the adolescent is to master literacy skills, the better prepared he or she will be to move into the adult world of college and work.

In view of how important school is for the mental development of adolescents, it is unfortunate that so many teenagers in our society drop out of school. Some drop out by choice. They don't see school as being important or relevant to their lives. They may be low achievers who are simply bored or tired of school. Others may have less of a choice. They may need to assume a full-time job to supplement their family's income. Teenagers who have babies are more likely to drop out of school. They may not want to combine their parenthood duties with going to school, or they may need to get a job in order to support their family. Whatever the reason, on the average, school drop-outs achieve less education, are less skilled, and earn lower incomes as adults than do those who stay in school. Staying in school increases the adolescent's chances for healthy mental development.

DEVELOPMENT IN ADULTHOOD

When do you stop being an adolescent and start being an adult? There is no simple answer. Society says when you turn 18, you are legitimately an adult for certain purposes. You may get married without parental consent, bear children, and vote in elections. However, you must be 21 to enjoy other privileges of adulthood, such as the purchase and consumption of alcoholic beverages. Others may consider you to be an adult as soon as you move out of your parents' home, regardless of your age.

For our purposes, we will consider adulthood to begin any time after age 18, when the individual has achieved an appropriate level of emotional and financial independence from the parental home. This may occur at age 18, when the high school graduate leaves home for college, or at age 20, when one leaves home to marry and take a full-time job.

Human development does not stop with childhood or adolescence. Just as children move through various stages of growth and development, so do adults. The one thing you can count on as an adult is *continued change* in yourself as a person.

Figure 9-4

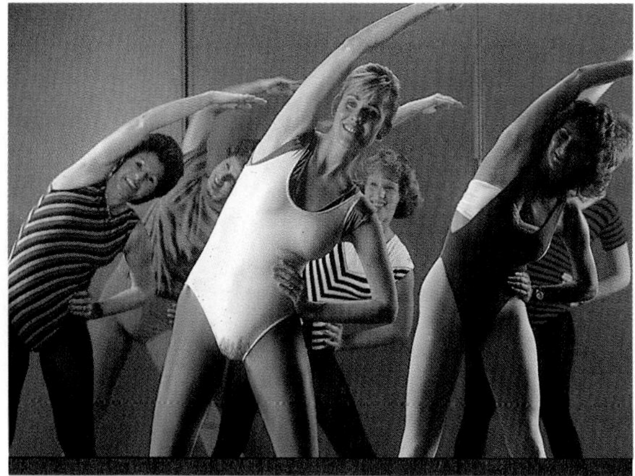

Aerobic exercise is quite popular among adults who are concerned about their health.
Steve Chenn/Westlight

PHYSICAL DEVELOPMENT IN ADULTHOOD

By the late teenage years, one has reached the peak of his or her physical growth potential. While pounds may be added or lost in one's weight, maximum height and growth in one's bone structure have been reached. Young adults often peak in physical fitness. This is demonstrated by the fact that professional athletes reach the "top of their game" during their twenties.

In our society, we have seen a remarkable increase over the past several years in the number of adults who exercise on a regular basis. Jogging, running, swimming, bicycling, and other types of "aerobic" exercise have become quite popular (see Figure 9-4). This is due to our heightened awareness of diseases in the cardiovascular systems of adults: heart disease, high blood pressure, and strokes, for example. These conditions are made worse if the person is overweight, smokes cigarettes, consumes excessive amounts of alcohol, or has a diet that consists of large amounts of low-density cholesterol and saturated fats.

Aerobic exercise, combined with a sound diet, strengthens the person's heart and circulatory systems. A decrease in the number of adults who smoke cigarettes has also had positive outcomes for adult health. Scientific research leaves no doubt that cigarette smoking increases the incidence of cancer and heart disease in adults. All in all, proper exercise, diet, and regular medical exams promote the physical well-being of adults.

SOCIAL AND EMOTIONAL DEVELOPMENT IN ADULTHOOD

Social and emotional development in adults is tied to three major life events that people in our society encounter: work-for-pay, marriage, and parenthood. These three domains of adult life shape the course of adult development. Sometimes these life domains work together in harmony; other times they conflict with one another.

The Need for Gainful Employment

As we will discuss in greater detail in Part Five of this book, adults in our society must work in order to support themselves and their families. Income earned from working provides the food, shelter, and clothing necessary to satisfy basic physical and safety needs. Work and the income it generates also serves as a symbol of one's social status. The kind of job we have influences the status of our homes, neighborhoods, and position in the social world. Work is also a means to achieve personal fulfillment through productive contribution to society.

Work today is an important activity for the development of both adult men and women. A man's job or career has always been an important aspect of his social status and personal identity in our society. Prior to the 1970s, however, relatively few women considered their work outside of the home to be a significant part of their personal identities. This has changed. Many women today find personal fulfillment in their work. They wish to know themselves and to be known for more than being married and being mothers to their children. Furthermore, in today's society two incomes are often necessary for the family to live at the desired standard of living. Thus, whether it is for reasons of personal fulfillment or financial necessity, work is a significant activity in the development of adult men and women today.

Marriage

Getting married has always been a popular activity for adults in our society. In fact, we are one of the most "marrying" societies in the world. At least 90 percent of all American adults will marry at least once. The reason for this is that marriage is defined by society as a legitimate way for adults to satisfy their needs for sexual and physical intimacy. Marriage also legitimates the bearing of children.

Whether or not we marry and whom we select to marry have important consequences for our social and emotional development as adults. Research shows that happy marriages are those in which spouses remain compatible and satisfy the partners' needs for intimacy and love. Such marriages contribute to each partner's self-esteem and psychological well-being. They assist the person's growth toward becoming a fully functioning individual. Unhappy marriages, on the other hand, are those in which spouses fall "out of love," have unresolved conflicts, or are unable to satisfy each other's intimacy needs. These marriages are associated with such negative psychological outcomes as depression, anger, and unhappiness. The decisions of whether or not to marry, when to marry, and who to marry are very important, yet too many people take such decisions too lightly (as we shall see in our discussion of divorce, Chapter 13).

Parenthood

The vast majority of adults in our society who marry also have at least one child. Some consider having children as a major avenue to adult status. Children might also be seen as a personally fulfilling extension of one's self. Children can fulfill certain adult needs for companionship that a marriage partner or friends cannot satisfy.

The percentage of married couples who have children has gone down somewhat in the past few years. Also, the average number of children born per family has decreased. For example, in 1958 American women bore an average of nearly four children. In 1988, the average number of children born per woman dropped to below two. This is due to a change in childbearing values. While having at least one or two children is still considered by many to be important, having several children is more likely to be viewed as too costly in terms of time and money. Also, with the sharp rise in the number of mothers who work outside the home, having several children may prevent them from attaining work or career goals.

"Middlescence" in Adulthood

Adults go through changes, much like those of adolescents. While not all adults go through the same changes to the same degree, many do go through a middle-age type of adolescence known as **middlescence**. Middlescence refers to those times in an adult's life when questions such as the following are asked:

> "Did I really do the right thing in marrying this person?"
>
> "Should I have really had these children, when I wanted a career, too?"
>
> "Am I really happy in this job? Aren't there other jobs I'd like better?"
>
> "Have I advanced as far as I can go on the career ladder?"
>
> "What have I really contributed so far in my life? What do I want to do with the rest of my life?"

Just as the adolescent searches for answers to the question, "Who am I?" so, too, does the adult wrestle with questions of personal identity. These questions reflect the three major domains of adult life: job, marriage, and parenthood. It is a time for self-reflection. Adults examine where they have been, where they are now, and where they are going. Middlescence represents a sort of "crossroads" for the adult who questions the past and wonders about the future.

The key word for adults at this time is *change*. It is human nature to desire change in one's life. Without change, people feel like they are in a rut, doing the "same old thing," day after day, week after week, and year after year. Getting up each day at the same time, going to the same job, and coming home to the same spouse and children may become a stale routine of daily living. At some point, many adults begin to search for change in their lives—some way to move in a new direction that will add zest and restore the fulfillment that somehow has been lost.

Middlescence presents a dilemma for the adult. It is a time of uncertainty and, in all likelihood, anxiety. The outcome varies from one person to the next. For some, the outcome for personal development is negative. This may involve conflict with the marriage partner, alcoholism, divorce, or poor performance at work that causes the loss of one's job. At the extreme, more tragic outcomes such as suicide or mental breakdown may occur. Just as some adolescents have difficulty coping with life changes that occur in the transition between childhood and adulthood, so, too, do some adults have difficulty coping with the *lack* of change in their lives. Some recognize the changes that have to be made but are unable to make them happen (see Figure 9-5).

Middlescence can also have positive outcomes for the adult. It can lead to personal growth if the person is able to create the desired changes. A person can take advantage of being at a turning point in her or his life. One can "shift gears," seek more fulfilling activities, or take advantage of the opportunities that are presented to establish more meaningful and intimate relationships with the spouse or the children.

Figure 9-5

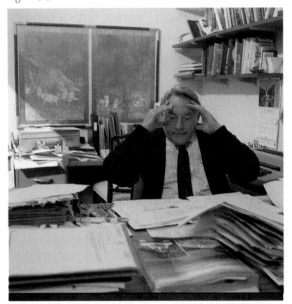

Middlescence can cause tension for some adults.

Consider the following case of one family's experience with middlescence.

CASE IN POINT

Maria was 39 years old. She and her husband, Andy, had been married for 20 years and had three children. Maria had dropped out of college when she gave birth to her first child. She had aspired to be a registered nurse. Maria stayed at home to take care of her first child, while Andy worked as a salesperson. Maria continued to stay at home as the second and third children were born. When she turned 35, Maria felt an "emptiness" inside. While she loved her hard-working husband and children, Maria no longer felt contented. She felt trapped at home and began to wonder if she really made the right choices in giving up college and a nursing career to marry and raise children. She was confused and unhappy. Her unhappiness soon spread to irritation with Andy and the children. At times she would lash out at them in anger, not realizing the resentment she was expressing toward them for the educational and career sacrifices she had made. She felt unappreciated, unfulfilled, and, worst of all, lost. Andy and the children did not understand what was happening to Maria. Eventually, she and Andy separated and considered getting a divorce.

Maria's situation turned out negatively for her and her family. However, it did not have to be negative. Decisions and adjustments in their lives could have been made to create a positive ending to this middlescent experience. Consider the following alternative ending that could have happened in this case.

CASE IN POINT

When Maria began to feel trapped at home and unfulfilled, she discussed her feelings with Andy. Andy agreed that Maria had made great sacrifices in her life. Andy suggested that with some adjustments in his work schedule, he could care for the children while Maria attended a local college in order to get her nursing training. They would have to take a loan to pay for college costs and find a person to care for the children when both Andy and Maria had to be away. Andy realized how strong Maria's feelings were about her "emptiness" inside, and tried to accommodate his work life to adjust to Maria's needs for change in her life. Although the two years it took to get her nursing degree were tough to get through, Maria did finish her college work and took a job with a local hospital. She felt great about her accomplishment. She also felt a renewed sense of love and gratitude toward her family for the sacrifices *they* made on her behalf. With a fresh outlook and a new career ahead of her, Maria was "on top of the world."

While middlescence poses challenges and stress for adults and their families, it can result in opportunities for personal growth and development.

Spotlight on issues

Differences in Middlescence for Men and Women

Gail Sheehy's popular 1977 book, *Passages: Predictable Crises of Adult Life*, shows how men and women differ in their experience of middlescence. She bases her work on the research of psychiatrist Daniel Levinson, author of *Seasons of a Man's Life*, 1978, and others who have studied adults moving through mid-life transitions.

For women who have followed the traditional sex-role pattern of being married, having children, and caring for the home, mid-life crises are more likely to be centered on family matters. As their children begin to leave home to begin their own adult lives, these women may fear the prospect of a major aspect of their lives coming to a close: *motherhood*. They have provided much time, energy, and love to their children. This will be missed by mothers who feel that they are no longer going to be needed in this role that is so important to them. What will give their life meaning once the children are gone? If they have not worked outside the home or if they have done so only periodically, they may lack the education and job skills required for meaningful paid work. They may wonder if their husbands still love them, or if they are still sexually attractive mates. These are "displaced homemakers," and they may begin to question the past and the present, in search of a meaningful future for themselves.

Women who have worked in careers or in steady employment may also experience dilemmas of middlescence focusing on marriage and parenthood issues. The single woman in a professional career may wonder if she should have married. Married women in a career may wonder whether they could have advanced up the "career ladder" more rapidly had they not married or had children. Some career women may regret *not* having children, or may feel that they had too few. Regardless of employment history, adult women can come to wonder about their own physical attractiveness and how they are viewed by men.

For men who have followed traditional sex-role patterns, on the other hand, issues in middlescence are more likely to be focused on job and career development. Traditionally speaking, men in our society have been responsible for being the primary breadwinners in their families. Middlescence means evaluating the career choices that have been made and pondering the uncertain future.

Did I select the right career path? Can I change careers at this time in my life? Have I reached the top of the "ladder" in my job or career? These are some of the questions that men in middlescence ask. After setting their sights high as young adults, some men are discouraged when they realize that they have gone as far as they can go in terms of promotions and income earned. They have reached a plateau in the work world. This can be a bitter pill to swallow in a society that judge's a man's worth on the basis of his income and occupational success. The "dream of youth" may become a "nightmare of middle age" for the man who is gaining inches around the mid-section, has graying hair, and an aging face. Men also are concerned over the loss of physical attractiveness during these years.

Such problems of middlescence are not inevitable. Not all men and women experience them, and those who do are affected by them to different degrees. Preventive measures are also possible. For example, women who have been full-time "housewives and mothers" might join voluntary organizations in the community in order to feel that they are making a meaningful contribution in their lives. Others go back to college, or seek advanced job training, in order to regain meaningful paid employment. If such steps are taken *before* the children leave home, then the woman has an alternative means of self-fulfillment in place once the children *do* leave.

For men, prevention might mean reducing their career goals; that is, not aiming so high or accepting that their dreams for the future are probably "impossible dreams." They might also consider a change in careers and seek retraining or additional education to shift gears in the work world.

Such preventive steps, whether taken by men or women, require a great deal of support from the spouse, children, and friends. It is a difficult task to undertake on one's own. Shifting career goals or going back to school require adjustments of family members. Time schedules must be shifted, housework schedules and responsibilities must be delegated, and financial priorities may have to be adjusted. As desirable or as necessary as these changes in adulthood might be, they are difficult to achieve successfully. For those who are able to do it, though, the benefits are well worth the effort.

Men and women often go through middlescence in different ways (see *Spotlight on issues*, pp. 195–197). For both sexes, however, the dilemmas posed by middlescence involve some combination of the three adult life domains of job, marriage, and parenthood.

DEVELOPMENT IN THE AGING YEARS

As with entry into the adult years, the entry into the aging stage of the human life span is gradual. For our purposes, we will consider age 65 to be that point when the aging stage begins. It is at this age that many people retire from the world of employment. While the aging years pose special challenges and problems for the individual, they can also be a time of great happiness and fulfillment.

People who are age 65 and over compose the fastest-growing segment of the American population. It is estimated that by the year 2000, this age group will include 30 million people, which will comprise nearly 14 percent of the total population. In 1900, there were slightly more than 3 million aging people, comprising only 4 percent of the total population. For a child born in the 1980s, the average life expectancy is about 75 years, 71 for males and 78 for females (see Figure 9-6). Our increasing life span has been caused by improved nutrition, exercise, and medical care (see Figure 9-7).

While we might think it is good that people live longer, there are some problems that our increased longevity has caused. Economic problems of the elderly have mushroomed about as fast as their population has grown. Living on retirement pensions or Social Security checks means that the elderly have

Figure 9-6

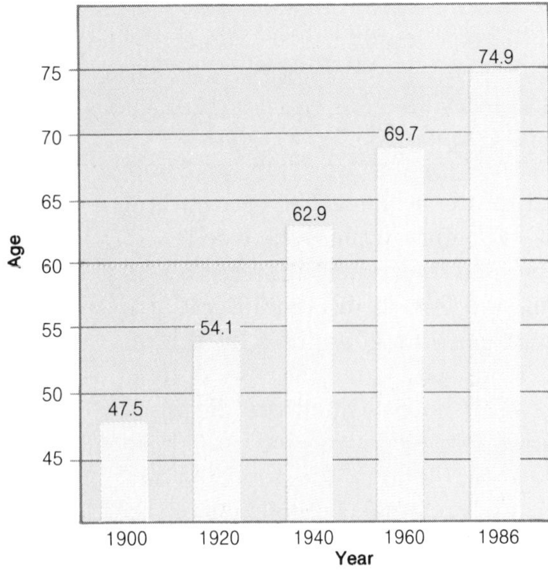

These are average life expectancy figures. In reality, each column differs by sex and by race. For example, in 1986 the life expectancy for males was 71.3 and for females 78.3. In 1988, life expectancy for whites (male and female) was 74.9, but for non-whites (male and female) it was 71.4.

Source: Statistical Abstracts of the United States, 1988.

Figure 9-7

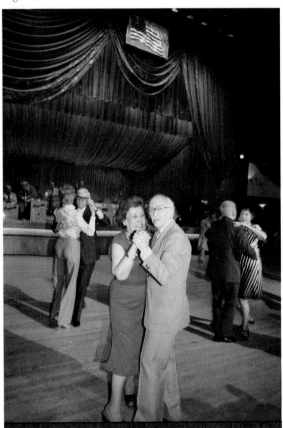

Improved nutrition, exercise, and medical care have expanded the aging population's life span.

Len Speier

fixed incomes. This means that their income does not increase, even though the cost of living increases. As costs for medical treatment, housing, food, and clothing increase, many elderly feel the pinch of inadequate income to pay for these necessities.

Living longer may also place an economic burden on the elderly's adult children. Having more aging people means a growing need for social and economic support from families. This situation can be stressful for those families where aging members are ill, cannot live on their own, or otherwise require much attention.

Understanding the Aging

Young people sometimes have difficulty accepting aging people as individuals. All people 65 and older are not alike. Though we can easily see the injustice of categorizing and stereotyping all youth or all young parents as the same, we fail to see the injustice and inaccuracy of treating aging people as if they were of one type. Aging people have individual likes, dislikes, traits, capacities, and physical and mental capabilities. Understanding that aging people have unique personalities, just as people in any life-stage, is important in interacting with aging people in our family as well as in our community.

Another aspect of aging that is sometimes misunderstood is retirement. To be sure, retirement is a difficult adjustment for some individuals. Leaving productive, financially rewarding work may be negative for some. Preparation for financial and social changes is necessary.

Aside from the uniqueness of aging people, other facts related to the aging years can help break some of the myths of aging. Focusing on facts rather than myths can help us face realistic issues related to aging family members.

Myth: Older people naturally withdraw from life.

Fact: Many older people play active, vital roles in community, political, family, and religious activities.

Myth: Most aging people live in nursing homes or health care facilities.

Fact: A small percentage—4 or 5 percent—live in such institutions.

Myth: In the aging years, people become irritable and hard to live with.

Fact: Such behaviors are based on life experiences, attitudes, and personality. Aging itself does not produce such behaviors.

Myth: People must retire at age 65.

Fact: Current laws allow older adults to choose retirement age.

Myth: The "golden" years of aging refer to ample supplies of money that aging people have set aside for this stage of life.

Fact: Some aging people may have large savings and investments available. Most aging people must carefully watch their spending. Poverty and the stress it produces are common among the aging.

Myth: Older people can't take part in physical exercise.

Fact: Continued exercise has more to do with physical ability than age does. Many people are physically active throughout their lives.

Myth: Most of the aged are disabled.

Fact: Only 7 percent of the aging are confined to their beds and their homes. Approximately 4 percent live in institutions; approximately 89 percent live in the community and are totally self-sufficient.

Myth: Older people suffer from serious mental deterioration; they become senile.

Fact: The confusion and disorientation referred to as **senility** may be more emotional than mental. Studies show that the ability to think and reason increases with age if these faculties are continually used. Boredom seems to be a factor related to senility.

Physical Development in the Aging Years

Many physical changes occur in old age. At some point, the process of **senescence** begins. This is the point in life when the human organism degenerates at a rate faster than it can regenerate itself. Body cells break down faster than they can be replaced. This is a long-term, gradual, and normal process that is *not* the same as *senility* (which is a mental disease).

Senescence means that the immune system of the body becomes less effective. Older people are therefore more susceptible to disease and infections. The bones become more brittle and are easy to break if the person should fall or have an accident. Physical injuries take longer to heal. Blood vessels begin to thicken and harden; the person develops a greater risk of heart attacks and strokes. The senses of taste, hearing, sight, smell, and touch all decline with aging.

Senescence is a normal and inevitable process in our lives. All of us will experience it. Yet, there are steps that people can take to slow down its arrival and minimize its effects. As with earlier stages of the life span, sound nutritional habits and regular exercise contribute to a healthy body. Such habits must have been started years earlier if their beneficial effects are to be felt in the aging years. People live longer and are less likely to feel the effects of senescence if they have established a continuous program of self-care throughout the years of adulthood. In addition to a sound diet and regular aerobic exercise, healthful living habits such as not smoking or not consuming alcohol to excess are included.

Social and Emotional Development in the Aging Years

Old age can bring a sense of completeness to life. The person can enjoy leisure activities that had to be delayed when he or she was employed full time before retirement. Playing golf, engaging in a favorite hobby, or traveling are favorite activities of the elderly person in our society. Great enjoyment can come from being free from the daily competition, demands, and struggles of the work world. More time may be spent with one's own children and grandchildren.

Personal well-being in this stage is related to a number of factors. These include:

- Good health
- Regular exercise
- Satisfying relationships with children, grandchildren, and friends
- Sound nutritional habits
- Adequate income and housing
- Satisfying marital relationships

If the above conditions are met, social and emotional development in aging is enhanced.

Development suffers, however, among those who find themselves isolated from social contacts. Loneliness is an issue that many elderly people face. Poor health and inadequate income create extra hardships. In the mid-1980s, around 15 percent of all persons 65 years and older lived below the poverty line. Older people are more likely to live in poverty if they are unmarried (single or widowed) women, reside in rural or small towns, or if they are black or of another minority. The stress of inadequate income is increased by expensive medical care that illness or accidents in old age can require. Health insurance often is not adequate to meet the high costs of doctors, hospitals, and medicine. If an elderly person is to manage, careful financial planning and budgeting are required.

Mental Development of the Aging

A common belief among the general population is that older people lose their ability to think. To the contrary, research shows that older people maintain a high level of mental sharpness up to the time of their death. Provided that elderly people are involved in interaction with others and are given opportunities to exercise their mental facilities, they do not become senile or lose their mental abilities. However, isolation from others and boredom can lead to a certain degree of disorientation and withdrawal.

It is also in cases of illness, such as a stroke or Alzheimer's disease, that older people experience a loss of mental functioning. Alzheimer's disease afflicts approximately 5 percent of the elderly, or between 500,000 and 1.5 million people in 1988. This disease causes the nerve cells in the brain to become twisted and tangled. The ailing person suffers memory losses and possibly severe disorientation and hallucinations. Sometimes these people recognize their family and friends, while at other times, they don't. For these reasons, Alzheimer's disease creates a heavy burden on family members. At the moment, scientists have found no prevention or cure for Alzheimer's disease.

Meeting the Needs of the Elderly

The increasing number of aging people in our country presents some major issues that will affect community and family life in the United States. More products and services focusing on the needs of the aging must be available in our society. Some of these needs include the following:

- Housing/community planning to provide small, easy-to-care-for dwellings that are easily accessible to shopping and entertainment
- Transportation availability for people who cannot or choose not to drive a car
- Health facilities that are readily available and focus upon needs of the aging
- Opportunities for aging people to have interaction with people of various age groups
- Services for people who can no longer attend to all of their household chores but who choose to remain in their own homes
- Opportunities for aging persons who reside in institutions to become part of a broader community of people
- Facilities for intensive health care when aging people can no longer care for themselves
- Recreational and entertainment facilities that emphasize less strenuous physical exercise and meet the needs of aging people
- Financial management assistance geared to the needs of the aging
- Opportunities for aging people to utilize their skills and expertise to the betterment of themselves and the community as a whole.

These needs will not easily be met. Combined efforts of educational, religious, medical, and community groups are needed. Progress has already been made in some areas. Adult day care centers, outpatient care centers for aging, special transportation facilities, and programs utilizing "grandparent" tutors and aides in schools (Figure 9-8) are already

Figure 9-8

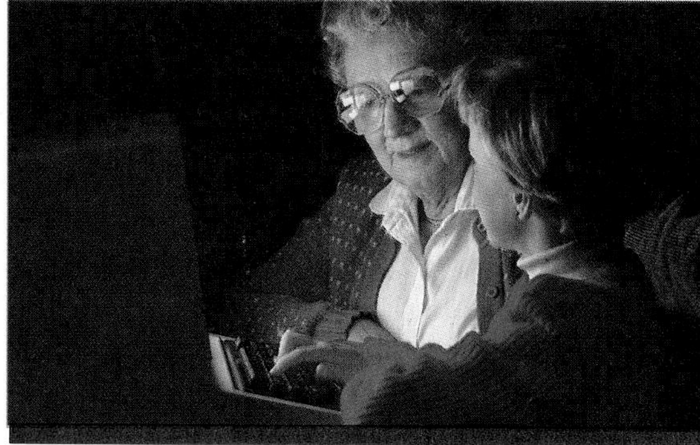

Elderly people can share a lot of knowledge with teenagers, children, and other adults; likewise, teenagers and children have knowledge.

Peter Beck/The Stock Market

available in some communities. Programs such as "Meals on Wheels" and community-sponsored outings are also promising steps forward. However, too few communities provide such services: too many aging people are without products and services to meet their needs.

Today's young people are directly involved in meeting these needs. The high school and college students of today will be the decision makers and community leaders when the aging population reaches the 30 million and beyond level. Greater realization of issues of aging and a greater understanding of aging people will be helpful in making these decisions.

Spotlight on issues

Aging People in Society

The percentage of aging people in American society is growing. As this aging population grows larger, it also is becoming more diverse, with a variety of backgrounds and experience. The extended life spans of individuals have created an aging population that cannot be clustered together in terms of personality, needs, or behavior.

In early America, elderly persons were those over 60, who were conservative in dress and thought, often reliant on family members, and who received most of their pleasures through the experiences of others. Today many aging people, well beyond 60, have an independent lifestyle in which they are involved in society and aware of changes in current thought and behavior.

The variety in ages and subsequent variety in the aging population have underscored the special needs of aging people in our society. Aging people will continue to need material items and services such as food, clothing, shelter, transportation, and health care. But these needs will continue to increase with the growing number of aging people. The aging population also will require a greater variety of goods and services to meet these needs. For example, health care services will have to be adapted for those who are mobile, relatively healthy, and financially stable as well as for the immobile, sick, and poor.

As their numbers increase, the aging population will move beyond *wanting* these goods and services to *demanding* them. Aging people already constitute a large percentage of the voting population. The aging may begin to make demands on business and industry as their spending dollars grow. It is likely that goods and services will change to accommodate the needs of the expanding aging population. The following are examples of some possible changes that may occur:

- More and better representation of aging people in the media, including advertisements
- Increased attention to human sexuality among the aging population
- Increased interdependence among aging people
- Combined consumer efforts among the aging that may lead to changes in restaurants, food packaging, entertainment, clothing, and printed material
- Increased public dependence on aging volunteers
- More part-time employment among the aging population
- Increased public transportation and assistance with this transportation (for example, assistance with baggage and mobility at airports)
- More specialized psychological and counseling services for the aging population
- More and better medical facilities for preventive and intensive health care

Some of the needs, desires, and demands of this wide aging population may conflict with those of other age groups. For example, the increasing number of aging people who seek part-time employment may compete with teens who also seek the same jobs. Concerns, empathy, and understanding will be needed to cope with this new social challenge.

WRAPPING IT UP

Human development does not stop with childhood. It continues through the stages of adolescence, adulthood, and aging. Development in any particular stage is influenced, to a significant degree, by how the person developed in previous stages.

Adolescence represents a time of great physical, social, and emotional change in the individual. Mental development also occurs in this stage. It is a time of transition between childhood and adulthood. For this reason, adolescence is both an exciting and troublesome time for most individuals.

During adolescence, the body undergoes physical changes that propel it toward a fully functioning adult form. These changes are accompanied by a growing orientation toward friends in the peer group. Interaction with the opposite sex and dating become important events in the adolescent's life. Peers of both sexes are an important source of status and social interaction for the adolescent.

The degree of influence by peers on adolescents' thinking and behavior increases relative to that of the parents' and other family members'. Teens strive for independence and autonomy from parents. Parents may view this effect as a loss of love from their child. This can create conflict between teens and their parents. However, parents continue to be the major influence on adolescents' core values and goals for the future. With regard to major life issues, parents and teens agree more than they disagree.

The stresses of adolescence can lead to certain problem behaviors. Adolescents who become involved in sexual activity run the risk of pregnancy. Teenage pregnancy rates in our society are quite high relative to other parts of the world. The consequences are generally quite negative for all involved: the teenage mother, the teenage father, and the child that is born.

Peer pressure may combine with the stresses of adolescence to lead to alcohol and drug use. The consequences of this behavior are negative. It can lower school performance, lead to serious health problems (perhaps even death), and cause serious conflicts with parents and friends. Such behavior is also illegal and can result in problems with the police.

Adolescent suicide is on the increase. Some teenagers are less able to cope with the changes of adolescence than are others. Social rejection, isolation, or difficulty in coping with emotions lead some teens to attempt to take their own lives. Teens in trouble usually give some warning signs. They can be helped if others are able to recognize the signals. Teen suicide is a tragic and unnecessary waste of human life and potential.

Human development in adulthood also includes a number of changes. The primary realms of adult life in our society involve some combination of marriage, parenthood, and work outside the home. These realms may operate in harmony, or they may conflict with each other. Adult decisions concerning what job to take or career path to pursue, whether or not to marry, who and when to marry, whether or not to have children, and when and how many children to have, are all important for social and emotional development.

Middlescence is a period in adulthood that highlights the conflicts arising from work and family decisions. It is a time when the adult questions past decisions and struggles with issues of personal identity for the present and the future. Men and women in our society tend to face different issues relating to work and family at different times. Middlescence poses challenges that can result in either positive or negative outcomes for the adult, depending on how they are handled. The person may regret decisions that have been made, but yet lack the ability or resources to effect the changes that are desired. Support from family and friends is important to assist the adult facing the dilemmas of middlescence.

The aging years conclude the human life span. The number of aging people in our society has grown significantly during this century. This has resulted in a number of social and economic problems for this rapidly increasing population. Social and economic burdens of the aging population are also felt by the younger segment of the total population, including the family members of the elderly. Aging persons differ from one to the next in terms of their personalities, problems, and behavior.

During the aging years, the body begins to degenerate faster than it can regenerate.

Physical deterioration can be slowed down with proper exercise, nutrition, and good living habits throughout the adulthood and aging years. Social and emotional development of the elderly is enhanced by positive relationships with friends and family as well as adequate income and good health. The mental abilities of the elderly remain strong, provided that they engage in adequate social interaction and mentally challenging tasks. Social isolation, low income, and poor health all lead to potential mental deterioration for the elderly.

Because of the growing numbers and influence of our older population, society must face the challenge of meeting the aging's needs. At present, the availability of community services to meet the needs of the elderly are woefully inadequate. Much of the potential for productive contribution of this age group is lost because their needs are unmet.

Exploring Dimensions of Chapter Nine

For Review

1. What is adolescence? In what ways does this stage of human development differ from that of childhood? adulthood?
2. What are the major consequences of adolescent pregnancy? of drug and alcohol use by teenagers?
3. What are the three major domains of life that affect the social and emotional development of adults? In what ways might two or more of these conflict with each other?
4. What is middlescence? What can be done to prevent middlescence from being a problem for adults?
5. List five of the myths of aging and give information to correct each myth.

For Consideration

1. Your friend, Tony, seems different to you somehow. He doesn't joke around and have fun like he used to. One day in the lunch room Tony

turns to you and says, "Why is life so rotten?" What would you say to Tony? What other actions might you consider taking?

2• Pamela has been a good friend of yours for several months. One day she says to you, "Jimmy and I are finally going to do it. We're going to have sex this weekend!" While she seems excited about this plan, she also seems to be a little worried. What would you say to Pamela? How would you react if, two months from now, Pamela came to you and said, "I'm pregnant! Please help me decide what to do!"?

3• What is the relative impact of peers and parents on adolescents today? In what areas do parents have the greatest influence? the least influence? Do you think parents or peers should have more or less influence on the values and behavior of teens today? Explain your answer.

4• How do you plan to avoid or work through the dilemmas posed by adulthood? Discuss your answer in terms of whether or not you plan to get married, when you plan to get married, whether or not you plan to have children and when, how many children you would like to have, and what type of job or career you aspire to have.

5• In what ways can society reap the greatest benefit from what our aging population has to offer? How is our society failing to make use of the productive potential of the over-65 group, many of whom are retired from the labor force? What are the major changes that will be necessary in our society to positively accommodate the increasing number of aging individuals in our population?

For Application

1• Write an essay concerning both the problems and particular benefits pertaining to teenagers in your school and community. Give suggestions on how to better solve these problems. Identify the changes that would have to be made in order to promote adolescent development in all areas (physical, social, emotional, and mental).

2• With the assistance of your teacher, invite a panel of professionals to discuss the problems and perils of drug and alcohol use. Include on your panel a police officer in your community who deals with these problems, a drug and alcohol abuse counselor, a medical doctor, and a person who has had a problem with drugs or alcohol. Ask each to present his or her own individual perspective on the issue of drug abuse, particularly as it relates to teenagers. Then have them react to each other's thoughts.

3. Volunteer at a local nursing home or residence for the elderly. Before your first day on the job, write a brief essay about your attitudes toward older people and your own thoughts about growing old. Keep a daily log, or diary, of your experiences as a volunteer. After one month, write another brief essay evaluating how your attitudes toward the elderly have changed, and how your attitudes toward your own aging have changed.

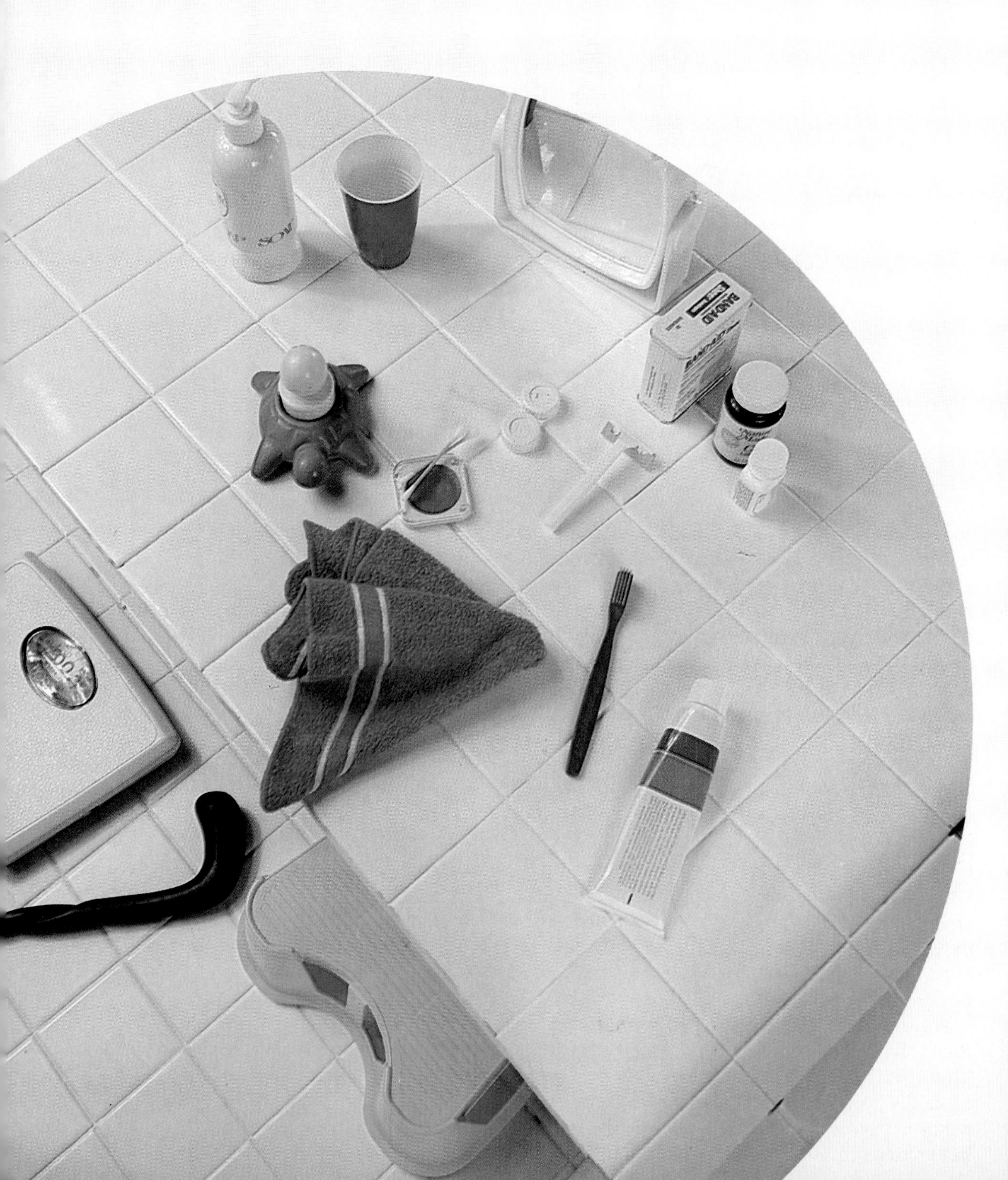

part four

Exploring Family Life

The family is the most basic and universal of all groups in society. Throughout the history of the world, and in all known cultures, family units of one form or another have provided essential functions to guarantee the survival of the society. Families are universally recognized for their functions of human reproduction, care and nurturance of the young, transmission of cultural values and beliefs, and the meeting of physical and emotional needs of all family members, both young and old. It is in the context of the family that so much of our personal identities, interpersonal skills, and social and emotional development are shaped. With rare exceptions, family life is one thing we all share in common.

Because of the vital role that families play, it is important to know about different types of families and how they function. It is also important to understand that living in families today is quite different than it was 100, 50, or even 20 years ago. The form and functions of families have changed in response to drastic changes in our society.

What impact have these changes had on the people who live in families? Some families are better able to meet the needs of members than others. For some people, the family exerts a positive influence on individual development; for others, the family may exert a negative influence on development. Some families have special needs—such as a physically or mentally handicapped member—that create additional stress on their ability to function in a positive manner.

Positive family life is enhanced when family members successfully establish their own personal identities and form healthy interpersonal relationships. These individual skills of personal identity and relationship formation are basic to family relationships. Yet, these skills will not guarantee strong, stable, or positive families. Living in close family relationships with a high level of interaction requires a variety of management, communication, and coping skills.

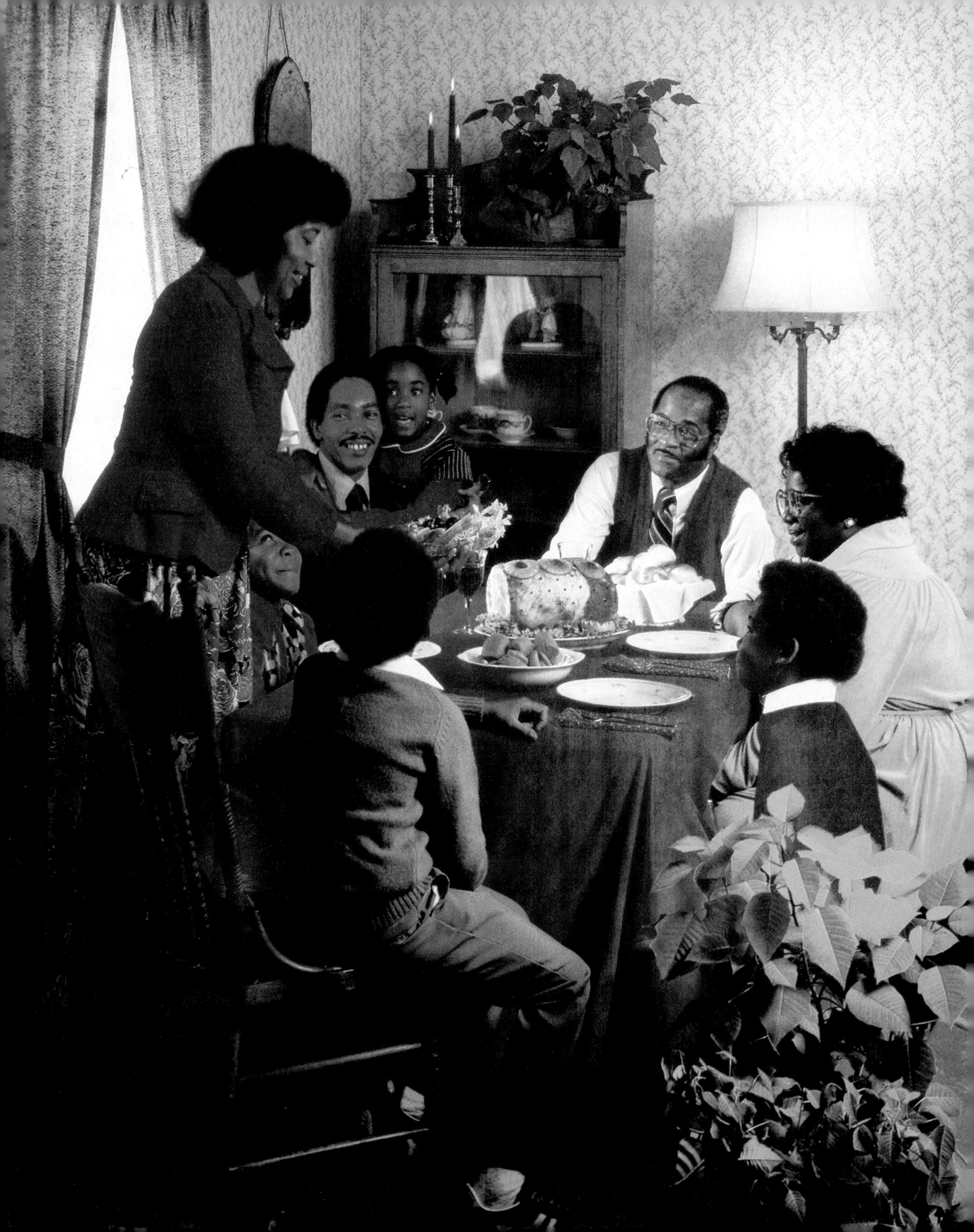

ten

LIVING IN FAMILIES TODAY

This chapter provides information that will help you to:

- Understand various definitions of the family.
- Be aware of family functions and how they alter over time.
- Understand that various family patterns are established to fulfill family functions.

Living in families today is probably more difficult than it was in the past. The social and cultural environment in which families live is more complex than that of earlier time periods. Today, there are different levels of commitment to the family and different expectations of what should be gained from family life. Yet, many aspects of family life today are the same as those in past generations. This chapter explores current definitions of the family, functions of the family, and various family patterns that are established to carry out these functions.

Consider the many ways in which the term *family* is used. What meanings and implications come to your mind as you read the phrases below?

The amusement park has *family* rates.

She's using her *family* name now.

Our chicken dinners are served *family* style.

I bought a copy of *The Family of Man*.

The Klotzmeir *Family* Reunion will be held the first Sunday in July.

They are thinking of starting a *family* business.

Squirrels and rabbits are members of the rodent *family*.

The theater is showing a good *family* movie.

They plan to sell the *family* farm.

Grandmother was pleased to learn that Edward's wife was in the *family* way.

DEFINING FAMILY

When young children are asked to explain the word *family*, they usually describe their own family situation. Answers such as "Daddy, Mommy, and me" or "My mom, my sister, and me" reflect a child's thinking that all families are like the child's own. But with maturity and experience, people learn that there are many types of families. This variety in types of families makes a single definition of family difficult. Consider the groups of people in Figure 10-1. Can you establish common factors that describe all of these groups? Are all of these groups families?

Some definitions of family would include all of the Figure 10-1 groups as families. Other family definitions would eliminate some of these groups. Refer to these groups as various definitions are discussed.

Probably the most common definition of **family** is *a group of people living together who are related by blood, marriage, and/or adoption*. This clear, simple definition is used by the United States Census Bureau. It is helpful for gaining an accurate count of individuals in families without counting people more than once. However, the definition may not include all the groups of people that you commonly think of as families. Compare the definition to the groups highlighted in Figure 10-1.

Groups G and K would not be families since the individuals are not related. Likewise, not everyone in Group F is related. The Census Bureau considers these groups households. Not all of the members in Group L are considered part of the family. The census definition considers Nancy Crosston and the two children a family because they reside together. Mr. Crosston, however, is not a part of this family because he resides alone. The children spend as much time with their father in his home as they do with their mother in her home. Yet, by the census definition, their family includes only the children and their mother.

The census definition would include Group E. Yet, the son actually lives on a college campus 1,000 miles away. Although he spends only a few days a year at his mother's home, he legally resides with his mother. All persons in Group I would not qualify as family since

Figure 10-1

Groups of Families

GROUP A	GROUP B	GROUP C
Mr. and Mrs. Garza; their two sons	Mr. Kelso; his son and daughter	Mr. and Mrs. Greene; their adopted son
GROUP D Ms. Smith; her aging father; their cat	**GROUP E** Mrs. Fuller; her son, who is a college student	**GROUP F** Peter and Emma Farthing; Peter's daughter from a previous marriage; Emma's son from a previous marriage; Peter and Emma's son
GROUP G Miss Morrow and Mrs. Fentwell, retired lawyers	**GROUP H** Mr. and Mrs. McKennsa, who are retired; their adult son	**GROUP I** Mrs. Grayson; Mrs. Grayson's mother; a foster child
GROUP J Mr. Griffin; his young grandson	**GROUP K** Paul Dolari, a young bank teller; Sol Sidman, a college student; Sol's dog	**GROUP L** Nancy Crosston; her son and daughter; Nancy's former husband and father of the children, who lives alone
GROUP M The Doltons, a young couple without children	**GROUP N** Sara Valton; her two sons	**GROUP O** Peter Falbrow and Jane Marlot, a middle-aged married couple

the foster child is not related by blood, marriage, or adoption.

It's clear that the definition used by the Census Bureau may not be enough to express our meaning of the term family. Feelings and relationships within groups of individuals often go beyond the limiting factors of residence or blood and legal ties.

There are several broad definitions of family. Within these definitions there are types of family structures. These structures are described below:

Nuclear Family:

A nuclear family consists of a mother, father, and one or more children. It is a common family structure in our country.

Single-Parent Family:

Single-parent families consist of one parent and one or more children. Until recently, almost all single-parent families included a mother. Fathers were seldom given custody of children in divorce cases. Now custody decisions are awarded more equitably. More fathers are now involved in this family structure.

Extended Family:

Extended families include one or more relatives in addition to the nuclear or single-parent family. The extended family may reside together. The extended family also includes members who do not reside together.

Blended Family:

A blended family includes stepparents and/or stepchildren.

Foster Family:

A foster family includes one or more non-related or nonadopted children. Through special arrangements with government or private agencies, a child may live with an unrelated family for a short period of time or for extended periods of time.

A broader definition of **family** is a *group of people who reside together or come together periodically and are related by blood, marriage, adoption, and/or a common purpose.* This definition could include all of the groups in Figure 10-1 as families.

Some people prefer to include a sharing of income, wealth, and/or exchange of goods and services in a family definition. Other earlier definitions of family stipulate two or more adults living together and rearing their own or adopted children. This definition which requires both children and multiple adults would eliminate all but A, C, F, and H of the groups in Figure 10-1. These definitions may be helpful for certain purposes and under certain circumstances.

How do you prefer to define "family"? Are you comfortable with any one definition? Do you feel that people can form long-lasting, caring relationships and yet not be related (Groups G and K)? Do you feel that related people can provide meaningful, caring relationships yet not reside together (Group E)? Perhaps the meaning of family can be strengthened by considering the various structures and functions of family units.

Spotlight on issues

Single-Parent Families

Single-parent refers to marital status of the parent, rather than to the number of parents a child has. While a child's parent or guardian may be single, that does not necessarily mean that the child has only one parent. A separation or divorce may create the following possibilities for a child: two parents who are single, one parent who is single and one who has remarried, or two parents who have remarried.

It is estimated that 60 percent of the children born in the early 1980s will live at least one year in single-parent homes before they complete high school. Today, 14 million American children live in single-parent homes. These numbers reflect a great increase in the number of children in single-parent families in just a few years. In 1970, only 7.4 million American children lived in single-parent families. Over 70 percent of these children in single-parent families today have experienced the divorce or separation of their parents. How has single-parenthood affected these children and how will it affect the growing number of single-parent children in the future?

Social attitudes about single-parenthood have changed over the years. But, the effects of such a large number of single-parent homes cannot be determined until more long-term studies can be completed.

Some studies of single-parenthood may be misleading because they often reflect situations that *seem* to be caused by single parenthood. Actually, many situations that seem to be the result of single-parenthood may have been present prior to the divorce, separation, or the death of a parent. For example, financial problems present in many single-parent homes may have begun prior to the divorce or separation and may have even been one of the causes for the divorce or separation. Other factors related to, but not necessarily caused by, single-parenthood include an overworked parent, increased home responsibilities of children, and greater self-reliance on the part of the children.

It is important that children realize that positive developments can result from their parent's divorce. Often children create stronger and deeper relationships with individual family members. Increased responsibility often assumed by children can help build self-esteem and pride. Both children and parents may experience personal and family growth from remarriage. For example, stepparents may be able to offer the child a new resource for advice and support.

Children in single-parent families do show higher levels of stress while they are adjusting to single-parenthood. When family members become accustomed to the new single-parent lifestyle, the stress level is similar to that of a two-parent home.

Positive family interaction and general family strength are not determined by the structure of the family. Strong and positive families can be found in all types of family structures. Likewise, unstable families with low levels of interaction can be found in all types of family structures.

CHANGING FAMILY STRUCTURES

At one time in our society, the nuclear family structure was by far the most common (see Figure 10-2). However, as shown in Figure 10-3, this has changed. Today, fewer than one in three American households are composed of a married couple with children under the age of 18. Also, a growing proportion of these households are "blended families" headed by married couples in second or later marriages, following a divorce in the first marriage. We also are seeing a growing number of single-parent households, along with households with people living alone.

Figure 10-2

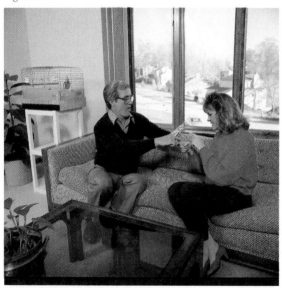

The nuclear family structure was at one time the most common family structure in our society. Today alternatives to the nuclear structure abound. The family pictured here consists of a widowed father, his divorced daughter, and their pet.

There are many reasons for this growing diversity of family structures in American society. Compared to past years, we are seeing today somewhat greater levels of:

- Delayed marriage, where people are waiting until they are older to get married
- Permanent singlehood, where people are choosing not to marry
- Divorce, creating a growing number of single-parent families, remarriages, and step-parenting situations
- Delayed childbearing, where couples are waiting to have children until they are older
- Permanent childlessness, where couples are choosing not to have children

These trends mean increased diversity in the structure of American households. Each trend will be discussed in this Part Four on "Exploring Family Life." In the meantime, it is important to understand that no particular family structure is inherently better or worse than another. Any family structure is capable of fulfilling important functions. It is not so much the structure that matters as it is the process of family relationships which occur within any given structure.

FUNCTIONS OF THE FAMILY

A function is an action that meets a goal or a purpose. The family fills particular functions for individuals. These functions allow individuals to live and behave in a manner suitable to themselves and society. Over time, the functions change in levels of importance. Cultural and subcultural differences will also

Figure 10-3

Changing Structure of the American Family: 1970–1986

Household Composition	1970	1975	1982	1986
Family Households	81.2%	78.1%	73.1%	71.9%
Married couple only (no children under 18)	30.3	30.6	30.1	29.7
Married couple with children under 18	40.3	35.4	29.3	27.8
Single parent with children under 18	5.0	6.7	7.8	8.0
Other (such as extended families)	5.6	5.4	5.9	6.4
Nonfamily Households	18.8%	21.9%	26.9%	28.1%
Persons living alone	17.1	19.6	23.2	23.9
Other	1.7	2.3	3.7	4.2

SOURCE: U.S. Bureau of the Census. Household and Family Characteristics, March, 1982. *Current Population Reports*, Series P-20, No. 381, Washington, D.C., 1983b.

U.S. Bureau of the Census. Household and Family Characteristics, March, 1986. *Current Population Reports*, Series P-20, No. 419, Washington, D.C., 1987.

affect the importance and operation of the functions.

Another way to think about family functions is to consider why families are found in all cultures throughout all stages of history. Families fulfill functions that people desire or need.

The Protective Function

Families provide protection from the time children are infants until they can manage in a home of their own. Even after leaving home, young people may return for a time to the protection of their original family. As parents age, their children may provide a family protective function. The protective function meets the individual's most basic needs for safety and security.

The protective function has changed over time to become less demanding for the family. Families throughout history as well as in prehistoric times provided protection from wild animals, the elements, and lawless people. This type of protection is seldom needed today. Police and fire fighters have taken over some of these functions. Insurance programs and public assistance provide some financial protection. Yet families continue to provide protection to individual members in various ways. Consider the following examples of the protective function:

Five-year-old Jason holds his younger sister's hand to prevent her from getting too near the traffic.

Nine-year-old Stephanie led her family in a home fire drill after a school program during fire prevention week.

Katie intercedes when her younger brothers are harassed by bullies at the swimming pool.

Juan's father met him at the police station as soon as he heard of Juan's accident.

Mr. Thompson removed all household cleaning materials from the lower cupboard to prevent his toddler from getting into harmful chemicals.

Mr. and Mrs. Phillips added dead-bolt locks to all their doors and have encouraged their children to keep the doors locked for safety.

Figure 10-4

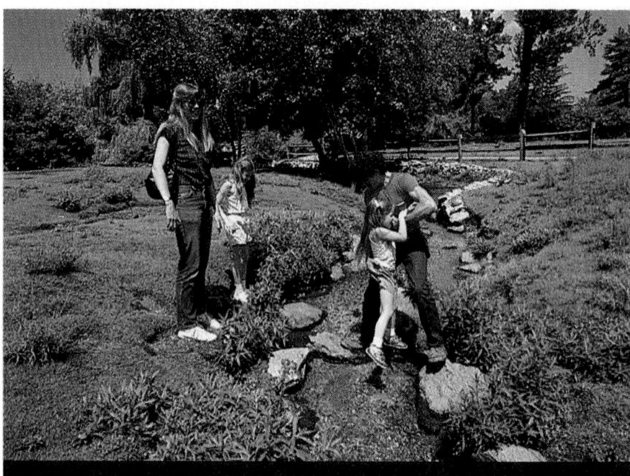

Protection is an important function performed by the family.

The methods of protection and the elements from which family members are protected have altered over time. Yet, the protective function continues to maintain an important place among family responsibilities (see Figure 10-4).

The Economic Function

In earlier periods in American history, families were primarily production units. That is, parents, children, and often grandparents worked together to provide their own housing, furnishings, food, and health and household goods.

Today, family members (or a single family member) earn money with which the family buys goods and services. A family income—resources earned by family members—has replaced the need for production of goods and services by family members. The dollars earned by family members are used to purchase the food, clothing, shelter, health care, services, and furnishings for the family. Most families today are consumption units rather than production units. That is, they consume more than they produce.

In recent years, the American economy has caused families to again consider production of some goods at home. Though there has been some increase in home gardening and household do-it-yourself projects, families still basically produce only a small amount of their own goods and services.

Families carry out their economic functions differently than they did in the past. Yet, the economic function is still a major aspect of modern family life.

The Procreative Function

Procreation is the bearing of children—the production of future generations. The family unit has always been the accepted mode for bearing and raising children.

Families in the past had large numbers of children primarily because many family members were needed to produce goods. Also, the land was underpopulated and our country needed more people. Because diseases prevented many children from reaching adulthood, parents produced larger numbers of children to assure a generation to follow.

Many families today are concerned with overpopulation and are less dependent on family members for production of goods and services. Most childhood diseases have been eliminated. Current economic situations highlight the cost of each additional child. All of these factors affect parents' decisions to have smaller families. The average size of families has been reduced to 3.19 people in 1987, while it was 3.58 in 1970, 3.70 in 1940, 4.10 in 1930, and 4.80 in 1900 (see Figure 10-5).

The average number of people per household also has decreased greatly since the earliest census reports were taken. Some of this decrease is because of more single-person households and fewer children per family.

Though the number of children per family has decreased radically, the procreative function is still important. Procreation is a vital aspect of most families. Between 80 and 90 percent of married couples in America today will have at least one child. The number of children does not dictate the degree to which parents love, appreciate, or are devoted to their children. By removing the economic need for having children to help earn income, parents are more likely to have children because they want to and not because they need to.

The cost of raising children may be one of the reasons fewer children are born in American families today. In 1983 it cost approximately $93,000 to raise a child from birth to age 18 (using 1983 dollar values). Figure 10-6 lists average total costs of raising a child to age 18. (These figures are for urban families in the western United States, in 1983. Figures will vary by region of the country and rural or urban setting.) By dividing each of these numbers by 18, you can determine the *average annual* cost of raising a child.

Figure 10-5

Average Household Size (Families and nonfamily households)

Year	Number of People
1790	5.40
1900	4.20
1940	3.30
1970	3.10
1975	2.94
1980	2.75
1987	2.66

Figure 10-6

Average Cost of Raising a Child to Age 18, 1983

Transportation	$15,042
Education	1,740
Medical Care	5,796
Food at Home	18,609
Food away from Home	2,632
Clothing	6,006
Housing	30,800
All Other	11,964
Total	$92,589

The Recreation Function

Leisure time and relaxation are a part of family life. Values and attitudes can be taught during recreation time. Playing games and enjoying leisure time provides an opportunity to communicate and relate to each other (see Figure 10-7).

Figure 10-7

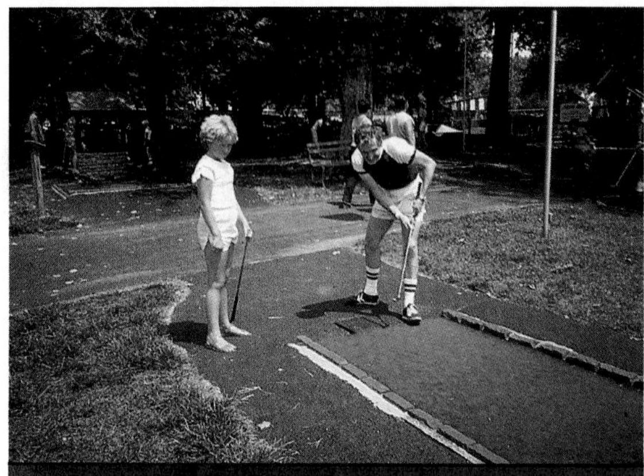

Leisure time and recreation are an important part of family life.

Like other family functions, the recreation function has changed over time. On the one hand, the amount of leisure time has increased from that of a century ago, thus providing families with more opportunity for recreation. On the other hand, increased transportation and children's greater reliance on peer groups have made recreation less family-centered.

CASE IN POINT

Carolyn has much more leisure time than her grandmother. She can spend many more hours with her children picniking, camping, shopping, playing board and card games, and enjoying family sports.

Benji also has more relaxation and leisure time than his grandparents. Yet the amount of recreation time spent with his children is less. He enjoys bowling, tennis, and classical music—none of which his children enjoy. His son loves swimming and football. His daughter enjoys canoeing and running. Benji's family shares few recreational activities.

Spotlight on issues

Family Recreation

The term *family recreation* has become very popular among salespeople. Camper-trailers, thermos bottles, home computers, board games, outdoor grills, and tennis shoes are some of the items that salespeople often claim make family recreation time more enjoyable. While these items may indeed bring enjoyment, they are probably not necessary for family fun and recreation.

Consider the word recreation, or re-creation. If we analyze the term, we can see that it implies renewal or creating a fresh beginning. Families as well as individuals frequently need the opportunity to refresh themselves and make new starts. The stress and strain of daily work, family, and school life can bring about the need for renewal or rebuilding of family interaction.

How can families achieve such periods of renewal with limited time and finances? Families that enjoy and seem to benefit from recreation indicate that the activities need not be extensive or expensive. There are several features of family recreation that seem to encourage positive outcomes. Beneficial family recreation often includes a change in the environment, group efforts, nonfamily members, setting aside stress, and limited costs.

A CHANGE IN THE ENVIRONMENT • Removing the family from its usual surroundings can help refresh and renew family interaction. Different surroundings can foster new ways of viewing and relating to family members. Changing the environment can be as simple as taking a walk around the block or as complex as a lengthy boat cruise. Surroundings within the home can also be altered to encourage recreation. Eating dinner in a different part of the house, or rearranging a room to accommodate a toy train can provide a change in environment without leaving the home.

GROUP EFFORT • Many families suggest that group efforts help to build a spirit of togetherness and cooperation that encourages renewal. This cooperative attitude, they believe, extends beyond the recreation period into daily family life. Group games, whether physical, mental, or both, foster this group feeling. The cooperation needed to sail a boat, pitch a tent, or plan and carry out a bicycle outing are good examples of dependency on family members. The teamwork and cooperation involved in a basketball game, card game, or hiking expedition encourages a common goal as well as family fun.

NONFAMILY MEMBERS • Family recreation can include other persons or families. Adolescents particularly like to include friends in family outings. Several families can come together to provide the renewal experience of recreation. Provided that group interaction is maintained, this inclusion of friends can allow family members to get to know persons important to particular family members. Such situations allow for sharing of different views and approaches to family life.

SETTING ASIDE STRESS • Most families indicate that the best family recreation allows members to put aside the stress of daily life. For some people, stress is best alleviated by strenuous physical exercise. For others, stress is lessened by quiet, sedentary activity. Stress is not always set aside on vacations and other activities, however. Frequently, plans and activities become so extensive that stress is increased rather than lessened.

LIMITED COSTS • Often when families recall recreation that they most enjoyed, they find that pleasure and cost are not strongly related. Some of their best activities were no-cost or low-cost. Families seeking such activities can consult local directories for festivals, fairs, and other events that provide family fun at little expense. There are many possibilities for no-cost and low-cost family recreation that are often overlooked.

- visiting a park
- camping
- swimming
- going to a museum
- going to an antique show
- listening to a concert
- going to the zoo
- attending a sports rally
- bicycling
- going to a bazaar
- going to a fair
- skating
- visiting the library
- hiking
- watching a parade
- canoeing
- going to a pet show
- going to an arts and crafts show
- folk dancing
- going to the theater
- participating in or going to a sports event

Whether a family enjoys these low-cost, no-cost activities or becomes involved in extensive and costly excursions, family recreation is a bargain. It provides an opportunity for family members to share time, experiences, and, in general, to relate to each other while having fun.

Certain types of recreation and leisure *appear* to be family-oriented because family members are physically close. Television or movie-watching, for example, brings family members together. Yet there may be no family exchange of words or ideas: no interaction takes place. In some homes, families watch television, make comments, and generate discussions on important topics as well as enjoy humor or drama together. Such use of television or movies could enhance family sharing and could be considered family recreation.

The way family members manage their leisure time will determine the importance of the recreational function for the family.

Decisions about the amount of family-oriented recreation and the type of recreation are important decisions.

Religious Function

The family fulfills a religious function whether or not it is part of a specific organized religious group. Attitudes and values related to beliefs about a supreme being are conveyed to children through their parents and other family members. Church and synagogue attendance, meditation, prayer, and formal and informal religious observances are ways in which families convey their beliefs about religion.

Current studies reveal that attendance at organized religious services has declined for both families and individuals in the United States. There are fewer religious observances in the home. Families that are members of a specific religion usually rely on the clergy to relay the teachings of the religion. In many ways, the religious function of the family has decreased. Yet, for many families it is still a prime function.

Love and Affection Function

Providing love and affection is one of the most important functions in today's family. The love shown to a child by family members relays the child's worth. This self-worth allows a child to function positively within and outside the family. As children mature outside the family, teachers, peers, and close friends can assist in providing love and affection that establish a positive self-concept. Still, the foundation is laid for receiving and giving love and affection in the home family surroundings.

All family members—siblings, parents, grandparents, and others—can provide acceptance, support, and security to other family members. This mutual reliance on family members continues throughout adulthood. You might have received warm hugs from a parent when you scraped your knee. You may receive the same hug or embrace when you receive a college rejection or fail to be selected for a job. A similar embrace may be given when you celebrate launching a new career. Families provide the stabilizing, supporting influence throughout the life cycle.

CASE IN POINT

Mark had a very rough time during his senior year. A friend of his was killed in an auto accident. Mark was really depressed. His grades suffered, and he had a hard time thinking about his future. If it hadn't been for his family's support, he is not sure he would have made it through this crisis very well. His family members were always there when he needed them—to listen, to help put things in perspective, or just to tell him they love him.

Ed and Ai-lien rely on each other's love and affection. Ai-lien's job is physically exhausting. Ed's job puts him under much mental stress. They give each other support and assurance by physically displaying their feelings for each other. They show their affection and concern by listening to each other's troubles and frustrations; by giving a hug, a kiss, or a touch of hands; and by allowing their physical presence to give each other strength.

The love and affection function is probably more important today than it was a century ago. Today's society seems to increase the individual's need for comfort, affection, and love. There are many causes of stress that impact on family members. Competition in school and on the job is often intense. Concentrated urban populations and increased mobility leave people feeling isolated and alienated. High technology adds a level of impersonality to our daily lives—some people interact more with computers and other machines than they interact with other people! The large array of consumer choices available for both goods and services can be a stressful daily factor. All of the current situations combine to make the need for love and affection necessary to a greater degree than it was in the past. The family is a major supplier of this love and affection.

What happens when the family does not supply love and affection or does not supply it to the degree that an individual needs? Often an individual will "act out" negative behavior in order to receive the love, attention, or affection even if it is received in a negative way. The unfortunate result of limited love and affection can be unruly behavior, shoplifting, irresponsible sexual behavior, drug abuse, and alcohol abuse.

The Nurturance Function

To **nurture** is to provide all of the influences that modify genetic potential of an individual. That is, nurturance is all the input to an individual other than what the individual was born with. It is the provision made for promoting the well-being and development of family members.

Family members are nurtured by deliberate means and simply by experiencing life in their home. Nurturances include education related to factual information and skills, values, beliefs, and attitudes, and basic socialization.

FACTUAL INFORMATION AND SKILLS • For centuries, the home and family have been an important center of learning. In earlier times, the teaching of all academic skills was also the responsibility of families. Reading, writing, arithmetic, and other subject matters were taught by family members. This aspect of the education function has been lessened in most families. Today, most children enter public or private schools by age five or six. Preschools and nursery schools provide an even earlier education outside the home for many children. Family members continue to be interested in children's academic education through participation in school activities and by their voting responsibilities related to educational issues (such as voting for school board members or a bond issue to build a new school).

Families continue to teach children many skills necessary for present and future life, although much of the teaching of information and skills is carried out by schools. Brushing teeth, tying shoes, knowing left from right, and writing the child's name are only a few of the many skills and facts families teach their young. At later stages, families teach care of clothing, grooming, choosing and preparing foods, managing money, driving a car, and thousands of other skills. Still later, family members may provide information about selecting a car. They may teach skills in purchasing or renting a home. Throughout the life cycle, facts and skills are taught in the family.

VALUES, BELIEFS, AND ATTITUDES • A major aspect of the nurturance function is carried out in the areas of values, attitudes, and beliefs.

A family conveys to its members those things that the family feels are morally just and right or morally wrong. Attitudes about honesty, truth, and concern for society and humankind are relayed to children through their family. Beliefs about the rights of individuals and political thought are conveyed by the family. Schools and other institutions add to the learning of values, beliefs, and attitudes. Yet, families supply the basic groundwork for this learning. Parents have a major responsibility in nurturing children in this area.

BASIC SOCIALIZATION • **Socialization** is the process of learning what you need to know in order to exist in a social setting. Families are the primary socializers of children. Children continuously learn socially acceptable behavior from observing and participating in various experiences. Families also make deliberate efforts to socialize their children. For example, a parent may tell a child the following: "We are quiet in church." "We write on paper, not on the walls." "We must wait in line until it's our turn." These are basic social skills individuals must learn in order to get along in our society (Figure 10-8).

To gain a better perspective on the importance of the nurturance function, consider the following questions. Who taught you to ride a bicycle (a skill)? Where did you learn to make a peanut butter sandwich (a skill)? Who taught you to value honesty (a value)? How did you learn that the sun rises in the east and sets in the west (knowledge)? Where did you learn the appropriate way to greet people (socialization)? Family members were probably influential in your learning all of these things.

Other institutions in society can perform a number of the functions discussed above. For example, schools teach knowledge and skills, and churches provide a religious function. However, no institution provides this combination of functions. Only families, in various forms and structures, offer this collection of functions.

Figure 10-8

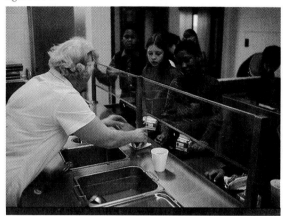

Learning to wait one's turn in the school lunch line is a basic socialization skill that many children learn by observing and participating.

FAMILY PATTERNS

Families have unique ways of fulfilling their functions. Individual families carry out functions by means of various behaviors. You can participate in the same activity in different families and find different behaviors. Expectations of one family may be totally different from expectations of another family. Patterns have developed in families that create unwritten rules or modes of behavior that develop into a unique family culture. Consider how the following families conduct themselves during the evening meals.

CASE IN POINT

Mr. Carson sits on a kitchen chair reading the newspaper. Mrs. Carson does all of the food and table preparation. When the meal is ready, the children are called. The television is turned on, and all watch the screen while they eat. Conversation is limited and centers around the television show or requests for food to be passed.

The Alvarez family prepares the meal quickly. All family members participate. The food is hastily placed on the table or on the kitchen counter where family members stand and eat. The rush is usually because of evening activities. But even when there is nothing planned for the evening, haste is a part of the meal. Though rushed, the family members usually manage to gather in the kitchen at the same time and converse briefly while they eat.

Members of the Sanders family appear in the kitchen at 5:45 p.m. Each member takes a plate, fills it from the pans on the stove, and sits at the kitchen table. Conversation is continuous, often with several conversations occurring at once. The meal is usually a noisy, boisterous occurrence with much laughter. The members eat immediately with no delay for those who are late. As members finish, they take their plates and utensils to the sink and leave for their evening activities. A rotation of clean-up and food preparation is followed.

The Gillettes always have a sit-down meal. They hold dinner until all family members arrive and are ready to eat. Ms. Gillette usually prepares most of the food, but the children often assist. Conversation is a major part of the meal with discussion of various events of the day. Grievances and issues are often brought out at meal time. These frequently accelerate to arguments and sometimes to fighting and crying.

The Sanders family would be frustrated by the arguing of the Gillettes. The Gillettes would find the hasty dinner time coming-and-going of the Alvarez family and the Sanderses to be an irritation. The Carsons would miss not having their television during dinner, while the Avarez family would be surprised that only Mrs. Carson prepares the food. These families clearly have different expectations about behavior during the evening meal. Yet, all of these families are in the same socioeconomic class with family members of approximately the same age. What brings about the different patterns of family behavior? What causes the different expectations of families? If one small situation (such as the way families eat their evening meal) can vary so much among families, then what about major events (Figure 10-9)?

Family patterns may be established purposefully with particular goals in mind. More often family patterns develop from the parents' families and the patterns experienced throughout life. If an individual grew up in a noisy, fun-filled, active family, this will likely continue to be a pattern within the family the individual creates. Patterns from the homes of all adults, modified by community expectations and social changes, will influence the

Figure 10-9

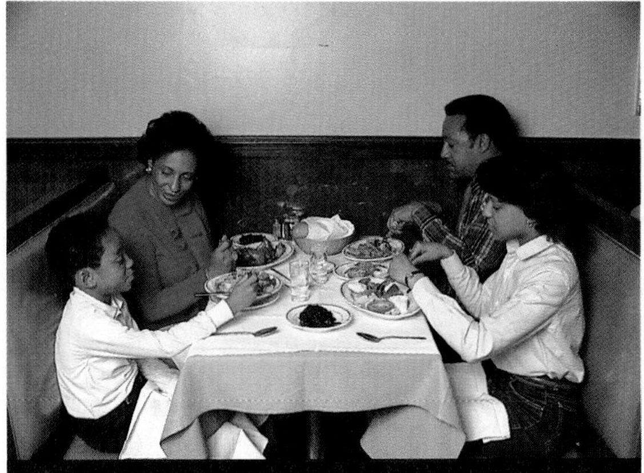

The way families conduct their meals is one way in which they establish modes of behavior that develop into unique family cultures.

patterns of a family. There are several basic dimensions to family patterns. By considering these dimensions, the patterns of your own family become more clear. You may see opportunities to change patterns that are inappropriate or ineffective. Awareness of family patterns is helpful in establishing patterns in your future family.

Focus

One dimension of family pattern is the family focus or theme. A family's focus—the areas, topics, or issues on which a family places emphasis—is related to what the family wants out of life. Goals, values, attitudes, and beliefs give direction to the focus. Although the focus is usually established by the parents, children add new aspects and alternatives to the focus. Often the focus of a family goes without much thought and seems to evolve automatically.

CASE IN POINT

The Lozanos family has an avid interest in conservation of natural resources. The family members have participated individually and as a family in political action to conserve public lands and endangered species. This interest is reflected in their appreciation of natural beauty. The philosophy of unspoiled natural beauty is a focus for this family.

The Noltons are a competitive family. They have a desire to win no matter what area of competition is involved. They encourage and support individual competition. Each person is involved in some type of competitive sport: golf, tennis, soccer, and baseball. Being the best or nearly the best in any given category is a focus for individual and family activity.

Giving of self to help others is a focus of the Estrada family. Numerous family activities as well as individual actions have a basis of helping individuals or groups who are in need. Planting flowers at the entrance to the local park, delivering groceries to aging persons, and providing care for flood victims are examples of family endeavors to aid others.

Each family has a different focus or several focuses. For example, values may dictate an emphasis on saving or on a "get-it-spend-it" philosophy. Other values may stress reaching out and extending toward others or a "keep-to-ourselves" attitude. Realizing your family focus can assist you in better understanding your family and family members.

Spotlight on issues

Families and Television

Americans spend more time watching television than they do on any other activity except sleeping. By the time most young people graduate from high school, they have spent more time watching television than they have in the classroom. They will have logged 20,000 hours of television viewing and 13,000 hours in school. Young children watch an average of 30 hours of television a week. What impact does this amount of television viewing have on families?

Habitual television viewing prevents other family activities and worthwhile endeavors. General conversation as well as family games and sports are neglected when people watch television. Studies have shown that students who were heavy television viewers were able to raise their grades by decreasing their television-viewing time. Other research indicates that elementary school students who were heavy television viewers are not as physically fit as students who watch less or no television.

Children who watch a large amount of television may tend to overlook other family members as role models in establishing goals and forming values. These children may be forming their values and goals based on what they see on television. And what they see on television may be unrealistic and violent.

Television tends to be unrealistic in its portrayal of life. The characters and people on television and what they do are meant to entertain, to inform us, and to hold our interest; therefore, the characters may be more beautiful and wealthier than average, and the plots may involve more crime, more violence, and more sexual activity than exists in real life. Television was never meant to be a mirror of society, but children as well as adults may make that assumption.

Researchers indicate three possible effects of television violence. Children may become less sensitive to suffering and pain of others; they may become afraid of the world around them; and they may behave in a more aggressive and sometimes harmful manner toward others.

Persuasive television commercials may cause tension among family members. Television advertisers target the young because children are more impressionable; that is, easier to influence. Young viewers may be deceived by advertising that encourages buying merchandise beyond a parent's means or items not worthy of purchase.

What can families do to curb the influence of television? Families can take action to counter the effects of television viewing. The following are suggestions on how to limit the quantity of television viewing:

- Establish a maximum number of hours per day or per week that television can be watched.
- Complete all homework before watching television.
- Spend time with a focus on games, conversation, or reading before watching television.
- Break the habit of turning on the television for "noise."

To improve the quality of television viewing, try these suggestions:

- Turn on the television only when a specific program is wanted; avoid random viewing.
- After viewing an interesting program, find articles or magazines which elaborate on the topic.
- After viewing a television program, discuss it with the family.
- Encourage conversation about particularly disturbing aspects or major issues of a program.
- Make clear to young children that many things are not real, are only pretend, and that stunts are used to create an image on television.
- Seek new and educational television viewing.
- Become involved in local and national advocacy groups for positive television programming.

Family Pace

Families have a particular pace at which they move. Pace is how slowly or swiftly life is carried out. Life in one family may move like a whirlwind with members coming and going rapidly. Life in other families may move at a steady, slower pace where members take their time in accomplishing things. Patterns of arising and going to bed, the timing of energy and efficiency peaks, and family values related to being on time are part of a family's pace.

The pace of activities may vary throughout the year. Holiday seasons, vacation time (as shown in Figure 10-10), and the weather will affect the pace at which a family moves. Yet, though there are these variations, most families have a typical pace which is part of their established family pattern.

Figure 10-10

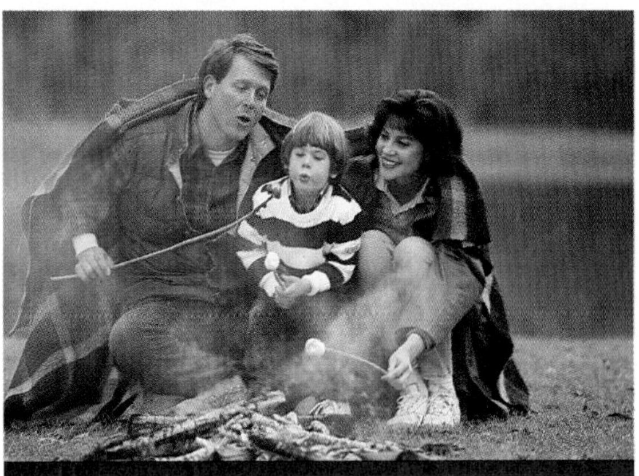

Family pace affects vacation choices. Some families, preferring to get away from it all, may choose to spend their vacations camping where they can enjoy moments of quiet relaxation.

CASE IN POINT

The Amos family moves at a slow, leisurely pace. Ed Amos and his sons enjoy quiet relaxation. They usually have a leisurely evening meal regardless of how elaborate or simple the food. Weekends usually hold some activities, but seldom are they spaced so closely that the members cannot take life easy. When too many activities are scheduled, the Amos family members begin to feel uncomfortable and robbed of their relaxation time.

The Clayborn household moves like a cyclone. Each member has activities tightly scheduled. The evenings and weekends are a marathon of activity. Though they sometimes complain about how busy they are, the Clayborns like the rapid pace at which they move. Too much relaxation seems to make the Clayborns upset and ill-at-ease. They wonder what they may be missing.

Family Boundaries

Another dimension that helps establish the pattern for a family is family boundaries. **Family boundaries** are the lines that separate the family from other people outside the family. This boundary is strong in some families. Here, emphasis is placed on being together and activities are family-centered. Some guidelines that operate in a tight boundary family are listed below. These guidelines may never be written or even stated, yet are a definite part of the family pattern.

- Relationships with nonfamily members have limited importance
- Children bring friends to the home only after getting permission from the parents
- People seldom drop in unexpectedly
- Guests in the home are planned in advance
- Family members protect their family privacy

Other families have loose boundaries with friends and neighbors coming in and out at all times of the day. Such families would operate with the following guidelines:

- There are often nonfamily individuals in the home
- Children feel free to bring friends home at any time
- Friends and neighbors stop by often and know they will be welcome
- People visiting are always welcome to share a meal
- Relationships with nonfamily members are highly important
- Family members do not feel the need to protect family privacy

Families with loose boundaries find it difficult to understand families with tight boundaries. This may be especially true for adolescents who are highly influenced by their peers. Interactions in the homes of friends may present problems when family boundaries are different.

CASE IN POINT

Jim and Sid are good friends. Sid's family, which operates with a loose boundary pattern, always welcomes Jim and others into their home. Jim enjoys the casual coming and going of family and nonfamily members. Yet, sometimes Jim feels that Sid's home is a little confused and chaotic.

Jim's family is less welcoming of Sid and others into their home and is uncomfortable with outsiders present. Sid often feels out of place at Jim's home.

Jim and Sid will maintain their friendship more easily if they understand that families have different boundary patterns. Accepting a pattern different from their own may be necessary.

Family Rules

Another family trait that helps determine family pattern is **family rules**. This does not refer to only those rules stated clearly or written on paper. Family rules are often unstated but highly important guides for behavior. Sometimes families do not recognize their rules. These rules may have been intentionally established. They may have been borrowed or adapted from the families of the parents. These rules may or may not be based on logic. Consider the following family rules that are open and spoken:

- No feet on the sofa unless shoes are off
- If the children don't want to buy their school lunch, they pack their own lunch themselves
- The books on the living room bookshelf are handled with care
- Television is not turned on until all homework is done
- The glass pitcher that belonged to Great Grandma is not to be used

These stated rules are clear and easy to understand. The following rules are not stated but are understood by all members of the family:

- Family arguments and disagreements are not discussed outside the family
- Change can be taken from the money box in the kitchen, but money is never taken from purses or wallets
- Grandma gets a kiss on the cheek whenever she visits
- A family prayer is said at dinner but not at breakfast
- Mother always checks to see if the doors are locked before going to bed
- No one sings or hums at the dinner table

When rules are clearly understood by all family members, the rules can be helpful guides to the interaction within as well as outside the family. Too often, a rule may not be commonly understood by all. Assumptions are made based on a rule not clear to all members. Members assume that all other members know what they know. For example, you may have a general rule in your home about the use of the telephone in the evenings. You may interpret the rule as "Don't make too many phone calls." Your parents may consider the rule as, "Don't be on the phone so long." These different interpretations can easily bring about conflict with your parent angrily saying, "You know the rules." Gaining clarity of the family rule—a specific amount of time or a specific number of phone calls—can prevent many conflict situations.

A family's focus, pace, boundaries, and rules establish a particular pattern. This pattern makes the family unique and different from other families. The pattern establishes how the family will carry out its functions and which functions it will emphasize.

WRAPPING IT UP

Living in families today is made more complex than in past years due to our changing technological and cultural environment. Yet, whether we refer to today's families or families of 100 years ago, common functions have been fulfilled by them. The functions met by families have been important to the survival of cultures all over the world throughout history.

The protective function of families helps to meet the needs for security and safety of individual family members. The economic function provides for the essential needs for food, clothing, and shelter. The procreative function replenishes the population of the society, and assures that it has a future. The recreation function helps to maintain the morale of individual family members, and cements the bond of affection among them. The religious function of families shapes the values and attitudes that family members have toward such issues as life and death, and also helps to shape moral development.

The love and affection function also satisfies important human needs for human contact and establishing meaningful interpersonal relationships. It is in the family that the person first experiences acceptance and love. The nurturance function is the means by which families instill in their members important knowledge, attitudes, and values necessary for functioning effectively in the society. When these many functions are viewed together, it is clear that society asks families to assume a great deal of responsibility for maintaining the well-being of its members.

Families fulfill these functions to varying degrees, and in their own personal ways. Families establish certain patterns of relating among family members. These patterns reflect different paces, and involve *family boundaries* that call for privacy and which separate them from outsiders. Families also establish their own rules, some of which are explicit and some of which are implied (unspoken, but in force). The degree to which families are able to function effectively, and to meet the developmental needs of individual family members, is influenced by the unique set of family patterns that are established.

Exploring Dimensions of Chapter Ten

For Review

1. What is the definition of family used by the U.S. Census Bureau? What groups of people commonly thought of as families are not within this definition?

2• The nurturance function includes education in what three basic areas? Give several examples of each area.
3• Family patterns become established by means of a family's focus, pace, boundaries, and rules. Explain these four dimensions of family patterns.

For Consideration

1• Create your own definition of family. Explain how this definition is suitable for some purposes yet unsuitable for other purposes.
2• Choose one of the family functions and consider it in depth to determine how and why it has changed over time. Consider if its importance has strengthened or lessened. Make a prediction for this function related to families in the future.
3• The love and affection function operates throughout the life cycle. Consider how this function alters as you mature. Explain how love and affection is gained and received throughout the life cycle.

For Application

1• Consider classroom rules in order to understand how stated as well as unstated rules operate. List unstated and unwritten rules in your classroom. Have classmates do the same. Then list stated, written rules. Are there some different interpretations of the unstated, unwritten rules? How might these differences cause frustration and conflict? Consider how different interpretations among family rules might cause frustration and conflict.
2• Create a class mural depicting family functions. Show how each function has changed over time. Depict increases, decreases, or stability in importance of the function.
3• Discuss with your family members how family patterns operate in order to fulfill functions. Discuss focus, pace, boundaries, and rules. Try to determine how your particular family patterns developed. Consider which patterns members might like to alter. Consider why it is important to have mutual awareness of patterns.

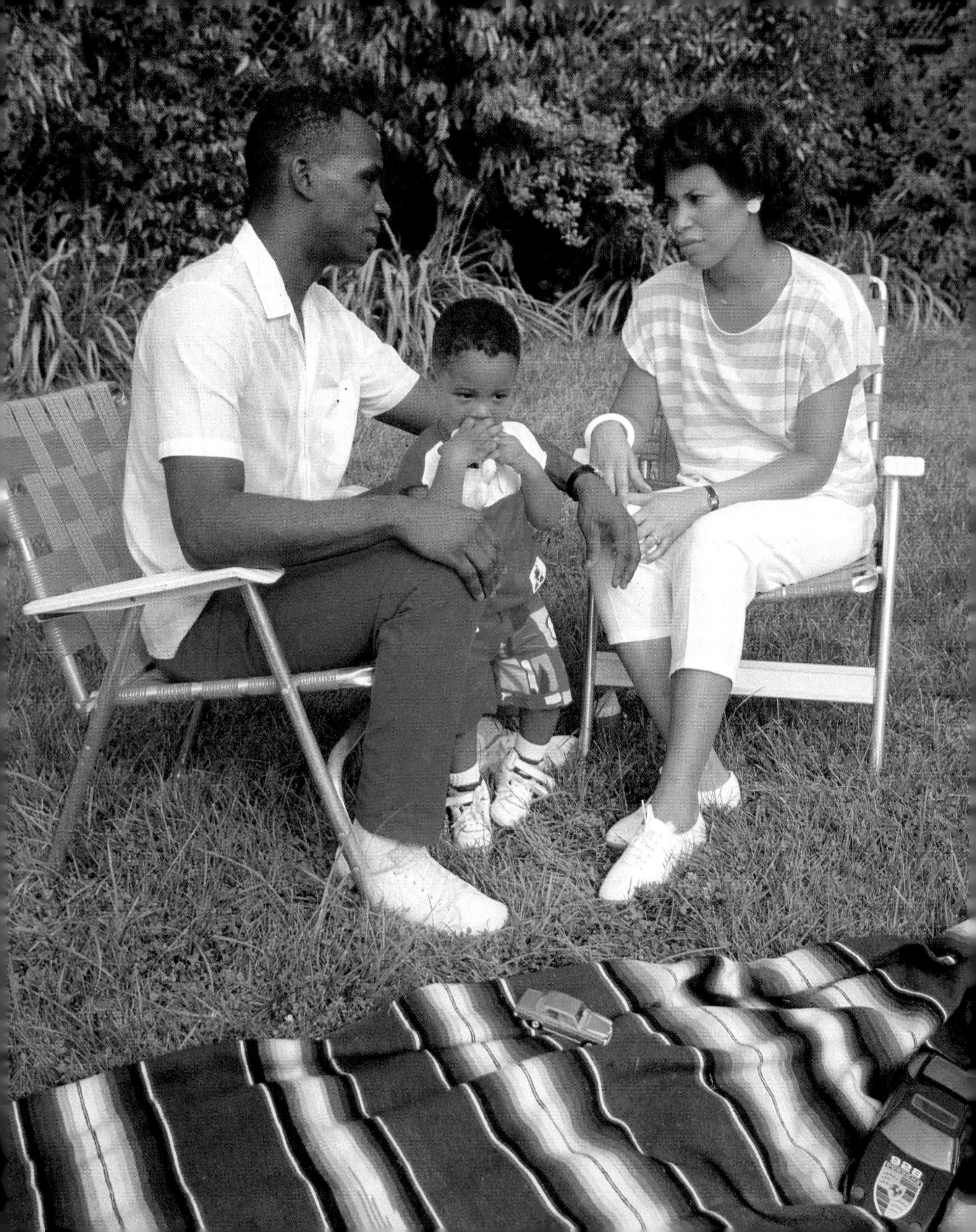
928

eleven

DEALING WITH ISSUES ABOUT MARRIAGE

This chapter provides information that will help you to:

- Understand why many people today are choosing to remain single.
- Recognize male/female differences in and the pros and cons of singlehood.
- Prepare for marriage by asking and thinking about certain pertinent questions.
- Understand the legal aspects of marriage.
- Recognize the complications and difficulties in the divorce process.
- Become familiar with measures of divorce prevention.
- Understand the traumas caused by desertion.

Families are dynamic, ever-changing units of people. The family develops and changes from stage to stage while individuals in the family move through their own developmental changes. This multidimensional process creates situations that are frustrating and disturbing while at the same time joyous and exciting. The stages of the family make up the *family life cycle.* These stages are: the beginning family; the childbearing family; the family with preschoolers, schoolagers, and adolescents; families as launching centers; and aging families. These stages can be viewed as the entry period when a couple plans for family life; the period in which the family members play parenting roles; and the period in which the family contracts in size and faces later stages in life.

In this chapter we will focus on the institution of marriage. We will address such important questions as, "Does everybody get married?" "Who and when should a person decide to marry?" "How can one prepare for marriage?" We will also look at the process of ***unmarrying***, or divorce. Marriage marks the entry into the beginning stage of the family life cycle.

Few decisions in life are more important than the decisions of whether or not to marry, when to marry, who to marry, and what to do to stay happily married. These decisions need to be approached rationally. You may not currently be making these decisions. Indeed, for some of you these decisions are many years in the future. However, thought should be given to these issues in order to plan and prepare for your future.

SINGLEHOOD

Issues related to singlehood are major lifetime decisions. Thought, consideration, and decision-making processes need to be involved in deciding if and when you move from singlehood to married life. Singlehood can result from death of a spouse, divorce or separation, as well as from not marrying at all. Our discussion focuses on the decision to move or not move from the initial single status. Many factors discussed will pertain as well to decisions related to movement from singlehood to remarriage.

In the past, people who chose to remain single were sometimes considered odd. It was usually assumed that single people could not find anyone to marry them because people felt no one would *choose* to remain single. Women who never married were labeled old maids and were often considered a lifelong burden by married siblings. Single men were referred to as old bachelors and were often considered to have odd, hermitlike behaviors. Since men traditionally did the choosing and women were chosen, the single male had less stigma attached to single status than did the single female.

Attitudes have changed about people who choose not to marry. Single life has gained a more respectable status. The public is beginning to be aware that not all people find fulfillment in married life. There is a growing realization that alternatives to marriage may bring greater fulfillment for some people. Careers, life goals, and desired lifestyle may take precedence over married life. People feel less pressure to marry. Current economic situations may also lead some people to remain single (or to postpone marriage).

Though only about 10 percent of our young adult population today is likely to remain single throughout life, many people currently have chosen to postpone marriage and extend their singlehood. Some wish to develop a stronger personal identity, firmly establish their career, or experience independence from parents before they make a commitment to marriage.

Statistics show an increase in the number of people who have never been married. This does not necessarily mean a dramatic increase in life-long singleness. Many of today's never-married people are young (twenties and early thirties), and will marry eventually. We currently have no evidence that many more people will choose to remain single throughout life.

Male/Female Differences in Singlehood

There are some differences between men and women with respect to singlehood choices. More men and women are choosing to delay marriage or permanently remain single than in previous years. However, a greater percentage of young females are making singlehood choices than ever before. From 1960 to 1986 the percentage of never-married women, ages 20–24, increased by nearly 30 percent. See Figure 11-1.

Figure 11-1 shows that an increased percentage of both males and females are remaining single during their twenties. Figure 11-1 also shows that for all age categories except the oldest, in 1986 fewer percentages of women were never married. Do you think these percentages will change? Will more people remain never married? Will marriages be postponed until people are in their late twenties or thirties? Do you think this will change? Will a greater percentage of women remain never-married? When today's 16-year-old females reach age 45, will a greater percentage of them never marry? Though we can only speculate about these questions, what factors influence your answer?

Today, women have much greater opportunities for education and careers than they did in the past. They can now experience independence that was not available to their

Figure 11-1

Never-Married Americans by Age and Sex, 1960 to 1986

Age	Male				Female			
	1960	1970	1980	1986	1960	1970	1980	1986
Total	17.3	18.9	23.8	25.3	11.9	13.7	17.1	18.3
18 years	94.6%	95.1%	97.4%	96.2%*	75.6%	82.0%	88.0%	88.4%*
19 years	87.1	89.9	90.0		59.7	68.8	77.6	
20–24 years	53.1	54.7	68.8	75.5	28.4	35.8	50.2	57.9
25–29 years	20.8	19.1	33.1	41.4	10.5	10.5	20.9	28.1
30–34 years	11.9	9.4	15.9	22.2	6.9	6.2	9.5	14.2
35–39 years	8.8	7.2	7.8	11.3	6.1	5.4	6.2	8.4
40–44 years	7.3	6.3	7.1	8.5	6.1	4.9	4.8	5.5
45–54 years	7.4	7.5	6.1	5.9	7.0	4.9	4.7	4.7
55–64 years	8.0	7.8	5.3	5.9	8.0	6.8	4.5	3.9
65 years and over	7.7	7.5	4.9	5.1	8.5	7.7	5.9	5.2

SOURCE: U.S. Bureau of the Census, "Statistical Abstracts of the United States," Washington, D.C., 1988, p. 40.

*Data for 1986 combines 18- and 19-year-olds.

mothers and grandmothers. Many young women see the need for launching a career early and adding family life later when their careers have been established. Still, other women, as well as men, find their careers exhilarating and fulfilling enough without marriage or children.

There also seems to be a difference in levels of happiness between males and females who remain single. Studies among never-married individuals show that women indicate higher levels of happiness than men do. Single men are less healthy physically and mentally than single women. They die earlier than either single women or married men. Never-married women are more successful in their work than their married female counterparts, while never-married men are less successful than their married male counterparts. These career differences have been explained by noting that married women may have their families blocking their careers, while married men have wives enhancing their careers. These possible sexual biases may continue to affect male/female singlehood decisions.

Pros and Cons of Singlehood

Single life is often portrayed in the media as a never-ending, fun-filled social life (see Figure 11-2). Several periodicals have been developed for the increasing audience of young as well as mature singles. Emphasis is usually given to career advancement and social endeavors. Seldom are the less glamorous activities such as washing windows and doing laundry discussed. How accurately is single life portrayed by the media? What motivates people to remain single? What are the pros and cons of singlehood? These are necessary to know in order to make a decision about remaining single.

Figure 11-2

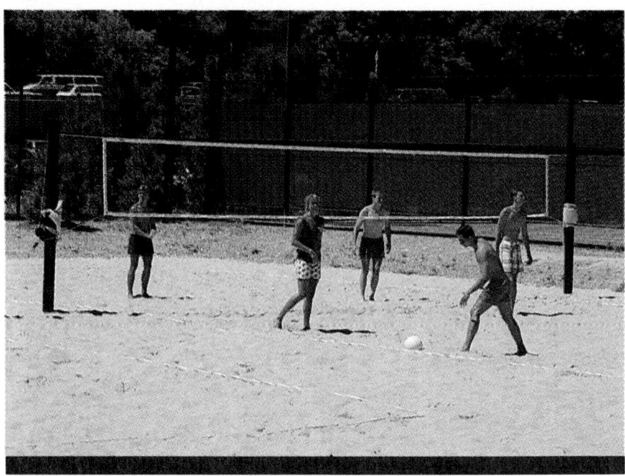

Single life is often portrayed as fun, exciting, and glamorous. Is singlehood really all fun and no work?

What are the rewards or positive features of singlehood? When asked this question, most singles indicate that they find *personal fulfillment* and *independence* are major gains of remaining single. Consider the following statements from never-married individuals:

> I just don't think that I could accomplish all I have or all I want to if I were married. I want to continually learn more, do more, experience more. I don't think I could do that with a husband and children.

> Maybe I'm too self-centered. I know I always think of me first, and I don't think a good marriage can allow that. Maybe I just need time. Right now I've got too much to do.

Both of these people are expressing feelings of personal fulfillment that they feel could not be gained in married life. Needs for independence and freedom are expressed in the following statements:

> I have to be free to go where I want when I want. My parents always seemed to hold me back. I certainly don't want to have a wife do the same. I may marry some day, but so far I've found my freedom too enjoyable.
>
> My uncle once sang a song called, "Don't Fence Me In." That's how I feel about married life. Don't put me inside a fence. I need to be free.

Other people might argue that with a sensitive marriage partner, you *can* have personal fulfillment and independence. Mutual respect, some people would say, allows for individual needs in married life. Yet, it is clear that many single people have not found or are not seeking such a partner. They feel that the costs of marriage outweigh the benefits. They also feel that personal fulfillment and freedom are positive aspects of life that, for them, can only be found in singlehood.

The positive aspects of singlehood are balanced by some negative aspects. Loneliness is clearly the most often mentioned drawback by those who remain single. Even those people who are the most positive about singlehood find loneliness to be a facet of being single. After leaving the security of family life or college community life, people often find that living alone is uncomfortable. People miss companionship and someone to share conversation and household chores. Intimacy and stability needs must be met in other ways—through social activities, good friends of both sexes, and an active work life. Those who choose to remain single must make concerted efforts to interact with others and form new, meaningful friendships (see Figure 11-3). This is especially true as more and more peers become married and fewer friends are left to share singles activities.

Another negative aspect of singlehood is the continually disapproving attitude that many in our society have toward single people. Social norms which state that marriage and parenthood are virtues can lead to social disapproval of those who choose to remain single. Singles may be stereotyped as having character deficits and personality flaws, or as being selfish "jet setters" and "sexual swingers." Such attitudes can lead to single people being avoided by potential friends and left out of social activities.

Whether the positive aspects of singlehood outweigh the negative aspects is a personal decision. The pros and cons of singlehood are totaled and balanced differently for each person. The balance sheet may change as a person grows older. Marriage may seem more desirable after career goals and independent life have been experienced. Marriage may seem less desirable after achieving rewards and fulfillment in other areas.

Whatever your choice, little is lost by experiencing singlehood for a time. Many marriage and family counselors feel that living alone and forming an identity is a positive experience for most people. One reason young married couples have difficulty in adjustment is that the individuals have not yet formed a personal identity. These young married people are therefore trying to achieve an identity at the same time they are trying to achieve the tasks of a newly married couple. Experiencing a period of singlehood appears to be good preparation for marriage.

PREPARATION FOR MARRIAGE

Nearly everyone who enters a marriage today does so with the idea that it is *permanent*;

that is, a lifetime commitment of love and loyalty to another person. Few enter marriage thinking that they will divorce or separate if it doesn't work out. Marriages that do survive the test of time may last anywhere from 50 to 75 years. "Till death do us part" is still a part of marriage vows today.

The decision to marry or stay single is not made in a vacuum. Seldom do people pose the question, "Should I marry?" or "Should I remain single?" Few people really think of marriage as a 50- to 75-year commitment to another person. Rather, people ask, "Should I marry him?" or "Should I marry her?" or "Should we marry now or wait until later?" What is really being asked is whether or not a person is really right and whether or not it is the appropriate time to marry. These questions pose concrete decisions to be made, yet too many people take these decisions too lightly. They enter marriage without adequate forethought or preparation, and without an adequate understanding of the responsibilities involved.

We learned in earlier chapters that people are drawn together because of common experiences and interests (Figure 11-4). One factor that affects which people are drawn together is **propinquity** or nearness to others. You can't grow to love someone who isn't there. People in your school, at your job, and in your neighborhood are likely marriageable candidates because they are nearby. Homogamy is also a factor in the choice of individuals. **Homogamy** is the similarity of individuals' backgrounds. Homogamous people are likely to adjust well since they tend to think similarly and have similar values and philosophies. These points explain why many people are drawn together. Yet, they do not help people decide who they should not marry, when they are ready to marry, or if they should remain single.

Consider this simple solution to the issues of who and when to marry:

- Feed data about you, your partner, and your relationship into a programmed computer.
- Ask the computer, "Is the person right for me?"
- The computer will respond "Yes" or "No."
- Ask the computer, "Are we ready for marriage?"

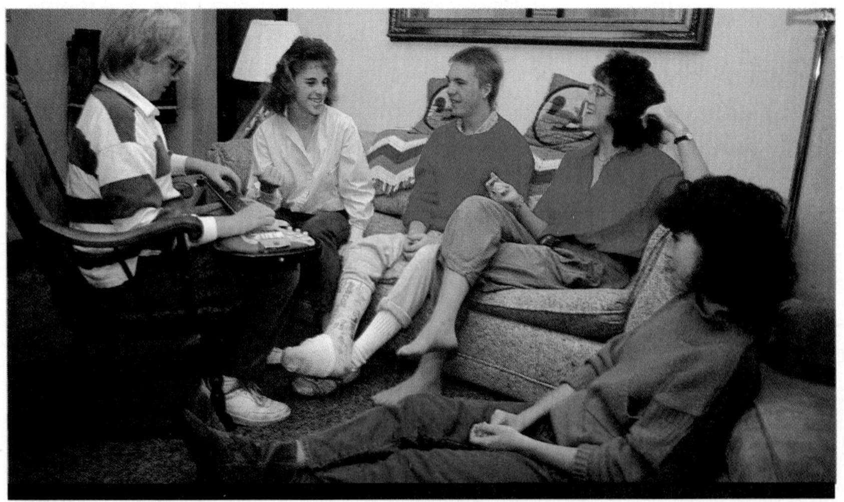

Figure 11-3
Similarity of interests or proximity can determine whether or not single people become friends.

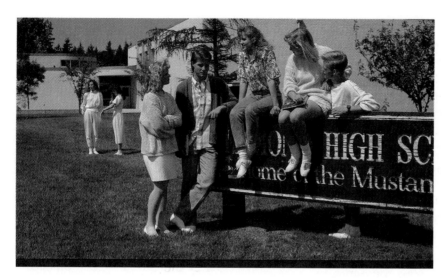

Figure 11-4
What are some of the reasons that explain why people are drawn together?

- The computer will respond "Ready" or "Not ready."

Unfortunately, such an easy system is not available. The questions we are asking are highly complex, personal, and laden with personal feelings and values. Programmed answers do not allow for the complexity of personal qualities in these decisions. There are no 100 percent reliable answers that can be provided by computers or by well-meaning people. There are, however, some guidelines and points for discussion that can help you consider if a particular person is right for you. There are some points to consider in deciding if and when you are ready for marriage. These are not answers. Rather, they are additional questions and issues to help stimulate your thinking and discussions. They do not give you a solution. They are merely guidelines to help you find a meaningful solution for yourself.

Is This the Person for Me?

There are basically two ideas about the choices people make regarding a mate. One idea stresses that we choose people who are similar to us in characteristics, ideas, and philosophies. A second idea stresses that we choose people who are different or even opposite from us in many characteristics in order to complement our needs. For example, if you are shy you might be attracted to an outgoing person who can balance your need to relate to others. Both of these ideas about marriage partners may be valid. However, it seems to be most common to choose a partner similar to yourself. Fewer couples build a strong relationship relying on opposite characteristics to balance their personalities. Therefore, it is beneficial to consider similar aspects of your and your partner's personality, goals, and philosophies when asking, "Is this the person for me?"

Some people feel that opposite personalities attract. This may be true. But in selecting a mate, commonalities in major traits seems to be a more accurate determiner (predictor) of successful pairing. Opposite qualities within similar qualities may be attracting forces. For example, two people may like music but like different types of music, two people may enjoy athletic, outdoor life but like different sports. These opposites are structured within similarities and can promote healthy, positive interaction. Major traits that are completely opposite may indicate situations that could foster major conflict.

SIMILARITY IN AGE • In our society the husband is typically a few years older than the wife. This is not a key factor to the happiness or stability of marriage, however. Age similarity makes little difference in the success of a marriage. Many successful, happy couples have wide ranges in their ages. However, people experiencing the same or similar stages of development and growth share more mutual feelings and experiences. For example, consider one couple where those involved have achieved some level of independence, have managed on their own, have met some challenges of young adult life, and have had similar experiences and achievements. Consider a second couple in which one person has achieved major independence and the other has been totally reliant on others. These two people function at different levels of achievement. There is a greater likelihood that the first couple will form a successful, long-term relationship. Similarity of the developmental stages in which individuals function may be more important than age itself. Use these two guiding questions for self-assessment:

1. Are you both at similar stages of development?
2. What skills have you each developed for adult life?

SIMILARITY OF INTERESTS AND ATTITUDES • When individuals reach the later teen years, they have already developed a personality and habits, interests, attitudes, and philosophies about life. When these interests and attitudes are different with respect to some factors, there are few problems involved. In fact, different attitudes and interests add spice and variety to a relationship. Individual ideas about reading, music, or entertainment are healthy differences in a relationship.

When major, overriding issues and attitudes are highly different, it is difficult to maintain a common way of life. Major religious and political philosophies, major attitudes related to leisure time, and issues related to relationships with others are some of the critical differences that can affect a relationship. A couple can override these differences by deliberate means, such as professional counseling and determined efforts to accommodate these differences, and a high level of positive communication. Any couple contemplating marriage (like the couple in Figure 11-5) should know, however, that these basic differences require additional long-term efforts throughout their life together. Use these guiding questions:

- How dependable is the person? How important is time and punctuality?
- How important are sex roles to the person? How does the person view sex roles related to the breadwinners? to household chores?
- What are the person's career and life goals?
- How do this person's parents treat each other? What behaviors and attitudes of marital relationships has this person experienced?
- How self-sufficient has the person been thus far in life?
- What attitudes does the person have about children? Is there a desire for children? Is the person patient or impatient with children?

Figure 11-5

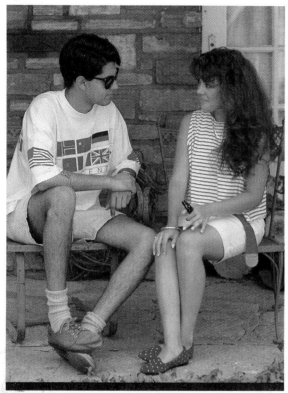

A couple preparing for marriage can overcome differences through a high level of positive communication.

- What attitudes does the person have related to earning, spending, and saving?
- In what stress situations have you seen the person? How is stress handled? How is conflict handled? How is anger vented? How willingly or unwillingly is the stress and/or anger discussed?
- How is leisure time spent? Is there a leisure time activity enjoyed mutually? How willingly does the person see a need for you to maintain other friends?

SIMILARITY OF EDUCATION AND OCCUPATION • Similarity in educational level seems to be an increasingly important factor in successful relationships. Until recently in our culture, it was common for men to have more education than the women they married. Though this is still true in some subcultures, couples increasingly have similar education levels. More women are continuing their formal education before and during marriage, thus closing the education gap that once existed.

Attitudes about education throughout life are also of importance. Life-long learning—courses and classes for individuals throughout the life cycle—is becoming more common and more necessary. For example, many women today are entering college or a trade school after several years of marriage and raising a family. Also, either women or men may seek additional education or training should they decide to make a major change in occupation. Conflicting ideas about such growth experiences can interfere with successful relationships.

Similar occupational background of young people may seem to be of little importance since the jobs you are currently holding may be temporary positions that have little similarity to the occupation or profession you may desire. Occupational background, however, includes the occupations of your family and the ideas and thoughts you have gained from and about occupations.

Some people who work with their hands ridicule and show disrespect for those who work in professional fields. Professional people may look down on the unskilled worker. It may be difficult for two people of different occupational backgrounds to respect and understand each other unless efforts are made to clarify feelings and gain understanding. Use these guiding questions:

- How similar are your educational plans? Do you each accept the termination plans for each other's education? Do you each respect the occupation the partner is striving for? To what degree do you see the need for life-long education? Have your parents and/ or partner's parents had recent educational experience? How do you each react to these experiences?

- How similar are the occupation levels of your fathers and mothers? How do you each feel about the differences? In what way can you reconcile these differences?

SIMILARITY IN LEVELS OF LIVING • Similar levels of income and similar ideas about gaining and spending resources are important to a successful marriage. Though it is clear that two people of widely different social status and income levels can marry successfully, the marriage usually involves some major efforts to deal with these differences. The story of a pauper marrying into a family of great wealth and being easily accepted and accommodated into the wealthy income group is most commonly limited to television and movie dramas. Altering your level of living requires adjustments on the part of both partners as well as family and friends. People involved in such adjustments should be aware that most people can adjust more easily to a higher income level than they can to a lower income level. It is an unusual person who can move from a luxurious style of living to a very low-income level.

Couples must also realize they cannot begin their new family at the same income level as that of their parents. Nearly all couples have an economic adjustment when moving from lifestyles of their middle-aged parents to that of young adults. Use these guiding questions:

- How different are the levels of living of your families? Can you both accept these differences?
- How will you or your partner adjust lifestyles if a major difference in level of income exists?
- How do you both feel about receiving financial assistance from one set of parents? What reactions will this cause? How will you deal with this?
- In what particular situation do you foresee differences in levels of living surfacing? What customs and traditions will highlight these differences? How will you deal with these situations?

SIMILARITY OF RACE, RELIGION, AND ETHNIC BACKGROUND • In our society, we are free to marry people of different race, religion, and ethnic background. Such marriages were and may continue to be objected to by parents and friends. Though the frequency of marrying someone of a different race, religion, or ethnic background has increased, special concerns and issues must be addressed. Concerns center around changing your faith and belief, dealing with cultural differences, and difficulties of raising children in a multi-cultural/multi-racial environment.

Successful marriages are shown to be more successful when partners are of the same religion, race, and ethnic groups; that is, they are homogamous. However, couples that vary in one or more of these characteristics can have a successful relationship if they deal with these differences. The likelihood of success will depend on the degree of differences involved, the customs of the community involved, the maturity of the young people, and the level of cultural differences to which the couple has been exposed. Use these guiding questions:

- What concerns related to children will be involved in these differences? How will you raise your children? in one of the cultures/

religions? in a combination of the two cultures? How will your families react?

- To what degree have you talked with people who have encountered these same differences?
- How well are both sets of parents able to accept the differences involved?

Despite the guidelines provided in this section, you probably still have concerns and questions about the type of person that is right for you. You may continue to confront yourself somewhat like this: "This is a big step—a major decision in my life. How can I be sure I'm making a wise choice? I think I love this person. But I know that's not enough. I've been in love before (I think). How can I tell if this is the right person for me?"

There are three overall guiding questions you might use to determine if you've taken the best possible steps in facing this major issue.

1• *Have you taken advantage of the freedom available in the American dating system?* That is, have you gotten to know many people? Have you dated enough people to experience your feelings and reactions to various personality types? Or, have you only dated one person? Have you allowed yourself to know too few people and therefore know yourself only in relation to these few personalities? By only knowing one or two eligible people, you are making a decision with little basis for comparison.

2• *Have you carefully evaluated yourself, your partner, and your relationship?* Have you considered traits, interests, commonalities, and differences as pointed out in this section and in other resources? When major differences have surfaced, have you openly communicated these differences with consideration of future differences, consequences of the differences, and ways to accommodate the differences? How would you assess your ability to communicate under such circumstances? Were these communications helpful? If necessary, have you sought counseling assistance?

Spotlight on issues

Education for Marriage

The decision to marry affects not only the marriage partners but also extended family members and future children. Many people struggle to gain the proper training and education for a job or career. Yet, few people take the time to prepare themselves for marriage. Why not train and educate for marriage?

Marriage is one of the most intense interpersonal relationships that a person can have. Therefore, all learning and experiences that help people relate to one another can help prepare for marriage. Usually, though, marriage education becomes necessary when two people have committed themselves to marriage. It takes place before and during marriage.

PREMARITAL EDUCATION • Prior to marriage, a couple may take classes or receive counseling to prepare themselves for married life. Religious groups may suggest or require prenuptial counseling. Private marriage counselors and psychologists also provide preparation for marriage. The quality of these sessions depends on the skills of the leader(s) and the level of commitment of the couple. Aside from those who attend brief sessions required by some clergy performing the marriage ceremony, only a small percentage of people participate in premarital education. Many professionals in the area of marriage and family counseling consider this situation unfortunate and believe that many marital problems and concerns might be solved before marriage.

Recently, there has been increased effort to provide premarital education within communities. Local mental health agencies provide group and individual sessions to assist couples in preparation for marriage. Teaching communication skills and clarifying expectations are major features of such classes.

MARRIAGE EDUCATION WITHIN MARRIAGE • Marriage education after the wedding ceremony is available in two types: remedial and preventive.

Remedial marriage education or counseling takes place after major concerns and issues have arisen. In many cases, severe problems have surfaced before people seek assistance. Although many marriages can be improved through remedial counseling, some may be too troubled to be helped. As in the field of medicine, marriage education can be more beneficial (and perhaps less costly) if it can be applied in a preventive way.

Preventive education for marriage refers to courses, classes, and counseling or other programs designed to assist couples who are not experiencing any major concerns or problems within their marriage. Religious and community groups frequently provide opportunities for workshops or retreats to improve stable relationships. Usually these sessions are group-oriented with 5 to 15 couples and group leaders.

Some groups operate on a long-term basis with monthly or bi-monthly meetings. There may be emphasis on mutual sharing and support.

Although these groups are considered preventive, they do not necessarily focus on prevention of specific problems or concerns. Recently, there has been an emphasis on marital enrichment—that is, emphasis on improving the quality of marriage in general. Growth of the marital couple is stressed. This growth approach seems particularly beneficial as the couple passes through various life stages. Entry into parenthood, the responsibility of caring for young children, the new freedom for children who are becoming increasingly independent, and the beginning of retirement are significant elements affecting marriage. Enriching the quality of the marriage at these periods is especially important. Focusing on growth of both the individual and the couple at these specific periods can be beneficial.

Education for marriage is not a "one time" situation. It continues throughout the lifetime of the couple.

3• *Have you been able to keep a balance between the emotional and intellectual appraisal of your partner?* Have you been able to objectively assess this person as a marriage partner? Can you overlook for a moment the romantic and sexual level of your relationship to consider more significant factors in long-term adjustment? Though the deep feelings of love, romance, and sex are of major importance to a successful marriage, they can sometimes overshadow other factors of compatibility such as family patterns, communication and conflict management skills, attitudes toward children, leisure activities, and other aspects mentioned in the guidelines above.

If you can answer a strong yes to the three criteria above and you feel good about the results, you may be well on your way to having located a person with whom you want to share your life. If you answer a no for one or more of the criteria, you may have some homework to accomplish. If you're not secure about the answers you've found, you may not have located a person for you. This does not mean the person is wrong for you. It may mean the person is wrong for you now. Time is on your side. Explore, meet people, enjoy many friends. There is no rush.

Are We Ready for Marriage?

If and when you and a partner have decided that you are right for each other, a question still remains. Are you ready for marriage?

Here is another question with no easy answer. Today in our culture, the typical age for marriage is 25 for men and 23 for women. Figure 11-6 shows the average median age at first marriage from 1920 through 1986. Age, however, may not be as important as the developmental stages which the partners have reached. People typically marry at times when they have accomplished a task—graduating or completing a particular segment of education, taking a significant career step, or achieving a particular aspect of independence.

RESPONSIBILITY • How carefully have you considered your responsibility to your partner "in sickness and in health"? How thoroughly have you assessed your ability to financially, physically, and mentally care for your partner in the case of illness?

Figure 11-6

Median Age at First Marriage

Year	Males	Females
1920	24.6	21.2
1930	24.3	21.3
1940	24.3	21.5
1950	22.8	20.3
1960	22.8	20.3
1970	23.2	20.8
1975	23.5	21.1
1978	24.2	21.8
1979	24.4	22.1
1980	24.7	22.0
1983	24.4	22.5
1984	24.6	22.8
1986	25.7	23.1

SOURCES: U.S. Bureau of the Census, "Statistical Abstracts of the United States," Washington, D.C., 1988.

U.S. Bureau of the Census, "Marital Status and Living Arrangements: March, 1986." *Current Population Reports*, Series P-20, No. 419, 1987.

WILLINGNESS TO SHARE SELF • Are you ready to share your life with another person? Are you prepared to compromise on issues? How well have you thought through altering your pattern of lifestyle behaviors to meet those of your partner?

Have you considered needs and wants of your partner and your ability to accommodate these needs? How willing are you to give of your personal time to meet these needs of your partner?

ECONOMIC INDEPENDENCE • How well-prepared are you to earn a living at a full-time job? Are you and/or your partner still training for a job or career? How stable is the job you currently hold? What means do you have to borrow money if necessary? Have you and your partner established credit? How much money do you have secured for crisis situations?

To what degree have you and your partner discussed the management of money? How well do you agree about spending patterns and budgets? How aware are you of the costs of housing, food, transportation, and clothing?

These questions may urge you to think further about your readiness to marry. They may point out that you and your partner have some areas which still need consideration and discussion. They may also reaffirm your feelings that you are ready for marriage. They may highlight that you have already done some careful thinking and consideration of mature issues involved in the marriage decision.

WHY MARRY? • People marry for various reasons. Most individuals marry someone for multiple reasons. In earlier chapters, self-concept, values and goals, and fully functioning individuals were discussed. These concepts are important aspects of the reasons for marriage discussed in this section.

MEETING NEEDS • Most people have needs that are met by marrying. In turn, they meet the needs of their partner. This mutual meeting of needs provides a healthy and positive foundation for most marital situations. Most couples establish romantic and sexual attachments which develop and become more fulfilled in marriage. Shared ideas and plans for future life together are part of the needs for most couples.

Some reasons for marrying include certain needs that may lead to difficulties if they are the only reason for marrying. Gaining social status, gaining economic security, desire for a baby, and liking a person's potential in-laws are poor reasons to marry if they are the only reason for marrying. These reasons, in conjunction with other meeting of needs mentioned above, may be adequate reasons. These reasons by themselves, however, may indicate personality problems that need attention. They are *not* a basis for marriage.

ESCAPE • Too often, marriage—especially young marriage—takes place in order to escape another situation. Marrying for escape is unhealthy. People often find that they leave one problem only to find another. People marry in order to escape loneliness, single life, financial problems, trouble with family, and school. Unfortunately these issues seldom disappear with marriage. Rather, they reappear along with additional problems.

If you think that you are marrying for escape reasons, stop and analyze the situation. Is there any way you can overcome the problem first and then consider marriage? This approach will give you a chance to grow and give your marriage a better chance.

It is difficult to determine when a person is ready for various steps of marriage. Such a decision involves considering personal values, environmental concerns, and individual and family issues. There are some guidelines to consider when each individual (and couple) weighs the decision. These guidelines are meant to trigger your personal thinking and open discussion between you and your potential partner.

PERSONAL INDEPENDENCE • Ask yourself the following questions to help determine the degree of your personal independence:

1• To what degree are you ready to or to what degree have you already broken away from your dependence on your family? Have you managed independently or semi-independently for a time?
2• To what degree are you ready to relinquish some of your relationships with friends and form new groups of mutual friends? How well do you enjoy being with your partner's friends?
3• How ready and willing are you to assume adult responsibilities in society? How ready are you to take your place in society?

LEGAL ASPECTS OF MARRIAGE

Many people fail to realize that marriage is a legally binding contract that involves specific rights and obligations of both husband and wife. Involved in this contract is the government of the state in which the married couple resides. Each state has its own set of marriage laws. These laws are quite different from one state to the next. Before entering marriage, it is important that both partners understand the laws pertaining to marriage in their state.

In order for a marriage contract to be legally valid, three conditions must be met. These are:

1• Both partners must agree to the marriage. This agreement must be accompanied by the man's and woman's signature on a valid marriage license.
2• There must be no force, duress, or coercion placed on either party. That is, no one can place undue pressure on a person to get married. Both partners must enter the marriage of their own free will.
3• The marriage ceremony must be witnessed by a legally recognized person who also signs the marriage license, and a legally

recognized person must officiate (justice of the peace, minister, priest, rabbi, etc.).

Laws will vary from one state to the next in several ways. However, all states are concerned that people marry in a responsible manner. Therefore, laws are established to protect, as much as possible, the legal rights and well-being of those involved. These include both the marriage partners and any children that might be born in the marriage. These laws also pertain to property and money that is accrued in the marriage (for example, real estate, houses, furniture, automobiles, etc.).

Laws vary in terms of:

1. The legal age at which people can get married, either with or without the consent of parents. In most states this is 18 years of age without parental consent. With parental consent, states vary anywhere from allowing 14-year-olds to 16-year-olds to marry.
2. Requiring a blood test and/or physician's certificate prior to marriage. This is done to verify that both partners are free of any sexually transmitted diseases (STDs). Some states require such verification, while others do not.
3. How property is divided in case of divorce. Nine states have "community property" laws. **Community property laws** state that property and money acquired by either marriage partner during the marriage belong equally to both. Should they divorce, both partners have equal claim to the property that has been acquired. Community property laws do not apply to property that either spouse acquired before the marriage, or property acquired during the marriage that was placed in his or her own name (such as the title to a car that is not shared or an inheritance given to one of the spouses). **Separate property laws**, on the other hand, pay much more attention to which spouse paid for property or earned the money in case of divorce. Such property does not automatically belong equally to both partners.
4. The waiting period required to get married. Some states require a 5-day waiting period from the time the couple applies for the marriage license to the time they can get married. As of 1982, residents of Hawaii had to wait 30 days! Other states require no waiting period.

There are many other laws that pertain to marriage. The few mentioned here simply illustrate how different marriage laws can be from state to state. Other laws pertain to child custody in case of divorce or separation (who is granted the right to keep the children, the mother or the father), as well as child support when parents separate (how much money each parent is legally required to pay to provide for the food, medical, clothing, and shelter expenses of children). As discussed in greater detail later in this chapter, it is a relatively easy thing to propose marriage and to get married. It is a far more complicated and legally difficult matter to get "*unmarried*," or divorced (Figure 11-7).

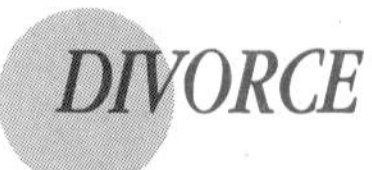

DIVORCE

People who are adequately matched to marry can grow to be sufficiently *unmatched* to *unmarry*, according to sociologist Nelson Foote. While most people enter marriage with the idea that it will last a lifetime, more than

Figure 11-7

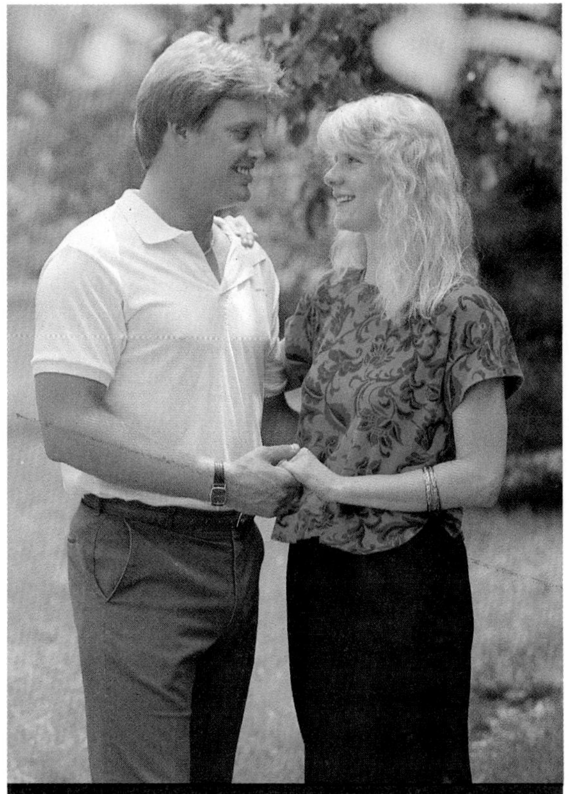

Thinking about and understanding the legal aspects of marriage as well as recognizing the complications and difficulties of divorce can help young couples prepare for marriage.

1 million American marriages are terminated by divorce each year. **Divorce** is the legal termination of the marriage contract.

Though divorce does not mean permanent severing of family relationships as in death, it means the altering of relationships and the changing of family composition and structure. Divorce is usually an uncomfortable, depressing process. Yet, it can provide the opportunity to alter and improve family relationships.

Divorce rates have had an upward trend for many years. Currently, there is a slowdown in the rise of divorces. That is, though the number of divorces continues to increase, they are not increasing as rapidly as they did from 1965 to 1980. During the past 20 years, the divorce rate has more than doubled.

1965 . . . . 10.6 divorces per 1,000 married women

1984 . . . . 21.5 divorces per 1,000 married women

Demographers (persons who study the statistics of human populations) estimate that approximately 50 percent of recent marriages will end in divorce. These include marriages among people in the 20- to 24-year-old range in the early to mid-1980s. This is an important figure to consider as divorce is discussed further in this chapter.

Divorce in Our Society

In past decades, it was considered immoral, sinful, and personally weak to consider ending a marriage. Individuals married for life and, regardless of the quality of the marriage, they remained married. This "commitment to permanence" in marriage was firm, and was an oath not likely to be broken for whatever reason.

Today, ending a marriage is common. Many of you have experienced parents, grandparents, and siblings who have divorced. The emphasis on personal growth and development and the increased contact with new people and interests are factors that have changed social attitudes about divorce.

This change in attitude related to divorce can be both positive and negative. On the positive side, people value the quality of personal and family life. They feel so strongly about this value that they will make major changes to gain a quality life. Americans apparently have high expectations of married life and refuse to accept a marriage that does not reach these expectations. The increasing divorce rate shows that people are not willing to live in an unhappy, unpleasant marriage.

On the negative side, the changed attitude related to divorce may foster complacent behavior toward problem-solving in marriage and families. It appears that few couples make concerted efforts to build a satisfying life together. Skills related to positive family relationships—communicating, exercising compromise, developing trust, sharing activities—have not been mastered or in some cases even attempted. Divorce may be used as a "quick-fix" to a troubled marriage, before the partners have made any serious attempt to solve their problems.

It seems that early American attitudes about divorce made it difficult to end a very negative relationship. Stability of the family and marriage were emphasized at all costs. Today's attitudes seem to increase the ease in ending a relationship that, with effort, may have become positive. Stability is sacrificed for the goal of happiness. Perhaps social attitudes and beliefs will begin to move toward a midpoint of these two approaches to ending a marriage.

Factors Related to Divorce

There are some factors of married and family life that relate to divorce. This does not mean these factors cause divorce. Rather, it means that these factors appear to be present in many families in which the couples seek and gain divorces.

High mobility in terms of occupation and living place is related to divorce. Mobility allows people to experience new values and beliefs. Mobility also allows less chance to interact with extended family and lifelong friends who have concern for a person's marital success.

Longer life appears to be an additional factor related to divorce. In earlier generations, a couple had few years remaining together after launching children before one spouse died. Even if the marriage was not satisfying, the couple may have chosen to continue the relationship. In the 1980s, a 45-year-old couple may have their children launched and have an average of 35 years remaining together as a couple. If their marital relationship is unsatisfactory, there is the likelihood that they may consider ending the marriage. Later years of marriage are often considered the most rewarding. If a marriage does not provide these rewards, divorce is an alternative for the many years of later adult life.

The number of women in the labor force seems to be related to increases in divorce rates. Employment provides self-sufficiency and encourages equality of the sexes. The employed female may be more likely to consider divorce when she has the means to earn her own living. Likewise, the male may be less hesitant to consider divorce when he knows support payments will be less likely because of an employed spouse. He may be more likely to consider divorce when he knows his wife can support herself.

Length of time married is related to divorce rates and trends. Approximately one-fourth of all divorces take place within the first two years of marriage and half of all divorces take place within the first seven years. The chances of divorce decline gradually with each additional year of marriage duration.

Age of people at marriage is also a factor in divorce trends. Couples who marry while in their teens compose the largest group of divorced people by age at marriage. Half of all teen marriages end in divorce within five years. Marriages of teenagers in which the bride is pregnant before marriage are even more likely to end in divorce.

Location of residence is related to divorce rates. Urban couples are more likely to divorce than small-town or rural couples. This may be because a person is more anonymous in a large city. In small towns and rural areas, there may be community pressure and reaction to divorce. This may prevent or delay divorce. Also, family support systems may be greater in the rural/small-town areas.

Education and income are related factors to divorce. People with less education and lower income tend to have higher rates of divorce. Lack of money is a difficult aspect of any relationship. Inability to meet the most basic physical needs has a strong negative effect on marriage. "Living on love" is poetic, but difficult on an empty stomach.

Religious affiliation of marriage partners is related to lower rates of divorce. Divorce rates are higher for couples without religious ties or with mixed religious affiliations than for couples with the same religious affiliations or ties. This may be because of religious beliefs that view divorce negatively. It may also reflect the shared values and beliefs as well as marital assistance provided by many religious organizations.

Divorce Process

Marriage is a legally binding contract between the husband, the wife, and state law. Only the state has the power and authority to legally terminate this contract. **Divorce** is the legal process that ends a marriage. What makes this legal process a complicated one is that, somehow, property (house, cars, furniture, etc.) must be divided by the divorcing couple. Also, any children born in the marriage must be taken care of, financially and socially. Legally, it is much easier to *get married* than it is to *get unmarried* or divorced. The legal entanglements of divorce add stress to what already is an emotionally stressful situation for parents and children.

Separation agreements are often forerunners of divorce. Legal separation contracts contain terms and conditions under which parties agree to live apart from one another. Couples may legally separate for purposes of divorce. They may also separate for an agreed upon need to have some time alone to reorganize their values and goals. Separations may lead to divorce or to reuniting the spouses. Separation often provides the means for decision making.

The state governing body determines the divorce process. Thus, states have different approaches for obtaining a divorce. As is the case with marriage laws, divorce laws vary from one state to the next. The two basic approaches to divorce are the adversary system and the no-fault system.

ADVERSARY SYSTEM • This system of divorce requires that one partner be faced with legal action. The adversary system assumes one party is innocent and one party is guilty. The various grounds for divorce are set by the state. The state indicates what grounds are sufficient to end a marriage. These grounds for divorce vary greatly from state to state. Most states consider desertion, adultery, insanity, sexual impotence, and mental or physical cruelty as adequate grounds for divorce. Each state may have a variety of additional grounds for divorce.

There are some strong criticisms of the adversary system of divorce. Though in some cases there may be clear cut patterns of "fault" in a relationship, most divorces appear to be outcomes of problems and issues related to both partners. The adversary system usually causes or increases hostility and encourages bad feelings between the partners. Since the "guilty" partner may suffer in property division, child support, and custody, both parties fight to present themselves as innocent and their partner as the sole cause of the divorce. Aside from being unrealistic, this process causes anger and bitterness. This process is especially detrimental in cases where children are involved. Seeing a parent labeled as guilty can be damaging for some children. The process is also detrimental to later interaction related to shared custody of children or visiting rights. It is usually difficult to manage a positive parent interaction after hostile and negative feelings have been aired in a courtroom.

NO-FAULT DIVORCE • Nearly every state has instituted some form of a nonadversarial means for divorce, known as "no-fault" divorce laws. Although couples may choose to enter an adversarial divorce proceeding, with the "no-fault" process a marriage can be ended with neither party having to prove that one party is guilty of any misconduct.

A no-fault divorce allows partners to claim that their marriage has broken down. Proof of this breakdown is usually a separation. That is, the fact that the spouses cannot bear to live together any longer shows that a meaningful relationship no longer exists.

A major problem with the no-fault divorce is with the granting of a fair property settlement. The no-fault system appears on the surface to grant equal property settlement. Yet, the economically dependent spouse is often less able to provide for himself/herself. Additional provisions may need to be made to the economically dependent person for a period of time in order to prepare for getting a job. Also, in many "no-fault" state laws, the divorcing spouses must agree on child custody, property rights, and who will pay any debts that have accrued in the marriage.

FINANCIAL ARRANGEMENTS • Financial considerations in divorce include alimony, child support, and property settlements. **Alimony** is the payment of money by the primary wage-earner, ex-husband or ex-wife, during and after the divorce. Alimony is awarded less often today than in the past. Some states do not even recognize alimony payments. In some cases, where a spouse has not been employed, judges award alimony to the nonwage-earning spouse for a short term in order to allow for job training and/or to find a job. This is the female partner in the vast majority of alimony cases. Still, alimony is awarded in less than 15 percent of all divorces. Since alimony practices differ by state, the receiver of the alimony award may have difficulty collecting payment if the former spouse moves to another state.

Child support is a more common award by the courts. Judges in most states have the right to force divorced parents to support their children until the children reach age 18. Child care and custody, historically, have been awarded to the mother. Today more fathers are gaining custody rights of the children, but still more mothers receive this award (about

90 percent). The major wage earner, typically the father, is more commonly ordered to pay child support. The amount of support, based on income and children's needs, is directed by law to the financial support of the child or children. Too often child support payments are stopped after several months. And high court costs and legal fees prevent the legal action needed to order the payments continued. However, this situation is changing today as states are enacting, and enforcing, "uniform child support laws." Parents who fail to pay child support are being arrested and forced to make payments.

Frequently, joint custody and joint support are a part of divorce action. In cases where both parents are employed and equally capable of child care, this is likely to be a more equitable situation. In joint custody and joint support, both parents provide economically for the children, and each has equal time to spend with the children.

In the case of property settlement, divorcing spouses frequently disagree about how much each deserves. Usually these matters must be decided in court. In community property states, the court may attempt to divide property equitably. However, this arrangement may not be completely *equal*. For example, the court may award the house and car to the wife if she is also granted custody of the children. The husband will usually be ordered to make monthly child support payments as well. The level of child support payments is determined by the judge. However, property settlements vary from one case to the next. There is always the possibility that either partner will be treated unfairly by the courts.

Separate property states are more likely to favor the spouse who has earned the most income during the marriage. This is usually the husband because of the greater income earning potential of men in our society. However, in most separate property states the judge will take into account the needs of the partner who earned less income as well. This means that if the woman is granted custody of the children and will be in financial difficulty after the divorce, she will be granted child support payments and perhaps additional property (house or car) in order to live at a comfortable level.

EMOTIONAL DIVORCE PROCESS • The above discussion focuses on legal aspects of divorce. Usually an emotional process has preceded the legal activities that terminate a marriage. A long period of conflict and discontent frequently occurs prior to discussion or action toward a divorce. Once a couple (or one spouse) has decided that the marriage does not work, the emotional divorce has occurred. The couple no longer feels the emotional, loving relationship that once existed. These feelings are replaced by emotional feelings of hurt and anger.

The emotional divorce is usually the first step prior to the legal divorce. Some couples appear to have an emotional divorce without following through with the legal divorce. They appear to continue in a situation that causes hurt and anger for each other. To keep a marriage legally intact without feeling love, trust, and affection or to end the relationship and gain a legal divorce is a decision based on personal values.

Impact of Divorce

Divorce has an impact on individuals and families long before and long after the legal divorce. Understanding the impact of divorce is important for both the adult experiencing divorce and the children experiencing the divorce of parents.

PSYCHOLOGICAL IMPACT • Many divorced people experience a period in which they must learn to think of themselves as individuals. People who married early in life may never have had experience as a single person on their own. The new, independent status may require developing skills and strengths. Fear and loneliness may be experienced, especially in the early stages of divorce.

The psychological impact is both positive and negative. The new independence may foster self-reliance, personal growth, and a newly found freedom.

COMMUNITY IMPACT • Divorce has a major impact on a couple's community of friends. Likewise, this community of close friends, fellow workers, and acquaintances as well as the larger community in which a person lives will respond in various ways. Some friends may ignore the divorced people since it may be embarrassing to talk about the divorce. Other friends will take sides in the divorce conflict. Still others seem to fear that a divorced person may be after their own spouse.

In most cases divorce means that individuals must begin to look for new friendship sources to add to the old community of friends or to replace former close friends. This growth process can have a positive psychological effect on divorced persons.

ECONOMIC IMPACT • Divorce has a strong economic effect on individuals and families. A divorce is the breaking of an economic partnership. In some partnerships, the money value may be low. It is clear that it takes fewer dollars for two people to live together than for two people to live separately. Housing, food, transportation, and daily expense are usually easier to afford for two people living together. For women, in particular, divorce often means a lowering of income and the standard of living. This is due to the fact that women earn less money than do men in the occupational system. Rarely is there enough money to suit the needs and wants for both parties, and each partner may think the other partner got a better deal.

IMPACT ON CHILDREN • In 1984, a total of 1,081,000 children under the age of 18 had parents who divorced in the United States. This is about the number affected each and every year. For parents, the divorce may be most difficult when dealing with children. Most parents weigh the impact of the divorce on their children long before the legal divorce begins.

There is disagreement among experts about the effect of divorce on children. Some sources feel divorce is damaging to children and should be avoided at almost any cost. Others point out that children are stronger and more agile than we realize, and that they will overcome negative impacts of divorce. Most authorities suggest that parents try to determine the least harmful environment for their children. Parents may need to weigh negative aspects of remaining in a high-conflict and hostile environment versus negative aspects brought about by divorce. If the marriage exposes children to parental anger, hostility, or open violence, then the divorce is the better action. If situations in the proposed divorce lead to unhealthy, negative, and otherwise detrimental environments, then a couple may wish to consider possible alternatives to divorce. Usually those marriages and families that are unhappy and held together for the children's sake do *not* provide the most positive environment.

Divorce and consequent changes in the family often create additional parent-child conflict. Child custody and visitation rights, new physical surroundings, changed household responsibilities, and alterations in discipline and behavioral guidelines are some aspects of parent-child conflict generated by divorce. Children who have experienced divorce often display symptoms that interfere with positive parent-child relations. Some of these symptoms include feelings of fearfulness, difficulty concentrating, extreme fatigue, and a drop in grades. Some people experience the mourning for the loss of the family of their childhood. Some young people have feelings of guilt that they may have caused the divorce.

Though problems faced by single parents are similar to those of parents with mates, the problems may be more difficult to solve. Conflict and frustration usually lessen as both parents and children adjust to new lifestyles. Time to adjust, patience, and increased understanding can bring about stable and positive parent-child relationships. Typically this is accomplished within a year or two after the divorce.

When a divorce occurs, parents need to work together objectively to remove ill feelings about the divorce process. Joint custody and visiting rights are situations that require interaction between parents. Though spouses may have negative feelings toward each other, they need to strive to be neutral and objective about each other when their children are involved.

The following guidelines related to divorce and parenting are helpful in understanding the impact of divorce.

- Children react to divorce in the same way as their parents. Parents who consider divorce a positive step to overcoming problems and building a new life will likely find their children doing the same.
- It is generally best if both parents together can explain the need or reasons for divorce to the child.
- Children should be reassured that the separation and/or divorce was not the children's fault. Be clear in explaining that they did not cause the divorce.
- Reassure children that they will not be deprived of their basic needs. Whatever the custody agreement, the child will be adequately cared for.
- Though the parents are divorcing, neither parent is divorcing the child. The child will continue to have two parents and will continue to have the same grandparents, cousins, etc.

Divorce Prevention

There are often sound reasons for ending a marriage. After a hurtful relationship is ended, all individuals involved in a family may function better. However, since pain, anger, and frustration are usually part of the divorce process, it would be better to prevent the need for divorce action.

Can anything be done to prevent divorce? Are there any approaches to prevent becoming a part of the 50 percent of today's marriages that will end in divorce?

Building a strong network of extended family, friends, and professional assistance is a good strengthener of marital relationships. More specific recommendations related to prevention of divorce fall into three categories. Each of the categories of divorce prevention is applicable to couple interaction prior to marriage as well as during the marriage. These actions are:

- Gain thorough knowledge of the marriage partner before commitment to marriage.
- Develop the ability to adapt and change to meet a partner's needs while maintaining your own personal integrity.
- Attempt to work out conflicts and crisis but seek outside counseling when necessary.

These actions can begin during the marriage preparation period. The engagement period is set aside for this purpose. These same processes carry over into active marriage (see Figure 11-8). The attempts to prevent divorce presented in Figure 11-8 are basically sound adjustment practices. They all require communication of the marriage partners. Without positive communication, couples have far less likelihood of maintaining a stable, successful marriage.

DESERTION

To desert someone is to withdraw, abandon, or fail in time of need. Desertion occurs frequently in our society and is not limited to adults deserting a spouse and children. Aging persons, young adults, teens, as well as adults leave their homes and families often without providing knowledge of their destination.

Usually desertion brings to mind a man leaving his wife and children. This stereotyped description is probably due to the traditional role of the man's responsibility to his family. However, all family members have responsibility to each other. The teenager who runs away from home and the wife who leaves her children and spouse have turned from their responsibility to family members. These individuals, like the father who deserts his family, have allowed pressures and stress to override their responsibility. Methods for dealing with such pressures need to be developed.

Difficulty of Dealing with Desertion

Unlike divorce, where figures, facts, and dates are plentiful, desertion is relatively unstudied. This is because there are no formal means to count the number of people who desert their families. No registration with the courts or definite social or legal process exists. Legal systems are vague about what constitutes desertion.

The vagueness of desertion makes it often more difficult to cope with than divorce. When a divorce occurs in a family, there is usually mutual consent. Even when one spouse does not want a divorce, there usually has been time to face the situation and accept the action. Desertion, however, has a heavy impact on the spouse and/or other family members without allowing them any voice in the decision-making process or time to adjust to the action.

Desertion creates uncertainty for all concerned. The deserter often loses all self-respect. The deserted family members may also lose self-respect. They have unmet

Figure 11-8

Divorce Prevention before and during Marriage

Divorce	*Action Before*	*Action During*
Prevention	**Marriage**	**Married Life**
• Gain thorough knowledge of marriage partner before commitment to marriage.	Matt and Sherry take long walks and talk about their goals, ambitions, and frustrations. They have also participated in premarital counseling where they learned more about each other's inner feelings.	Benji and Yoko have made a real effort to find times to exchange ideas and feelings. They feel this is important because they know they change as they mature, and they need to share these changes.
• Develop the ability to adapt and change to meet a partner's needs while maintaining your own personal integrity.	Sherry has never felt comfortable entertaining large groups of people. She realizes that this sort of entertainment is a necessary part of Matt's job. She has agreed to try to help Matt all she can, but she will not judge herself based only on this situation. She knows she possesses many other skills and abilities.	Benji is a worrier. He fusses and is anxious whenever Yoko is out of town on her job. After much discussion, Benji learned he would have to meet Yoko's need for a confident, trusting husband. Yet, Benji maintains his general protective and guarding behavior.
• Attempt to work out conflicts and crises but seek outside counseling if necessary.	Matt's mother has always had a tendency to boss and control others. Sherry began to feel frustrated and angry each time she visited Matt's home. Both Matt and Sherry realized that since they would be living near Matt's mother, this situation could cause major conflicts. Matt and Sherry met with a counselor at their church to work out some of their feelings.	As Benji and Yoko neared retirement, it became clear that their goals for the retirement were very different. Benji planned to retire in the South while reading and soaking up sunshine. Yoko wanted to explore a second career. This difference in goals has been worked through to the liking of both after meeting with a career-life counselor from Benji's office.

needs—often economic as well as social, emotional, and psychological needs. Children of a deserting parent particularly suffer a loss of identity and feelings of guilt. They question what they did to cause their parent to leave them. Desertion may be more damaging to family members than divorce.

Prevention of Desertion

Desertion of a family member does not occur because there are problems. All families have problems. Desertion occurs because too much time elapses before the problems are dealt with. This book focuses on dealing with individual and family issues, concerns, and problems. Facing issues, communicating openly, using problem-solving techniques, and developing a positive self-image are ways you can deal with pressures that seem insurmountable. When individual and family members have applied these techniques without success, professional help should be sought.

People who desert their families are usually running *from* something rather than running to something. The stressful situations have become overwhelming and unbearable. Factors in these unbearable situations include two basic issues. First are the issues related to independent-dependent behavior. Teenagers, spouses, and aging people may require more independence or feel that they require more independence than their family systems provide. Second, factors related to money—either lack of money or unfair distribution of money—are often involved. Focusing on solving problems related to these two issues may be vital to preventing desertion.

WRAPPING IT UP

America is a marriage-oriented society. Although the number of people who choose to remain single has grown somewhat, the vast majority of people in our society will marry at least once (approximately 90 percent at today's rates). Today many are delaying marriage in order to attain the desired level of education or work status, or to establish an adequate financial foundation to support a family. Thus, we have seen an increase in the average age at which people in the United States marry for the first time.

Anyone can choose singlehood. Whether singlehood is a permanent alternative to marriage or simply an extended period of independence prior to marriage, this lifestyle has certain advantages. Career and educational goals can be more easily reached. Values on autonomy and freedom can be realized without having to feel responsible for another person. A level of emotional maturity can be gained before entering a long-term commitment such as marriage. Singlehood may also have negative aspects. Loneliness and negative social attitudes toward single people can place stress on the person who chooses not to marry. Nonetheless, today, compared to past years, many people consider remaining single to be a more acceptable alternative to marriage.

Many important decisions must be made when considering marriage. Answers to "who, when, and why" questions have major implications for the future life of the individual. How do you know when you are ready for marriage? Who is the best person for you? How do you know when you really love a person enough to marry? These questions have no simple answers. Yet, given that people enter marriage with the idea that it is a life-long commitment—one that could last anywhere from 50 to 75 years—how we answer them has major importance for our future lives.

A number of considerations are important in marriage decisions. Similarity, or *homogamy*, between the partners in terms of age, interests, attitudes, and values fosters compatible relationships. Also important are educational, occupational, and standard-of-living levels. Added stress is involved in marriages that cross religious, racial, or ethnic lines. Although homogamy in these areas may make adjustment in marriage easier, it is still possible for those who are different in any one or more of these areas to establish a successful marriage. If differences do exist, partners must face an added challenge of dealing with them and anticipating the problems they might cause.

Marriage readiness involves dating a number of individuals in order to explore different personality types for compatibility. It also involves a careful assessment of yourself, your partner, and the relationship that has been established. How is the quality of your communication with your partner? Are decisions made effectively? Are conflicts and problems adequately resolved? Are we economically stable enough to live at our desired standard of living? Are we emotionally independent enough from our family and friends to make it on our own? Such intellectual assessment is important and should not be clouded by emotions or romantic feelings of love. Love is important but it is not enough to build a satisfying relationship in marriage that will last several years.

Marrying to escape from an unhappy situation is generally an unwise decision. Marriage involves a willingness to share yourself with another person and to assume responsibility for the other person.

While laws pertaining to marriage make it reasonably easy to get into, they make marriage relatively difficult to get out of. The rate of divorce in our society has grown over the years. It has reached a point where about 50 percent of young adults who marry for the first time are expected to divorce. Divorce may have both positive and negative aspects. It allows unhappy marriages to end, and gives people a chance to find a more fulfilling lifestyle. Yet divorce involves a number of legal considerations. These include *alimony, child support,* property settlements, and child custody. These legal concerns complicate the emotional divorce process.

Divorce touches many people each year. It has a psychological and financial impact on spouses as well as on their children. Usually an adjustment period of one to two years is necessary for adults and children of divorce to work through the problems that the divorce has presented. The most positive post-divorce adjustments are made when children are not blamed for the marriage break-up, and when the divorcing spouses try to reduce the level of anger and hostility between them when they are working through the divorce process.

Desertion also poses problems for families. Abandonment is a bitter pill to swallow. It lacks the finality of a divorce situation. Feelings of loss, guilt, and anger are more likely to occur due to the sudden nature of desertion. The chances of desertion or divorce can be reduced by concrete actions of family members. These include trying to work out conflicts and crises and attempting to adjust and adapt to each other over time as needs, expectations, and life circumstances change.

Exploring Dimensions of Chapter Eleven

For Review

1• What factors affect the decision to delay marriage?
2• What are the most commonly stated rewards of single life? What is the most commonly stated negative feature of single life?
3• List four areas of similarity that are important to a married couple.
4• Explain the two types of divorce processes and give implications for families for each.

For Consideration

1• Using television or movie dramas, find examples of people who did not attend to factors of readiness related to marriage and parenthood.
2• Create a brief description of an individual experiencing a most fulfilling and rewarding independent life. Create another description of this individual experiencing a rewarding and happy life of marriage and parenthood. How can a transition be made between these two descriptions? What steps and stages are necessary to reach the second description after experiencing the first?
3• Create an imaginary couple who are considering marriage. Help them through guiding questions that will assist them in making this decision.
4• Andrea's older brother has run away from home. Andrea's family is going through a very difficult time because of this desertion. Explain how this situation is difficult for the family. How might the situation differ depending on the age of Andrea's brother?
5• Ed and Marsha worry about divorce. Both have experienced the divorce of a parent and they do not want the same experience to happen to them. Give this couple guidelines for prevention of divorce. They are now engaged and plan to get married in ten months.

For Application

1• Interview three couples—one couple in early stages of marriage, one couple with school-aged children, one couple with older high school or college students—to determine what factors the couples used to decide if they were ready for marriage. Ask what social and economic changes have occurred that would alter the factors or guidelines they would use today in making such a decision. Ask them to suggest guidelines for use today.

2• Interview several friends, neighbors, and possibly yourself to determine how divorce has affected the lives of younger people. (Interview only those people who will willingly discuss this topic.) Consider how they were told about the divorce, their immediate reaction, their age at the time, and when they began to accept and adjust to the situation. Determine what factors helped or hindered in their adjustment. Ask their opinion about how parents, teachers, and others can help children accept divorce.

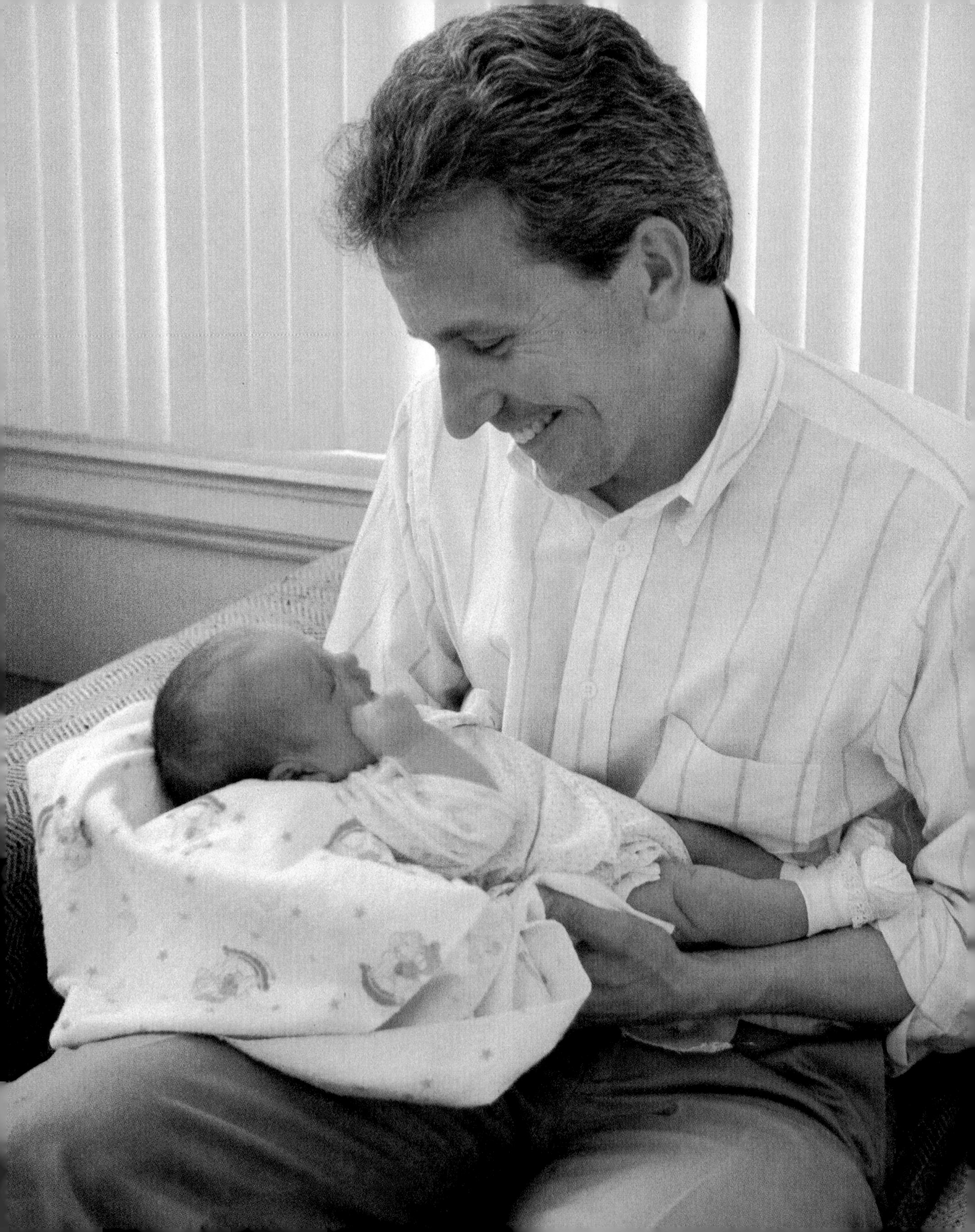

twelve

EFFECTIVE PARENTING

This chapter provides information that will help you to:

- Understand the decision to parent.
- Understand the process of effective parenting.
- Realize styles of parenting.
- Analyze the myths of parenting.
- Explore dependence/independence within the parenting process.
- Explore parenting education.

When we use the word *parent* as a noun it is easily understood; we all know what a parent is. When we use *parent* as a verb, however, it may be less clear. What does it mean to parent a child? What is effective parenting?

Effective parenting is a process of meeting the needs and wants of another human being. It involves guidance of children in a way that demonstrates respect and fosters movement from dependence to independence as the child grows older.

It is a process because it is continuous and it changes as children and parents grow and change. Effective parenting requires knowledge about the growth and development of children. Awareness of physical, social, moral, and emotional growth is needed in order to understand the behavior and attitudes of children throughout the life cycle. Effective parenting also means making the decision to become a parent when you have attained an appropriate level of readiness.

Parenting is not limited to parents. Many people perform acts of parenting for those who are not their own children. Various agencies and individuals help to parent children. However, the chief responsibilities for parenting remain with parents.

The years in the family life cycle in which children pass from fetus to infant to child to adolescent can be referred to as the parenting years. Families within this stage can be called **parenting families**. It is true that people are parents far beyond the age when their children are adolescents. Yet, after the age of 18 or after children leave the home, the parenting process becomes less intense. The parenting family—the family with children who are dependent on parents—will be discussed later in this chapter.

PARENTHOOD DECISIONS

One of the most important responsibility-laden decisions you will make in your life is the decision related to parenthood. The outcome of this decision will have far-reaching effects that will last throughout your lifetime. Moving from an adult, two-person relationship to an adult-infant, three-person relationship is a step to be considered carefully.

Most people in our society become parents, yet an increasing number of people choose not to do so. Whether these people continue in this way of thinking or if they eventually choose to parent will not be known for some years. It seems clear, however, that more young people are delaying parenthood. This delay is for some of the same reasons that people delay marriage: career goals, economic factors, and desire for individual and couple growth.

Many people who choose to postpone or permanently prevent parenthood find some of the rewards of parenting through the children of others. Often relatives, neighbors, community volunteer work, or professional work with children provide warm, loving, child-adult relationships.

There are reasons for becoming pregnant that focus on needs other than the desire to share a part of your life with another and raise a child in a loving, caring environment. These reasons include: to save a marriage, to prove masculinity or femininity, and to get away from an unpleasant job.

These reasons are usually considered inappropriate because they do not focus on the child. Also, these goals are seldom met by parenthood. Unstable marriages are rarely helped and insecure feelings about masculinity or femininity are seldom eliminated by the addition of a child. Unpleasantries of the job can be better alleviated by a job change or by confronting the employment issues.

For most people, parenthood brings great joy and happiness. For some, it can include sorrow, despair, and regret. Though all parents face some difficulties and frustrations as parents, many of the major difficulties can be prevented by attention to factors of readiness for parenthood.

These factors of readiness are *not* firm measures or formulas for determining if and when you should become a parent. There is no specific age or number of years as a couple that can be claimed as the right time to start a parenthood role. These factors are merely guidelines related to psychological, emotional, and material readiness for the responsibility of parenthood. Some people may review these guidelines and conclude that they will not be ready to be a parent for several years. Other people may need more time. Still others may feel they can never meet these guidelines and feel they will never choose to become parents.

Factors of Readiness

Readiness for parenthood involves physical, psychological, emotional, and intellectual factors. Consideration needs to be given to all as well as various combinations of these factors in order to determine if you are mature enough and ready for the major step of parenthood.

Knowledge of child development and child care procedures is a basic readiness factor. Being aware of normal developmental patterns will allow you to judge if you are ready to deal with the stages and processes which infants and young children go through. Accurate and realistic expectations of child growth and development can enable you to decide if and when parenting will be best for you. Likewise, clear and concrete knowledge of necessary child care procedures will permit you to make more objective decisions related to parenthood.

Such knowledge allows young people to gain another readiness factor—*patience with young children*. The early years of parenting involve diapers, bottles, and the continuous routines of eat, sleep, and wash. Such activities can become emotionally wearing on young parents. Prolonged, uninterrupted care of infants and toddlers by young parents who have not yet developed mature levels of patience can generate frustrations, child neglect, and child abuse.

The care of a child requires *high levels of energy at all times of the day and night*. The level of energy needed for parenthood, especially the early stages of parenthood, is often overwhelming to young couples. Parental energy to meet the physical needs of the child is demanding in itself. Young parents sometimes do not recognize the energy required to meet a child's emotional needs.

A major readiness factor is the ability to *put your personal priorities aside in favor of the needs of the child*. Infants are totally helpless: parents are responsible for an infant's total welfare. Individual needs must often be set aside for the needs of the child. Though clearly not all personal needs must or should be sacrificed, personal time and immediate personal goals and needs may need to be postponed. When parents are employed, work and child care consume most of a couple's time. Time for hobbies and personal activities becomes rare. Couples often have difficulty finding some time to spend alone as a couple. Going out to a movie or other entertainment may become far less frequent.

Issues may arise as to the *equality of the burdens as well as the rewards of parenting between the mother and father*. Postponement of personal gratification, physical and psychological drain of caregiving, and financial burdens may not be felt to be equally divided.

Spotlight on issues

Delayed Parenthood

Not all people are postponing parenthood, but it is not uncommon today to have a first baby at age 35 or older. According to recent studies, an increasing number of people are marrying later and delaying the birth of their first child.

There are several reasons why couples are delaying parenthood. Some reasons are:

- Maintaining dual careers
- Completing education
- Establishing financial security
- Gaining stability in marrige

Delayed parenthood presents several implications for our society:

- The additional childbirth risk to mothers and career interruptions seem to encourage couples who become parents at age 35 to 40 to have only one child. It may also be that couples who become parents after years of anticipation wish to devote their time and energy to only one child. Parents of only children make efforts to provide peer interaction for their child. There may be an increased use of such facilities as camps and youth clubs.
- Since many couples who delay childbirth do so in order to carry out career and job goals, it is likely that one or both parents earn above-average incomes. Thus, these families are normally more financially secure.
- Many parents, especially mothers, may choose to lighten career endeavors to devote more time to child care.
- There is a greater likelihood that parents may be in the retirement or preretirement stage while their children are in college or in late high school.
- These parents may become grandparents in their early 60s. This usually results in grandparents who have anticipated grandparenthood and who have increased leisure time to spend with grandchildren.

Delaying parenthood seems to indicate the likelihood of a nurturing environment for children. How do you think children in delayed parenthood families will function in society?

Such inequity—whether discussed openly or allowed to fester silently—can breed marital difficulties.

Material means for parenting are often the most obvious requirement when considering a parenthood role. Yet, the actual cost of raising a child is usually beyond most estimates. Immediate costs include medical bills, possible need to relocate or remodel to accommodate a child, clothing and child care equipment, and the possible cut in family income if one parent temporarily or permanently leaves employment. As shown in Chapter 10, the total costs of raising a child to his/her eighteenth birthday (in 1983 dollars) is around $100,000, or possibly more in higher cost areas. This amounts to about $6,000 per year.

It may seem from the information in this section that parenthood brings such overwhelming burdens that only the foolish or the overly brave could consider it. This is not so. The enjoyment, excitement, love, and companionship that parenthood brings can outweigh the burdens for *most* parents. Timing or readiness for parenthood is a key to gaining these positive outcomes. Many people have not found parenting to be as rewarding as they expected and began parenthood before they were ready for the experience.

Guidelines for Parenthood Decisions

The following readiness factors have been put in a guideline format for your consideration. None of them are limited to yes-no responses. They all require careful personal and couple consideration. Open discussion along with gaining additional information will be necessary to determine if and when you are ready for parenthood.

Knowledge of Child Development and Child Care:

How carefully have you reviewed child development books and pamphlets to learn of needs of an infant? Which needs do you feel you'll have most difficulty meeting? To what degree are you aware of child development stages?

How well aware are you of child care routines? Have you observed and/or participated in such routines with your partner? Have you had the opportunity to babysit with your partner?

How much (or how little) do you genuinely like children? Do you find them interesting and enjoyable? Do you find them irritating and a nuisance? Prospective parents should realize that parenting isn't always fun (Figure 12-1).

Patience with Young Children:

To what degree do you and your partner have patience to deal with monotonous routines of child care? How much have you been able to observe your level and your partner's level of patience with young children?

How thoroughly have you considered and discussed the commitment involved in parenting? What can you and your partner use as outlets from the frustration and routine of child care?

Energy Level:

How would you categorize your level of energy? Do you have significant limits to

Figure 12-1

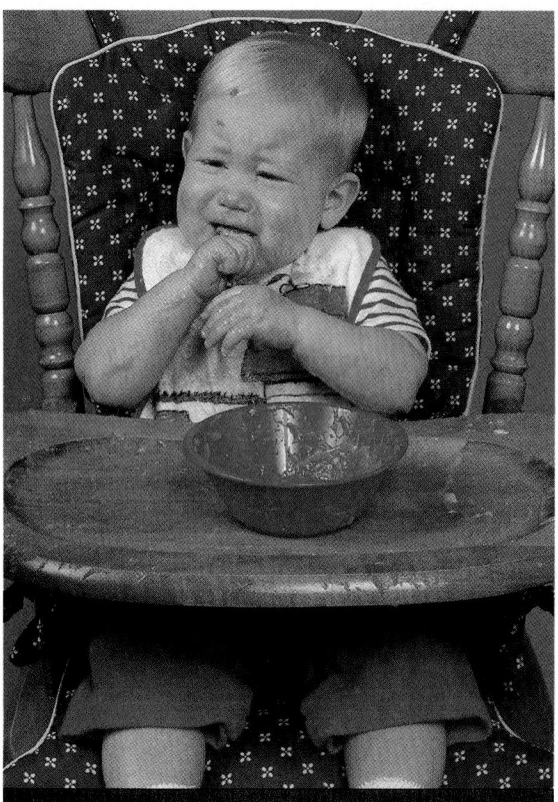

Infants and young children require high levels of care and attention from parents who may not always have sufficient patience or energy to cope with their child's frustrations.

your energy or in your general health that might hinder the caregiving you could offer a child?

To what degree does your normal workday drain you of energy to devote to spouse and child? Which type of energy do you find most taxing? physical energy? psychological, emotional energy? What methods could you and your partner use to assist with limited energy resources?

Relegating Personal Priorities:

How ready are you to put aside or postpone some of your personal gratifications? What activities and hobbies will you give up? How will you and your partner give priority to your activities?

How willing are you and your spouse to give up some of your time together as a couple in order to meet the needs of a child? In what ways could you provide low-cost, workable time together as a couple? How might you plan resources to maintain some personal and couple time?

Equality of Parenthood Role:

How well have you established mutually acceptable patterns of tasks? How equally do you and your partner feel these tasks are distributed?

How thoroughly have you considered the equality or inequality of changes that will occur with parenthood? If there is inequality, how will this be resolved? Is the inequality long-term or short-term?

Material Resources:

How financially ready are you for parenthood? What savings do you have for emergencies? What changes in insurance coverage will be necessary with parenthood? Will parenthood curtail a portion or all of an income? Will this be permanent or temporary? If temporary, what is the **opportunity cost** of this temporary leave? (What will this cost in terms of possible advancement, job tenure, etc.?)

To what degree are you aware of the costs of beginning parenthood? How well have you investigated the cost of obstetric care and delivery, provision of food, clothing, and equipment needed for an infant, and normal infant health care?

How satisfactory is your home in terms of the addition of a child? What changes would need to be made? How easily can these changes be made?

General Readiness:

How complete and how satisfying is the relationship between you and your partner? To what degree do you feel you have a satisfying communication pattern? To what degree have you established a mutually satisfying intimate relationship?

To what degree have you and your partner established workable relationships with friends, relatives, and the community in general? Do you feel you have a network of people from whom you could draw assistance if necessary?

Some parents would say that they never made a decision to become a parent. Rather, they just had a child with no decision involved. Others would argue with this saying that irresponsible sexual behavior indicates a decision to accept pregnancy if it occurs. That is, if two people choose to have sexual intercourse, they clearly run a risk of pregnancy. However you choose to look at this argument, one fact remains: sexual intercourse, whether within or without marriage, holds a risk of pregnancy. Even with precautions of birth control, some risk remains. The decision to be or not to be a parent can be dealt with more rationally and objectively if it is approached prior to sexual relationships. Concern about pregnancy needs to be considered, especially if a couple does not wish to have children.

Spotlight on issues

Child Abuse

One in every 40 children experience some type of abuse and/or neglect each year in the United States. This maltreatment may vary from tragic physical abuse, causing serious injury and death, to emotional neglect that prevents healthy development.

It is difficult to pinpoint the many causes of child abuse and neglect. Each incident is triggered in part by the particular social context in which it takes place. There are, however, usually three basic elements involved in a child abuse situation: the abuser, the child being abused, and a crisis situation that often sparks the abuse.

THE ABUSER • Usually the abuser is a parent of the abused child. Persons other than family members such as babysitters and neighbors may be involved. There are common characteristics among parents who abuse their children. Abusive parents are usually young, under stress, and may have been abused themselves. They are often isolated from family, friends, and community. They tend to be overly critical of their children and seldom give praise. They may show little concern about and reaction to their child's behavior, or they may overreact, becoming hostile and antagonistic. Frequently, the abuser is unemployed or has recently felt the effects of unemployment.

THE ABUSED • Children under six, children with handicaps, and children with behavior problems are most likely to be abused. Usually only one child in a family is abused; this child may be distinct from other family members in appearance, behavior, or personality. Abused children become wary of contact with adults. They may want affection and attention, but they have difficulty relating to people. Because their attention wanders and they have a hard time concentrating, they often become poor students.

THE CRISIS • Child abuse occurs when some crisis sets off the abusive person. The abusive action is seldom caused by a hateful parent or caregiver. Rather, it is usually the result of overreacting to a stressful situation. The child may refuse to eat, cry continually, disobey the parent, or wet the bed. The abuser, unable to cope with the many demands and too much stress, loses control.

Communities can provide an array of services to help prevent abuse and assist those who have abused their children. The following are examples of some low-cost or free services.

- Courses in parent education
- Counseling for mental health
- Financial and employment assistance
- Homemaker services
- Self-help groups
- Hot lines
- Day care for children
- Emergency protective care for children

These services will not be helpful without proper action. Potential abusers must be willing to seek help, and those able to provide that help must take action to supply it. Through such action it is possible to protect a child from further abuse or neglect. It may even save a life.

PARENTING STYLES

Through experiences with your own parents, parents of your friends, and through the media you know that not all people parent in the same way. Parenting styles can be categorized into three groups—authoritarian, democratic, and permissive. Each style includes typical parent behavior and typical child behavior.

The three parenting styles can be placed on a continuum reflecting control of the parent-child relationship.

AUTHORITARIAN——DEMOCRATIC——PERMISSIVE
(parent control) (child control)

Authoritarian Style

In this style the parent establishes rules and regulations and insists that the child obey. The parent does not allow negotiations with the child; the parent's decisions are firm. Power and superiority are part of the parent's role. The child plays a role of obedience and submission.

The authoritarian parent may use force, threats, and fear to bring about the desired child behavior. The situation makes a close, affectionate parent-child relationship difficult to achieve.

Children in authoritarian homes often become defensive and fearful of the parent. They may act out their feelings by being helpless, becoming hostile, or showing extreme anxiety. Typically, the child of authoritarian parents has difficulty learning self-reliance. Self-direction is difficult to learn when there is no opportunity for exploration.

Democratic Style

The democratic style of parenting emphasizes respect for the child and encourages a child's independence (Figure 12-2). Choices and decision making are a major part of this parent-child relationship. Children are given responsibility and are expected to contribute to family action. The democratic parent clearly defines the limits of the child's behavior and explains both the expected behavior and the reason for it.

Children in democratic homes express self-confidence and cooperation. They tend to be self-reliant and responsible for their own actions. They learn to make decisions and to be responsible for the consequences of those decisions.

Permissive Style

Permissive parents are the opposite of authoritarian parents. They seldom express

Figure 12-2

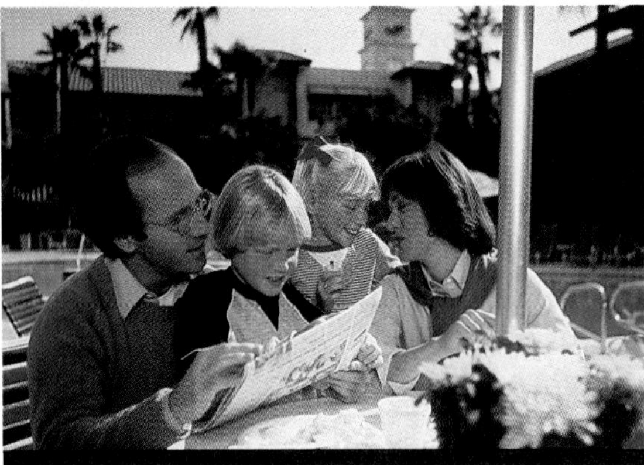

Allowing children opportunities to make choices can help them learn to be responsible for the consequences of the choices they make.
Holiday Corporation

CASE IN POINT

Sarah tells her parents that her friend Melanie is going to have a party next Saturday. Melanie's parents are out of town, but they said the party would be okay. After the party, Sarah and several other girls want to stay overnight with Melanie.

Authoritarian parent reaction: Parents tell Sarah that she cannot go to the party. No discussion of the party is permitted. When Sarah asks why she cannot attend she is told, "I have said you cannot go. Now let's forget it!"

Democratic parent reaction: Parents listen to Sarah's request and ask questions related to details. They ask what she thinks about an unsupervised party. They discuss some situations that might occur and the consequences of these situations. Together they reach some agreed-upon conditions for attending the party.

Permissive parent reaction: Parents tell Sarah she can do as she wishes but to be sure to let them know where she'll be.

their expectations for the child or for the child's behavior. They give few directions. They are indecisive when asked for guidance by their children. They portray an attitude of "anything is okay with me; you decide for yourself."

The child in a permissive home will frequently display high levels of creativity and imagination. However, the permissiveness without guidance frequently leaves children insecure and lacking in self-direction. The absence of parental guidelines may lead the child to impractical, dangerous, or illegal decisions.

The parenting styles may become clearer as you consider how each type of parent responds to a particular situation.

Variations in Parenting Styles

It is useful for purposes of discussion and analysis to place parenting behavior in styles and categories. Parents have a typical style which their children come to know and expect. It is important to remember, however, that parents do not always practice one style. They sometimes move from one parenting style to another. They may be typically democratic, for example, but become authoritarian in certain areas. When parents change their position on a specific area of parenting, their children usually become aware of this variation and function accordingly. When parents radically and illogically change from permissive to authoritarian to democratic behavior without any basis for these changes, children will likely become confused, over-anxious, and unsure of how to respond. When parents regularly follow one style of parenting, children know what to expect.

What causes a parent to follow a particular style of parenting? Usually an individual does not purposely choose a particular parenting style. Rather, a set of circumstances works together to determine the style followed by parents. The type of parenting an individual experienced when he or she was a child is a strong influence. For example, parents who grew up in strongly authoritarian homes may assume this is the only way to parent. They may be unfamiliar with other styles of parenting. Even if parents dislike the parenting style in which they were raised, they may follow it because this was the parenting model they experienced.

An individual's personal temperament also affects the style of parenting. People who have rigid beliefs about behavior and high standards of performance would be unlikely to follow a permissive parenting style. Highly communicative people who value others' opinions would be uncomfortable with the authoritarian parenting style.

The community in which one lives and pressure from friends and relatives will also affect parenting style. Current attitudes about parenting also influence the parenting style one follows.

Though these factors affect an individual's parenting style, concerted effort on the part of parents can change parenting behavior. No one needs to parent children in a fashion that is not to their liking. Consider the case of Dean.

CASE IN POINT

Dean grew up in a home with authoritarian parenting. He had never heard this word to describe the way his parents related to him and his sister. Dean knew that his family had "hard and fast rules" about behavior. He also knew that his parents punished him when he disobeyed these rules. Dean always knew what would happen if he did not meet his parents' expectations, and he felt good that the rules were clearly defined. However, there were some things about his parents' type of parenting that Dean disliked. He felt that he was not as close to his father or mother as he would like because their strictness prevented his being open with them. When Dean became a parent he decided that having a close relationship with his son was more important than enforcing absolute rules. Dean enrolled in a parenting class at the high school evening program. He is learning how to involve his son in the rules and decisions of their family. Dean also learned that different people need different parenting styles. The authoritarian style may have been right for Dean's parents but it was not right for him.

Current Trends in Parenting

Our society's philosophy and attitude toward parenting changes with time. During the 1940s and into the 1950s, a permissive style of parenting was popular. This seemed to be a reaction to authoritarian parenting styles of earlier periods.

What is the current trend in parenting? Current thought and action in both sexual and racial equality lead people to respect the rights of all individuals. The democratic parenting style allows for the respect and rights of children within a structure of guidance and nurturing. The nature of the parent-child relationship does not allow the child to have a voice in all aspects of behavior. Indeed, the law holds parents responsible for their children's behavior and in doing so expects parents to have authority over their children. Yet, many areas of the parent-child relationship provide opportunities for children to make democratic choices among various alternatives.

We might ask ourselves which parenting style is most practical in terms of realistically preparing children for adult life. In real life people do not function without rules or guidelines. Adults face many structures and limitations within which they must function. The permissive parenting style with its absence of guidance and rules does not realistically prepare children for adult roles. The authoritarian style is also unrealistic since it represents exacting standards with no opportunities to be a part of the decision-making process.

The democratic parenting style seems to lend itself to the needs of today's society. In real life, people have the right and responsibility to take part in decision making. People need to play an active role in society. In the future, young people will need to be able to make decisions in many areas and on many issues not yet known. They will need practice and experience in democratic decision making. Neither blind acceptance of rules and regulations nor total lack of rules will help children to function well in our society.

PARENTHOOD MYTHS

A **myth** is a widely accepted belief or set of ideas which is unrealistic or unfounded. Myths contain elements of truth and reality. It is sometimes difficult to separate the truth from the falsehood, the realistic from the unrealistic.

There are strong myths related to parenthood. Over the years people have romanticized parenthood and parenting. They have created a fantasy of what parenthood is all about. There is nothing wrong with maintaining a pretty picture of parenthood if we realize that the picture sometimes changes. Confusing the myths of parenthood with the reality of parenthood can be detrimental to the parent-child relationship as well as to the husband-wife relationship. Consider the case of Marla and David.

CASE IN POINT

For years, Marla had dreamed of being a mother. When she was in high school she liked to care for small children. She loved the dependency of tiny infants, she liked the curiosity of preschoolers, and she enjoyed the excitement for learning that school children seem to possess. David, too, liked children. He and Marla often watched parents and children in the park and in grocery stores. They discussed parenting, and they looked forward to the day when they would have their own baby and be part of the world of parenting.

Marla and David had enjoyable months of preparation. Their parents were thrilled with the idea of a grandchild. Baby clothes, furniture, and toys were collected. Names were chosen. Marla and David enjoyed the attention given by friends, neighbors, and relatives throughout the pregnancy. They were excited about bringing their new baby home.

As the weeks passed, Marla and David discovered that their new life was not as rosy as depicted in the baby magazines. They had not realized how physically exhausting parenting could be. They did not realize they would be so tied down with little opportunity to get out and enjoy themselves. The continuous needs of the baby began to make them feel trapped, and this made them feel guilty. They loved and wanted this baby, but somehow the whole situation was different from what they had expected.

The experience of Marla and David is an example of how the parenthood myth can be detrimental to family relationships. Books and magazines, television, family members, and friends can establish a glossy picture of what parenting is all about. Parents and friends may not mean to be deceptive. As they recall situations and incidents in their own parenting experiences, they probably remember the positive situations. Even the negative situations of parenthood that they relay may take on a whimsical or humorous aspect. Books and magazines may purposely portray a romantic side of parenthood. An advertisement with a handsome couple in a sunny setting with a beautiful, smiling baby will likely sell more diapers, soap, or baby food.

Television, particularly the daily soap operas, extends the myth of parenting. Only the lovely moments of parenthood are shown. The young child is frequently talked about but is napping or playing somewhere else. Seldom does the birth of a child have a negative effect on the lifestyle of the characters.

How can the realities be separated from the myths of parenthood? This is not an easy task. The difficulty is that there is some truth in most myths and we must guard against negating all of what the myths suggest. Consider the following myths of parenthood and the alterations that bring these myths closer to reality.

Myth: Raising children is fun.

Reality: Raising children is exciting, stimulating, and enjoyable. It is also a time-consuming and difficult job.

The reality of this myth is highlighted by the fact that parenting is a tough job. Few tasks in life are as extensive as that of parenting. Being with children is an enjoyable, stimulating, and exciting part of life. Children cause people to think and act differently. People participate and become involved in activities they might otherwise miss. Yet, to say that raising children is constant fun is inaccurate. Fun implies that there is the choice of participation. Tennis or fishing are fun because you can do these things at your leisure. A fun activity implies a take-it-or-leave-it situation. Raising children is not take-it-or-leave-it. It is a fulltime, 24-hour-per-day responsibility.

Myth: If you are a good parent your children will turn out well.

Reality: Parents are an important influence on their children, but there are many other influences.

Many people like this myth, especially those whose children have been successful. It is unfair, however, for parents to take total credit the outcome of their children's development. There are many outside forces that exert negative as well as positive influences. Schools, peers, media, and society in general are some of the forces that can assist or counteract a parent's influence. Parents must concede that they are not the only influence on their children. Furthermore, parents cannot guarantee the success and happiness of their children.

Myth: Children are sweet and cute.

Reality: Children can be cute, sweet, and adorable. They can also be irritating, unpleasant, and nasty.

In both the myth and reality, the terms cute and sweet refer to behavior and actions of the child rather than the appearance of the child. It is true that children are clever and their comments and behavior take on a charming and delightful style unique to children. It is necessary, however, that people also be aware of the less desirable qualities of children. They frequently behave stubbornly and display irritating behavior that requires high levels of patience and understanding.

It would be unfair to consider all adult behavior as warm and loving. Likewise, it is unfair to consider all child behavior as cute and sweet.

The dangerous aspect of the myth is that when parents see their child's unexpected, unpleasant behavior they may blame themselves. They assume that their own inappropriate parenting practices have caused this behavior. Further, parents may be unprepared to deal with their children's unpleasant actions. In their frustration, they may react with physically abusive behavior.

By clarifying these myths, we do not remove the joy and happiness of parenting. Rather, we reveal more realistic aspects—both positive and negative—of being a parent. The more realistic our expectations of parenting, the better we can meet the needs of children and the entire family.

WORKING TOWARD INDEPENDENCE

Throughout the parenting years, the child moves from dependence to independence. This is a gradual process. The process may include minor setbacks when children temporarily regress to more immature behavior. For example, the birth of a sibling, the death of a grandparent, or other changes in family lifestyle may cause children to regress to earlier, safer days of infancy. For the most part, however, children move toward managing more of their own affairs and making more of their own decisions.

Most parents attempt to guide their children toward responsible, independent adult life. Parenting behaviors that cluster around the democratic style of parenting seem best able to prepare young people for responsible adulthood.

Key components of parenting that can help young people to move toward responsible, independent adulthood include the following.

Modeling

Do actions speak louder than words? Your parents, and other adults, have been models for you. Which have you attended to most—their actions or their words? Telling children not to swear does little good if a parent uses

Spotlight on issues

Foster Care

What happens to children when a family crisis makes it impossible for them to remain with their natural parents? If extended family members cannot help, foster care may be the answer. Depending on the circumstances, foster care may be short-term or long-term, voluntary or court-ordered, in a family or an institution.

SHORT-TERM FOSTER CARE • Sometimes parents may need to reorganize their lives, to correct personal or psychological problems, or to regain financial stability. Consider the following situations.

Ed and Paula were experiencing some marital problems. They fought frequently and began to abuse their son, Nick. When a physician reported Nick's repeated and severe bruises to the county court, the boy was placed in temporary foster care. Ed and Paula received special counseling for their marital problems and for their abusive behavior. After four months, Nick was able to return to his parents.

Raquel is a 17-year-old single parent. Her father is dead, and her mother is not well enough to help Raquel care for her baby girl, Carmen. The baby's father left the community before the delivery. Raquel has been receiving some public financial assistance, and until recently she had been working part-time. She has to finish three months of school before she can graduate. She has agreed to voluntarily place 9-month-old Carmen in a foster situation so she can complete school, work with counselors to find employment and, in general, get her life in order. Like Ed and Paula, Raquel will be able to visit her child during the foster care period. In both of these cases, the outcome of foster care is potentially positive. This is not always the case, however.

LONG-TERM FOSTER CARE • Long-term foster care has generally had a less positive history. In some cases, children are unable to return to their homes yet are also unable to be placed in permanent homes through adoption. If the child's parents cannot settle their problems and are unwilling to put the child up for adoption, the child may have to be shuffled from one foster home to another. This is one of the worst aspects of long-term foster care.

In fact, the average foster child has been in the public care system for approximately eight years and has lived in three different homes.

FOSTER PARENTS • Foster parents are people who love and understand children. They must have strength and sensitivity to take in children who have lived with trauma and frustration and who have often lost trust in others. Regardless of the reason for foster care, the child experiences a dramatic and stressful change when entering a new environment. The child may feel and express anger, hostility, and/or depression.

Foster parents are supervised by social workers and are obligated to allow visits by natural parents. Foster parents must also promote the child's relationships in school, around the neighborhood, and with their own children. Few foster parents receive enough money to provide adequate care. Yet, many foster parents find that the presence of foster children strengthens their lives and their families. This much-needed service to others often brings with it rewards for the foster family as well as for the foster child.

profane language. "Don't ever let me catch you smoking" has little meaning if the parent has a cigarette in hand. Children model adult behavior far more than we realize. Parents must "practice what they preach" or their words will do little good.

Parents can do some of the best guiding and teaching through intentional modeling (Figure 12-3). Grooming, speech, patience, and confronting fears can be handled well through the modeling process. Observing a parent's responsible actions during a storm or other danger can provide an excellent model of behavior.

Guidance

Children need guidelines and rules. They need a structure or framework within which they can function. Most children do best when they have been given some basic rules but can choose among alternatives within these rules. A small child may be told he or she cannot bother the things on the top shelf, but he or she can choose to play with anything on the two lower shelves. A preteen may be able to walk to a shopping area or the movies, but must not go alone and must be home at a specific time.

Guidance and rules give people a sense of security. People are aware of their limits and can make decisions accordingly.

Consistency

Parents need to be consistent with their children. The guidelines or rules, the consequences of not following the rules, and parental behavior in general should remain consistent. If running across the street is

Figure 12-3

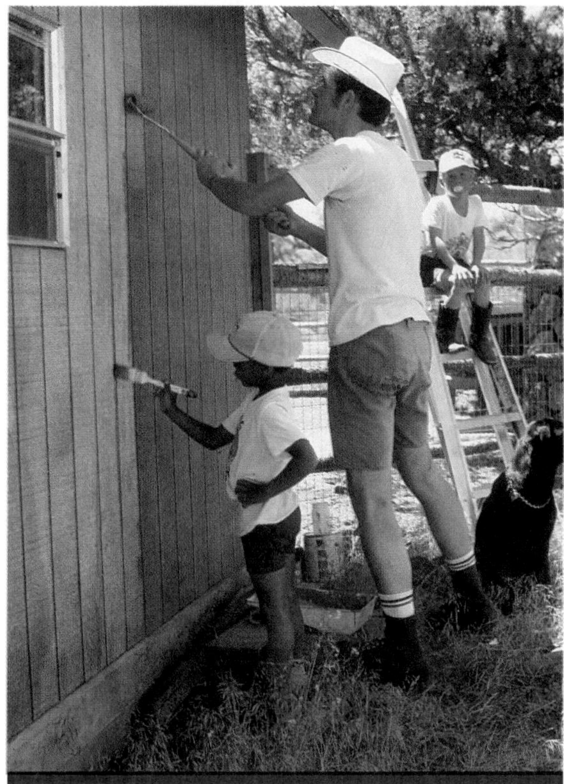

Parents model behavior for their children. This parent is showing his son that he values his son's ability to help with household chores.
H. Armstrong Roberts

wrong on Wednesday it should also be wrong on Friday. The discipline for disobedience should be the same for both cases.

As children grow older they can begin to understand variations in parental behavior. A particular curfew may be altered for a special occasion. Rules regarding use of the car may be overlooked when the neighbor's injury needs emergency medical treatment. Yet, even for adolescents, general consistency of treatment provides security and stability. We are more confident when we know what to expect.

Consequences

Allowing children to realize the consequences of their behavior can be a useful parenting tool. For example, if a child does not eat his or her dinner, there will be no dessert. If a young person stays out too late, he or she cannot use the car. Such consequences can be effective when made clear before the situation arises.

Consequences that are natural to the behavior are even more effective. If a child runs too fast down a steep sidewalk he or she may fall. If a child is continually late for dinner he or she will not be able to enjoy conversation with the family. Parents who allow the child to face such natural consequences are helping the child understand consequences that will be faced in adult life. For example, driving too fast may result in an auto accident; being late to work may result in being fired.

Respect

Regardless of the situation, the parent needs to communicate respect to the child. Though a child may have made a major error in judgment or has deliberately gone against a person's wishes, the parent must show respect to the child as a worthwhile person. This is particularly difficult in times of anger and frustration.

When children are shown unconditional respect they too develop this respect for the parent. Regardless of disagreements, differing points of view, and situations that generate anger, a parent and child can treat each other fairly and with respect.

Parental Needs

As you investigate the process of parenting, it becomes clear that the way parents feel about themselves will affect the method of parenting. Parents who have a personal need to make demands and have these demands met may follow the strict authoritarian style of parenting. Parents who need to be needed and have developed few interests other than parenting may discourage their children's independence.

Parents need to strive to be well-adjusted people who feel good about themselves and their way of life. They cannot depend on their children's achievements or limitations. But, as children grow, so must their parents. The parents' lifestyle must change as they enter new stages.

Support groups or growth groups are becoming more common. In these groups, parents of children of similar ages and stages share concerns about parenting and learn to grow in new areas of self-fulfillment.

SUBSTITUTE PARENTING

Earlier in the chapter, we indicated that the term *parenting* included people who were not necessarily the child's parent. Many people who are not parents perform parenting. Neighbors, day care providers, teachers, coaches, relatives, social workers, and baby-sitters are involved in parenting (see Figure 12-4). As the segments of our society become more interrelated and our lives more strongly affect those around us, it becomes necessary to think of all people in the parenting process.

What parenting style do you feel takes place in our schools? in our libraries? Is the respect for children maintained in the coaching of all sports? When children accept adult responsibilities as consumers are they treated with the same respect as adults?

Substitute parents—those people our society entrusts in various parenting roles—need to be aware of the important tasks they confront. Not only are they responsible for the jobs they perform (coaching a sport, teaching religion, instructing in dance, etc.) but they also are models for character. They

Figure 12-4

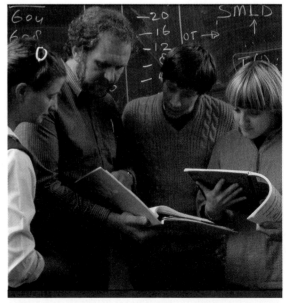

Teachers are one example of substitute parents.
IBM Corporation

help young people to grow toward independence.

Selecting Parent Substitutes

When selecting persons who will carry out substitute parenting roles, parents need to clearly state their philosophies of parenting. Some substitute parents' beliefs and practices may be the opposite of the parents' beliefs. For example, the combination of a permissive parent with an authoritarian child care worker or babysitter may cause frustration for parent, child, and employee. It is a parent's responsibility to avoid such confusion by selecting substitutes who are compatible with their own parenting style.

When interviewing people who may serve as substitute parents—a babysitter, a day care worker, or a household worker who may interact with children—it is important to learn about their parenting style. The following are examples of questions that parents can use to learn the potential substitute's methods and techniques of dealing with children.

- Do you think children should have rules?
- If so, who should establish these rules?
- What do you do when a child does something you cannot accept?
- What do you do when a child deliberately misbehaves?
- What would you do if a child questioned a rule you expected her or him to follow?
- What kind of choices does a child have related to behavior?
- Do you think a child needs to know what behavior is expected in a given situation?
- Do you think noisy children are bad children? Are quiet children good children?

Helping Children with Substitute Parents

Many substitute parents are not chosen directly by the parent. Parents do not usually select school teachers, park supervisors, police officers, and other public personnel. Such people, who act as parent substitutes, may have extremely different parenting styles. If this is the case, the parent can help the child by pointing out these differences in an objective and non-critical way. Regardless of these differences, the child will continue to be in contact with the substitute parent; a parent's critical or disrespectful comments will only aggravate the situation. Most children will accept the fact that different people have different ideas and ways of behaving. Parents can show respect for the substitute parents' beliefs and actions while explaining that their own actions and beliefs are different. The following statements are examples of how parents can help their children with differences in parenting practices.

- "I know that Mr. Garcia allows people to speak that way in his class. But I find it offensive, and I can't allow you to talk that way to me."
- "Ms. McFarland may let you paint without rules for clean-up, but when you paint here you need to wipe the counter and wash the brushes."
- "If you don't like the way we do things here at home you can tell us what's bothering you and we'll try to work it out. But Mr. Phillips is your teacher and he expects you to follow his rules in the classroom."
- "Even if Mrs. Carson doesn't make you wash your hands before snacks, I think you should wash whenever you sit down to eat. It is better to get rid of as many germs as possible. I'm sure Mrs. Carson wouldn't mind if you asked to wash your hands."

Sometimes parents can take action to change the parenting behavior of substitute parents. For example, if a teacher is too authoritarian or too permissive in the classroom, parents can take action to alter this situation. Conferences with the teacher, school administrator, and discussion with parent groups can assist in such situations. Participation in citizen groups can help assure well-coordinated parenting practices both at home and in society.

EDUCATION FOR PARENTING

Until the past several decades there was little study or deliberate learning involved in becoming a parent. People relied on their observations and experiences to gain parenting skills. Little thought was given to methods of parenting. People generally followed the pattern set forth by their parents.

Need for Parenting Education

Families today are probably of less assistance in providing parenting knowledge than were families of the past. Today, fewer people have had the opportunity to learn about parenting from their parents. With smaller families, the siblings are clustered close together in age. Young people with one sibling close to their age cannot usually recall observing many parenting practices for small children. Furthermore, today's increased mobility makes it less likely that young parents can rely on their families for guidance and assistance in parenting.

Parents of differing backgrounds may find they are good candidates for parenthood education. Two people who join together to raise children may find that their philosophies of parenting are not the same. Different experiences in family background and lifestyles, places in the family (first child, only child, etc.), and communities can create different expectations of parenthood. Parent education that allows both parents to bring forth their ideas, beliefs, and expectations of parenthood can help a couple reach a mutually acceptable idea of parenting.

Changes in society are another reason for parenting education. Increased numbers of working parents, earlier sexual involvement of adolescents, earlier schooling of children, and drug and alcohol abuse are some of the social changes that bring about new and unique parenting issues. These issues need to be considered carefully for their impact on parenting practices.

Though many of us respect and admire our parents and the job they did in raising us, we may wish to consider other ways of raising our children. The changes in society that alter expectations of parenting encourage many young parents to consider education for parenting a necessity.

Opportunities for Parent Education

There are many opportunities to learn about parenting, parenting styles, and the development of children. Organizations such as the Red Cross, PTA, YMCA, and March of Dimes sponsor national programs for parenting. Your local school system, religious organizations, and public radio and television may also provide parenting assistance.

These parenting programs focus on various aspects of parenting. (See Figure 12-5.) Classes

Figure 12-5

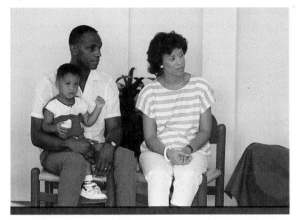

Parents who participate in parenting education classes report positive results. Classes help parents improve their parenting skills by providing information on infant care, discipline, and parent-child communication.

are available on infant care, child development, discipline, parent-child communication, values, sex education, and adolescence. Most parents who participate in parenting education report positive results. They feel they benefit from exposure to other techniques and philosophies within the process of parenting.

Helping a child grow from dependence to independence is the major task of the parenting family. Understanding this process and knowing the various styles and myths of parenting can make the parenting family stage an exciting and rewarding part of the life cycle.

WRAPPING IT UP

Parenting is the process of meeting the needs and wants of another person. The parenting family is one in which children are involved, from the prenatal through the adolescent stages of the human life span. ***Effective parenting*** involves deciding to parent at a time when you are ready to assume this difficult, yet rewarding, role. Effective parents respect the rights of their children, and meet their children's needs for love, acceptance, and guidance.

The decision to become a parent is as important as the decision to marry. Because of the costs involved in raising children, in combination with the heavy responsibilities that parents must assume in caring for children, more people today are choosing to remain childless. Many others are delaying parenthood decisions until they believe they are ready to assume this role.

Factors of readiness include knowledge of child development and child care procedures, acceptance of the fact that parenting requires patience and high levels of energy, and a willingness to set aside personal priorities in favor of the child's needs. All of these factors imply the importance of emotional maturity on the part of parents. In addition, readiness for parenting includes having an adequate income and an agreement between mother and father as to the equality involved in both the rewards and the tasks involved in the care of the child.

There are three major styles of parenting: authoritarian, democratic, and permissive. Authoritarian parents have rigid rules and demand strict child obedience and submission. Children have little power relative to parents. Permissive parents allow children to do whatever they want, with little guidance. Democratic parents combine aspects of authoritarian and permissive parenting but in a more balanced way than either of these extremes. Children raised in a democratic setting are more self-confident, well-adjusted, responsible, and prosocial in their behavior than are children raised in either the authoritarian or permissive contexts.

How you parent is a result of many influences. These include following the way you were parented, observations of friends and relatives in their parenting roles, and your personal temperament. It is important to understand that people have the ability to change the way they parent if they are unhappy with their current parenting styles.

Many *myths* exist in regard to parenting. Parenting myths are accurate in some respects, but inaccurate in others. Such myths as, "Children are always fun, cute, and sweet," lead to unrealistic expectations and, possibly, frustration and disappointment when children behave otherwise. Overly harsh treatment of children, including child abuse, is often the result of unrealistic expectations held by parents who are under stress.

As children grow older, they strive to achieve independence—to be their own person. In doing so, it is important to realize the role that parents have in fostering this development. Parents are models for their children. Children observe their parents' behavior and adopt those behavior patterns for themselves. Parents must establish fair and firm rules for effective child guidance and enforce them in a consistent and reasonable manner. Children must learn to understand that their behavior has consequences, either positive or negative. This is best achieved when parents have the knowledge, patience, and willingness to guide their children in a respectful manner.

Through contacts outside the family, children are exposed to many other adults who are *substitute parents* at one time or another. Teachers, coaches, day care workers, and others often must fill in for parents when the child is out of the home. These individuals are important influences on the child's development.

Many community programs exist today to educate parents to be more effective. We know much more today about how to achieve effective parenting skills than ever before in our society. Such social changes as growing numbers of working parents, earlier schooling of children, earlier sexual involvement of teenagers, and drug and alcohol abuse among children and adults also mean that parenting is more challenging than ever. Most parents who have enrolled in education for parenthood programs express satisfaction with the results. Effective parenting also means effective use of community resources.

Exploring Dimensions of Chapter Twelve

For Review

1• Explain four factors of readiness for parenthood.
2• Describe the three basic parenting styles.
3• List three myths of parenting and explain why they are myths.
4• Explain why parent education is needed today.
5• Give examples of substitute parents.

6. List and explain key components of parenting that help children move from dependence to independence.

For Consideration

1. Create an imaginary couple who are considering parenthood. Help them through guiding questions that will assist them in making this decision.
2. Explain the styles of parenting you hope to follow. What parts of the styles might you mix? Why?
3. Name several substitute parents who have been influential in your life. Why were they important to you?
4. Explain some important areas of life in which you've moved from dependence to independence. In what areas have you yet to move toward independence?
5. Some people think parenting classes should be mandatory. Explain why you agree or disagree.
6. Explain the importance of three key concepts of parenthood. Tell how you would implement these concepts.

For Application

1. Interview a couple with a young child. Ask them what aspect of parenthood has been most difficult, most surprising, most rewarding, and most detrimental to their marriage and to them as individuals.
2. Survey students in your school to learn the parenting style most hope to follow. (You'll need a good, brief explanation of the three styles.)
3. Survey your community to learn of available parent education programs. Who offers the programs? What is the focus of each program? What are the costs? How many people enroll? Describe the participants. (Males or females; low, medium, or high income; parents of infants, toddlers, young children, junior or senior high schoolers.)
4. Interview several substitute parents. Ask about their philosophies of parenting and how many parents request such information. Ask if their beliefs have conflicted with parents' beliefs.

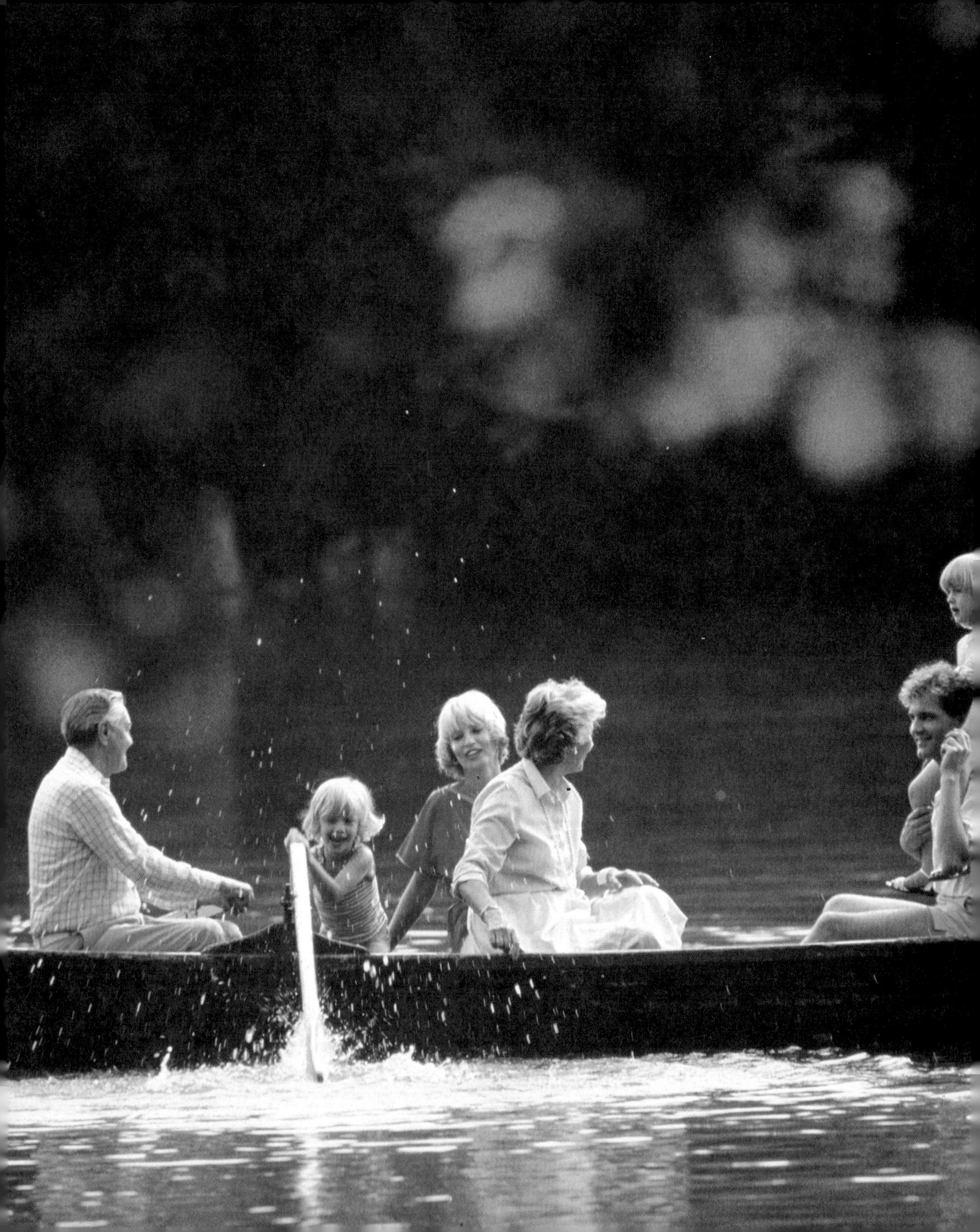

thirteen

EXPLORING FAMILY LIFE CYCLE ISSUES

This chapter provides information that will help you to:

- Recognize the various stages in the changing family life cycle.
- Understand the importance of the launching of children and the empty nest stage experienced by the married couple.
- Understand the problems and pleasures experienced by aging members in a family.
- Identify the five stages of accepting death and of accepting the death of a loved one.
- Know what makes a successful marriage and what leads to marriage instability.
- Recognize the process of disenchantment in a marriage.
- Understand the problems of infertility and methods used to correct such problems.
- Learn about blended families and the issues faced by members of such families.
- Recognize sexually transmitted diseases and their warning signs.
- Understand the crisis of domestic abuse in the forms of child abuse and violence in marriage.

In earlier chapters, we discussed the nature of change and development in the human life span. As is true for human development, families also move through a series of changes. In this chapter, we will examine some of the challenges and changes that contemporary families in the United States experience over the course of the family life cycle. These issues will affect you, the reader of this book, who will be an active participant in our families of the future.

THE CHANGING FAMILY LIFE CYCLE

Consider the following trends, each of which has been discussed in earlier chapters:

- People are marrying at older ages
- Married couples are delaying parenthood
- Married couples are having fewer children and are completing their childbearing at younger ages
- People are living longer

These trends have implications for the amount of time that adults spend in any one stage of the family life cycle. The **beginning family stage** lasts from marriage until the birth of the first child. Although postponing marriage until a later time would tend to shorten this stage, delaying parenthood has made this stage longer than it was in past generations. However, the **childbearing family stage** has been shortened by the fact that couples are having fewer children and are completing their childbearing at younger ages than ever before. This also means that the **parenting family stage**, where preschoolers, school-agers, and adolescents are present, is also shorter. Finally, the fact that we are living longer means that the last two stages of the family life cycle—the **launching family stage** and the **aging family stage**—are significantly longer than ever before in our society.

These changes result in an increase in the time married couples spend alone in the family life cycle; that is, without children present. In terms of the number of years added, the most significant of these changes involves the final two stages of the family life cycle: the launching and aging family stages.

LAUNCHING FAMILY MEMBERS

Launching is the process by which a family sends children forth in the world to establish independence from their parents, gain an education, earn their own living, and form families of their own.

The launching process is sometimes abrupt, such as when a child leaves home to live in a foreign country where the distance from home prohibits visitations. More often, the process is long-term and progressive. Such is the case when over the years a young person spends a portion of the summer away from home. Later, the young person lives away from home to attend college but returns home periodically. Still later, a job or marriage pulls the young person toward a new home and family. This slow, gradual process seems to be more easily adjusted to than the abrupt launching. The gradual process allows young people to experience independence by degrees yet continue receiving large measures of support from families. Parents, too, begin to relinquish their responsibility to their children in a gradual manner, thus easing the adjustment process.

Ritual and ceremony may be involved in this launching process. Graduation and weddings often serve as official recognition of the launching stage (Figure 13-1).

In the late 1980s, we are starting to see an increase in the number of young adults over the age of 19 who continue to live with their parents. More families are experiencing an extended amount of time with their adult children due to this delayed launching process. For example, in 1960, 43 percent of 18- to 24-year-old adults were living in their parents' home. By 1986, this number increased to 53 percent. Young men (59 percent) in this age group were more likely than young women (47 percent) to be living with parents. Sometimes this arrangement occurs because of financial difficulties experienced by the young adult who is unable to afford a separate household. It may also occur because young people today are choosing to marry at older ages. College students who continue to live at home while attending college also extend this launching period.

It is too early to tell if this arrangment is causing stress or hardship for a significant number of families. What do you think? What difficulties are likely to arise when young adults are not launched from the home until they are well into their adulthood years?

Figure 13-1

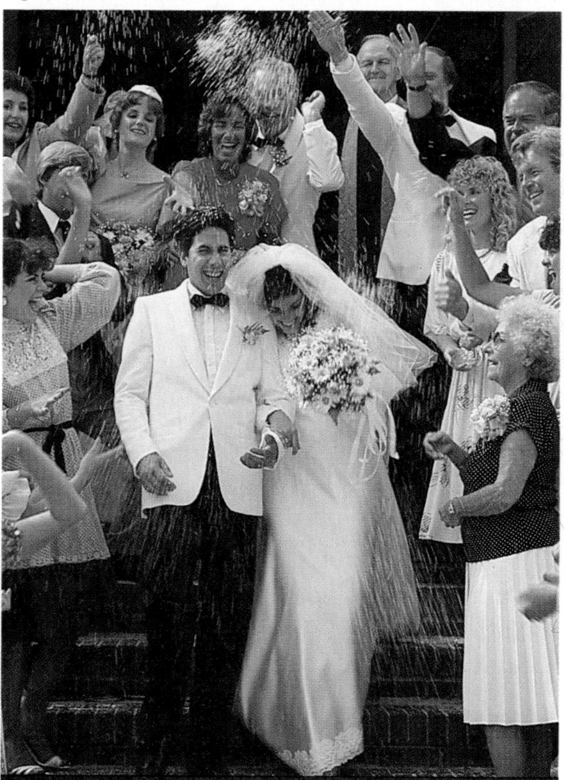

The wedding ceremony serves as an official recognition of the launching stage.

Roy Morsch/The Stock Market

EMPTY NEST

The **empty nest stage** refers to the period after all children have been launched. Parents return to being a couple or a single person without children in the home. The married couple faces issues of re-establishing their lives *as a couple* rather than *as parents*. The single parent faces issues related to remaining single or considering a serious personal relationship.

Fifty years ago, researchers reported that the empty nest stage was a stressful period for parents, especially for the mother. Most mothers at that time were full-time homemakers. Launching their children brought an end to the need for many of their services. For many people, the empty nest stage was stress-producing.

Today, as in earlier generations, some people may experience stress, frustration, or even depression as the stage begins. For the most part, however, this stage seems to be easily accepted by both men and women. This increased acceptance of the empty nest stage is related in part to fewer mothers having devoted themselves to full-time child care. More mothers today are employed throughout their children's lives or re-enter the work force when their children are school age. Therefore, though a mother's life changes when her children are launched, her daily activities may not be radically altered. This is also true for women who are highly involved in volunteer, community, or political endeavors.

Another factor related to greater acceptance of the empty nest stage affects both males and females. After launching children, most fathers and mothers are at the prime of their middle years. Middle age, usually considered from ages 45–65, appears to be a positive experience for most people. Typically, middle-agers are employed, have good health, and are beginning to enjoy some aspects of life which they could not financially afford earlier. In past decades, men and women were older when they launched their children and entered the empty nest stage. There was also a shorter life span. Thus, people had fewer years remaining after the launching stage. Now people can have many years of increased leisure, increased work and life pleasures, and increased years as a married couple after their children are grown (Figure 13-2).

Figure 13-2

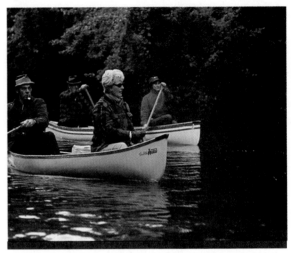

Married couples can have many years of increased leisure time once their children are launched and gone from the home.

The years after children have departed from the home are not only happy years for most parents, but they also are important in terms of tasks to be accomplished. Middle age is considered a preparation for the aging years. Developmental tasks completed during middle age are major determiners of a successful aging period. Some of these tasks include the following:

- Renewing and redefining the marital relationship
- Maintaining ties with children and their families
- Maintaining and strengthening ties with siblings, parents, and other members of extended families
- Preparing for retirement years both financially and emotionally
- Participating in community social life

AGING FAMILIES

The aging process is the passage from one stage to another. It continues from birth to death. However, most people refer to aging as the stage a person experiences from age 65 until death.

In Chapter 9, it was noted that people 65 and over comprise the fastest growing age group in our society. This means that a rapidly growing number of people are in this stage of the family life cycle.

The aging stage is difficult for many during the final years prior to death. At this late aging period, people may become infirm with some mentally and/or physically limiting factors, thus contracting in terms of abilities and functioning. For the most part, however, the aging years can promote growth and activities that are stimulating and meaningful.

Aging People and the Family

Many couples in the aging stage remain totally independent and live in their own family for many years. Even after the death of one spouse, the other spouse may continue living independently. For various reasons, other aging people live with their children or other relatives.

Regardless of their dwelling place, aging people can add much to a family's well-being. Their services and support to the family and community are often necessary. When grandchildren are present, strong and rewarding bonds are often formed between grandchild and grandparent. Grandparents may have the time and patience that a busy parent does not always have. Aging parents may provide both financial and moral support and assistance to a young family. Likewise, being needed by one's family can provide increased self-esteem in the aging family member.

Interaction in a three-generation family requires respect for the beliefs and values of others. Furthermore, when three generations reside together some basic understanding should be established in order for all members to maintain their self-respect and live in harmony. Successful three-generation families who reside together have the following common characteristics:

- The mother and father, *not* the grandparents, are the final authority in matters related to the children.
- There is a basic similarity of lifestyle of the family members.
- Each family member has clearly understood duties or responsibilities in the home.
- Communication between members is positive and meaningful.
- Mechanisms, such as family meetings, are used to coordinate activities.
- Each family member has a place belonging to him or her alone in order to retreat in privacy.

DEATH

We cannot consider individual or family life cycle stages without considering death. Death, as much as birth, is a part of the human life cycle. You must accept your own eventual death and the death of family members as a reality of life.

Facing and accepting death is not always easy. Our society seldom allows face-to-face contact with death. Most commonly, people die in hospitals and few of us experience the death scene. Death becomes distant and touches our lives less directly. People seldom talk about death, and when they do they use vague terms in place of the words *die* or *death*. Consider the phrases "he left us," "she passed away," and "gone to rest."

Yet, despite the shielding from death in our society, the result of death requires our dealing with grief and loss as well as eventually facing our own death. Being able to acknowledge and accept death is a major task of the life cycle.

It is considered most healthy to deal openly and honestly with the topic of death. When telling children or peers about death or when facing death ourselves, honesty is necessary in order to minimize the impact of death. Particularly when dealing with small children, dishonest though well-meant statements can be dangerous. Telling a child, "Grandmother has taken a long rest" indicates that Grandmother will later wake up. It also encourages refusal to sleep since the child may fear not waking again. Other statements such as, "Daddy went away," "Uncle Jim died because he was sick," or "She took a long journey," are deceiving. The child may interpret such phrases as the person deserted them, sickness always brings death, or travel and journeys cause death. Children, like adults, need honest, simple explanations of death. Providing experiences with pets and plants allows children to see death as a normal part of life.

Stages of Accepting Death

Experts in the study of death, **thanatology**, indicate that there are distinct stages a person passes through in the process of accepting an impending death due to illness. By studying people who knew they were terminally ill, the well-known thanatologist Elisabeth Kubler-Ross found that a person moves through five apparent stages in order to reach acceptance of one's death.

First Stage—Denial: The person denies that this is true and will say the statement is wrong or can't be true. This stage helps cushion the impact that death is inevitable.

Second Stage—Anger: The person resents and is angered by people who are in good health and are not dying. Sometimes the anger is vented on other people or on God.

Third Stage—Bargaining: The person realizes approaching death but bargains with self or God to do good things and thereby be saved. Often the bargain involves gaining time to live in return for good deeds.

Fourth Stage—Depression: The person grieves for the things not done in life and mourns the approaching death. This period of quietness and introspection signals that the person is getting ready for death.

Fifth Stage—Acceptance: The person calmly accepts the reality of death.

These stages are not neat and orderly. The person may move back and forth in an attempt to reach the final stage of acceptance and yet still fight this acceptance. Many people do not go through this process because they lack time or consciousness. Accidents, illnesses, coma, or sudden death do not provide this introspection.

Awareness of the stages can help family and friends accept the dying person's feelings and help with this process. In addition, awareness of the stages of a dying person's behavior can help family members respond appropriately. Figure 13-3 provides such guidance.

Figure 13-3

Guidelines for Handling the Five Stages of Dying

Behavior of the Dying Person	*Response of Family or Friends*
Denial Searches frantically for a favorable diagnosis. Dying person says, "It can't happen to me."	Understand why person is denying reality. Be patient and willing to talk.
Anger Shows deep anger. Bitterly envies those who are well. Complains incessantly about almost everything. Dying person says, "Yes, but why me?"	Treat with respect and understanding, not by returning anger. Realize dying person is angry over the coming loss of everything: family, friends, work, home, etc.
Bargaining Dying person says, "I'll bargain with God and get a time extension." Makes promises of good behavior in return for time and freedom from physical pain.	This stage passes quickly. If the dying person reveals "bargain," listen and act as a sounding board. Don't brush off the comments.
Depression The dying person grieves and mourns the approaching death.	Let the dying person express sorrow and grieve fully. Attempts to cheer the person will do little good. Be a listener.
Acceptance The dying person is neither angry nor depressed. Quietly and calmly has accepted approaching death.	It is time merely for the presence of close family and friends. Little talk is required.

SOURCE: Adapted from Elisabeth Kubler-Ross, *On Death and Dying*, Macmillan Publishing Co., New York, 1974.

Family Reactions to Death

Death of a family member usually makes us fearful. If our sibling, parent, grandparent, spouse, or child dies, it is concrete proof that we could die too and that death is final. Adjustment to a family member's death is only possible when we apply honesty and when we can share feelings. We work through this fear and discomfort through the grief process. **Grief** is the pain, discomfort, and feelings that most people have after the death of someone they love. The grief process follows basically similar stages as the stages for acceptance of death by the dying person. First the person goes through shock and denial. During this period the person denies that the death has taken place. The person may seem dazed and unable to comprehend the death. The second stage focuses on anger. Anger could be focused at:

- The physicians involved
- The person at fault in an accident
- Themselves, because they are living and the other person died
- The dead person, because they left the family member alone.

The third stage involves subconscious bargaining related to good work if the family member could be returned to life. Such bargaining includes statements such as "If only I could see her once more, I'd be the best husband to her!" Such a bargain, stated or thought, indicates that acceptance of the death is not yet complete.

The fourth stage is intense pain and feelings of real loss. This stage may appear to be unhealthy, but it reflects a psychological necessity if the person is to adjust to death. During this stage, people may dream of the dead person. Despair, hopelessness, and withdrawn behavior are part of this depression stage. Most people seem to need at least two or three months for this stage.

During the final stage of grieving, a person begins to accept the death and starts to put his or her life in order. Sleeping and eating become more normal; daily routines begin to fall into place. The person begins to think of the dead person with fondness, joy, and pleasure rather than pain.

Throughout the grief process the grieving person experiences many physical and emotional reactions to death. Sometimes we underestimate how our minds and bodies will react to the loss of a loved one.

Physical reactions can be an actual illness ranging from a cold to a major heart or respiratory problem. Other physical reactions are overwhelming tiredness or inability to sleep or eat. Some people report numbness or dazed response as if they are not quite sure of reality. An additional physical reaction relates to one's inability or unwillingness to cry or verbally vent anger. This results in a tight choking feeling in the throat. These physical reactions are very real during the grief process.

Emotional reactions are also strong. It is important that a person be able to express these emotions to others. Hiding, denying, or ignoring such feelings can be psychologically harmful.

A typical emotion felt at least to some extent by most people is **guilt**. Feelings that we could have done more to save an untimely death are common. Thoughts that we might have been nicer or a better person are frequently experienced. **Anger** against the dead person who "left me" or who "didn't prepare me for life alone" is also common. **Fear and anxiety** are also to be expected. Facing the world without a loved one is not easy. A new world and a new life await the grieving person, and the newness causes insecurity. Also, **relief and joy** may be part of the emotional reactions to death. When a loved one who has experienced long-term suffering dies, a person may feel relieved that their loved one's suffering has ended.

Understanding the stages of acceptance of death and the ways human bodies and minds react to death is helpful to us. We can begin to see death as part of the total life cycle. This knowledge prepares us to accept death. It cannot eliminate the pain of death. Some guidelines for working through the grief process include:

- Allow time to work through grief. Try to accept the death. Discuss the death with friends to help begin this acceptance.
- Accept the love and caring of friends and relatives. Allow them to help you and be near you.
- Recall the good relationship and the good times you shared with the dead person. Understand that grief is natural because of these positive times shared together.
- Postpone major decisions until thinking is clear and alternatives can be made clear.

The family structure contracts with the death of a family member. The roles formerly played by the dead person must be filled by others. Responsibilities and relationships will be altered. Some changes in the family will take place immediately. Other changes will not be complete for months or years.

The healthy family helps itself to bring about these changes. Family members are important sources of comfort during the grief period. They help each other by giving support and by providing a setting within which members can reveal their feelings and work through the grief process to acceptance and resolution.

ISSUES IN MARRIAGE ACROSS THE FAMILY LIFE CYCLE

In Chapter 11 we discussed the importance of marriage and the implications of divorce in our society. The majority of American adults marry at least one time, meaning that marriage remains a popular choice relative to permanent singlehood. People marry with the idea that it will be a permanent relationship ended only by the death of one spouse.

However, the rising divorce rate in our society signals that this commitment to permanence is not as strong as it was at one time in our society. Approximately 50 percent of today's young adults who marry for the first time can expect their first marriage to be terminated by divorce.

What is it that allows some people to establish and maintain satisfying marriage relationships over time? Why do others have difficulty doing so? How is it that men and women who are enough in love to get married somehow fall out of love over the years? The answers to these questions can be found in pressures and stresses that are faced over time in the family life cycle.

Is There a Key to Success in Marriage?

Few young people entering a marriage understand the difficulties involved in maintaining a satisfying marital relationship for both partners over the many years of the family life cycle. Some of the influences on a marriage are the *normal* stresses involved with work outside the home, bearing and raising children, moving to a new location, and launching children from the home. There are also unexpected crises that many families face at one time or another. Serious accidents or illnesses, loss of a job, death of a child or parent, and drug or alcohol abuse are just some of the unexpected stresses that families may face at some stage of the life cycle.

The simple passage of time further complicates matters. As shown in Chapter 9, adults change over the years. Hence, relationships such as marriage feel the effects of these changes that take place in marriage partners. Feelings of love may change as the newness of the marriage relationship wears off. A husband and wife may develop new interests that are not shared with each other. Marriage partners may come to take each other for granted, becoming disappointed with the loss of the intense feeling of romantic love that existed in the beginning stage of marriage.

SUCCESS VS. STABILITY IN MARRIAGE • In considering the changes that occur in marriage over the life cycle, it is important to define two terms: marriage success and marriage stability. **Marriage success** refers to the degree to which both marriage partners are fulfilling their goals and expectations over time. For most, this means feeling a certain degree of satisfaction with the way they communicate, make decisions, and share affection with their spouses. It is important to note, though, that goals and expectations are different from one marriage to the next. Thus, shared power in decision making may be a goal for one couple, whereas having one spouse or the other make the important decisions is a goal for another. Each marriage partner evaluates the success of marriage on the basis of what he or she expects to get out of the relationship.

Marriage stability, on the other hand, refers to whether or not the marriage remains intact over the years. Stable marriages are those in which partners stay together. Unstable marriages, on the other hand, are those which are affected by separation, divorce, or desertion. In considering the overall *quality* of a marriage, it is important to note that not all stable marriages are successful. That is, the partners may choose to remain together even if they are not happy or satisfied with the level at which they are achieving their goals in the relationship. For one reason or another, many poor quality marriages stay together—perhaps "for the sake of the children," or because of perceived social or religious disapproval if they were to divorce.

If we add to today's rate of divorce the number of couples in poor quality marriages who do not divorce, we are left with the fact that the number of truly successful marriages in our society is a minority of all marriages. Some experts estimate the number of successful marriages to be as low as 25 percent (one in four).

What distinguishes a successful marriage from an unsuccessful one? Why does marriage appear to be so fragile in today's society?

THE PROCESS OF DISENCHANTMENT • Recall from Chapter 11 the main reasons people today get married. We marry because we are romantically attached (in love) with another. We share common interests, attitudes, and values. The other person fulfills our needs for intimacy and acceptance, and we fulfill their needs. For these reasons, we choose to share our lives with each other through the commitment of marriage.

These very reasons for which we marry have a strong tendency to disappear over time. This is the **process of disenchantment**, and it poses a threat to the happiness and stability of any marriage. For one reason or another, those who marry because they have "fallen in love" experience a "falling out of love" as the years go by.

This process is depicted in Figure 13-4. Many studies show a "U-shaped" curve of marriage satisfaction as marriage changes over time. In the beginning stage, satisfaction tends to be high. This is because the marriage relationship is new and fresh. Feelings of romantic love are strong. Shared interests and activities create a strong bond between the married partners. However, the satisfaction curve begins to decline with time and the arrival of children. The happiness that people express

Figure 13-4

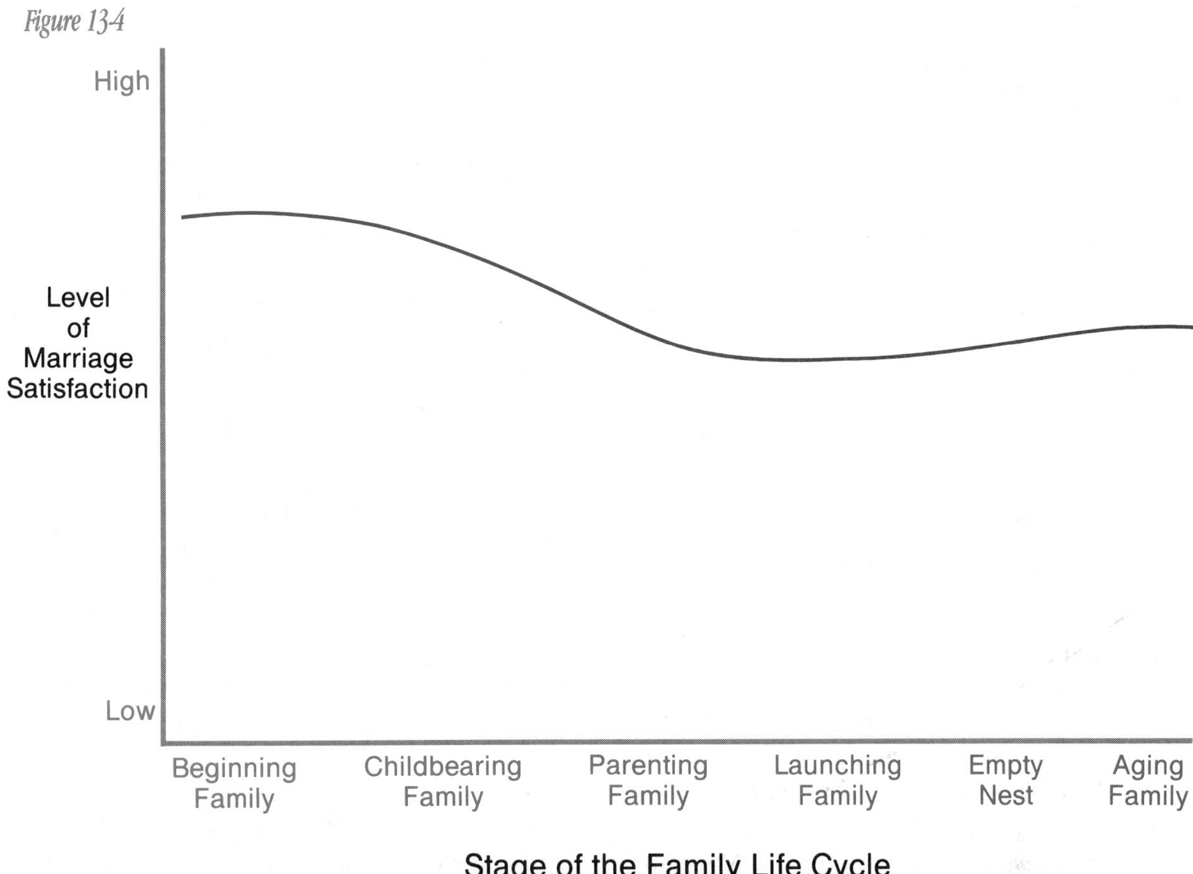

with the marriage gradually declines as children grow older. The curve reaches its lowest point when adolescent children are present in the family.

Then, with the launching years and movement into the empty nest and aging stages, the satisfaction curve reverses its downward trend. In these stages, the married couple has returned to the husband-wife relationship. The economic burden of the children tends to lessen. Retirement may bring a renewed opportunity to experience the fun of leisure activities that were forgone when growing children were present in the family. Note, however, that the level of satisfaction does not reach the high level of satisfaction that couples might have experienced in the beginning family stage.

The following factors, in one combination or another, contribute to this process of disenchantment:

- *Growing children in the home.* Children put a crunch on the parents' resources of time, money, and energy. With children present, and particularly as they grow older, it becomes increasingly difficult to maintain a high level of love, intimacy, shared activities, and communication that may have existed before the children arrived. The demands that children make on parents' resources reduce the availability of those resources that parents may need as *marriage partners* to maintain a satisfying relationship that is meeting their goals and expectations.

- *Role strain.* Along with the arrival and growing demands of children, parents are striving to balance the demands of work outside the home. As the family grows larger and children grow older, the financial needs of the family grow rapidly. Parents may find it difficult to keep up with rising costs. Also, today we are seeing a rapidly increasing number of two income families, in which both the husband and the wife work outside the home. The strain involved with work roles, in combination with demanding parenting roles, can place a tremendous stress on the marriage.

Spotlight on issues

Remarriage

The fact that more than 1 million married couples divorce each year means that some Americans are becoming disillusioned with the institution of marriage. Adding fuel to this belief is the fact that if today's rate of divorce continues, around 50 percent of young adults who marry in the late 1980s will be divorced some day. Yet, this belief that we are souring on the institution of marriage is not true.

One indication of this myth is the high rate of remarriage among those who divorce. Almost eight out of every ten people who divorce from their first marriage partners will enter a second marriage. In fact, most will do so in less than five years after their divorce. A growing proportion of all American marriages each year are actually remarriages of one or both of the partners (32 percent in 1977).

Not all divorced people are equally likely to remarry. Younger people are more likely to remarry than older people. Also, divorced men are more likely to remarry than divorced women. This means that young divorced men are most likely to remarry, while older divorced women are least likely to remarry. In addition, divorced parents are less likely to remarry than are divorced persons with no dependent children.

Hence, divorce is a temporary status for most people. Even after a negative experience with one marriage, contemporary American adults continue to prefer marriage over singlehood to satisfy needs for intimacy and companionship. But how satisfying and stable are remarriages? How do they fare in comparison to first marriages?

Studies show few differences in the overall level of happiness between people in first marriages and those in remarriages. The same factors which promote satisfying first marriages also apply to remarriages: exchange of love and intimacy, shared interests, companionship activities, and effective communication and conflict management. Divorce rates for remarriages are only slightly higher than for first marriages.

Nonetheless, remarriage partners face special concerns that those in first marriages do not face. Stress can be added if one or both partners bring children from a previous marriage into the remarriage. Stepparenting and blended family situations are challenging for all family members (as will be discussed later in this chapter). Remarried partners are less likely than others to be homogamous (similar) in terms of age, religion, education, and social class background. Also, stress may be added when ex-spouses of either remarried person live in the same neighborhood or community. Questions of continuing feelings for, and loyalty to, an ex-spouse may linger in the mind of a remarried person. Either partner may still be experiencing the trauma of the divorce from the first marriage partner.

The fact that a person entering a remarriage brings habits and patterns of interaction that were shaped in the first unsuccessful marriage further complicates matters. Some of these habits, such as ineffective communication and conflict management skills, may not be good ones. New patterns of household division of labor may run counter to a person's previous way of doing things. For example, a husband who was never expected to cook dinner in his first marriage may have difficulty when his second wife expects him to share the meal preparation responsibilities.

Despite the potential for problems in remarriages, many do survive without divorce and are successful. It appears that some people learn from mistakes made in previous marriages and strive to avoid repeating those mistakes. As long as the number of divorces in our society remains at its current level, the proportion of all marriages that are remarriages will continue to grow.

- *Decline in companionship and leisure time activities.* Many marriage partners experience a drop in the number of activities that they do together for fun and leisure. Such activities as going to a restaurant, going to a movie, dancing, or going to a sports or cultural event tend to fall by the wayside for some. This may be partly due to the married couple's attention being focused on children's activities. Married couples may also grow used to each other with the passage of time; that is, they begin to take each other for granted. Many couples in marriage counseling or entering a divorce process make the statement, "We just don't seem to have fun together any more."
- *Growing apart in interests, values, and expectations.* This is a gradual process that takes place as husbands and wives interact with different people and engage in different activities day-to-day. The wife at her job, and the husband at his; the wife socializing with her friends, the husband with his; the wife enjoying her hobbies, the husband enjoying his. Adults change and develop, and they may do so at different times, at different rates, and in different ways (see Chapter 9). There is a tendency for many husbands and wives to just "drift apart" in such a gradual manner that they may hardly realize it until it is too late to save the marriage.
- *Increased levels of conflict and disagreement.* Over time, there is a tendency for married couples to experience more conflicts. Unfortunately, there is not a growth in the ability to successfully resolve them. The most common source of conflict in marriage has to do with money management: how to earn it, spend it, and save it. Discipline and childrearing practices are also top on the list of marriage conflicts. In view of the role strain associated with the demands of children and work outside the home, it is not surprising that these conflicts increase. If unresolved or poorly managed, conflict leads to disenchantment.
- *Decline in exchanges of affection and communication.* As time goes by, married partners tend to reduce their frequency of holding hands, kissing, touching, and other signs of intimacy. The spark of excitement and romanticism of the beginning stage, what is known as the "honeymoon effect," wears off. Time takes a toll on love. The loss of intimacy and increased feelings of loneliness in marriage are made even worse by marriage partners not talking or listening to each other. Their frequency of self-disclosure and using each other as confidants declines.

PREVENTION OF DISENCHANTMENT • The process of disenchantment is a normal and natural tendency for any married couple to experience. Few can avoid its effects without taking concrete steps to prevent it. However, disenchantment in marriage is not inevitable. Some marriage partners actually grow stronger over the years, growing more and more satisfied with their relationship. Others may experience a more steady course by maintaining a relatively constant level of satisfaction. Still others may experience sharp rises or drops in satisfaction.

Here are some things married couples can do to reduce the potential effects of disenchantment:

- Set aside specific times, daily or even weekly, to spend on your own without children present. Use these times for communicating, sharing problems and concerns, or just engaging in a fun activity together.

- Seek out a marriage enrichment group in your community. Often churches and community service organizations offer such programs. Marriage enrichment groups involve couples who periodically spend weekends together to discuss mutual concerns and to share ideas about how to make marriages stronger.
- Make a conscious effort to continue exchanging signs of intimacy and affection. In all likelihood, these are what created a strong bond in the marriage in the beginning stage. To lose them is to lose a strong foundation for continuing the relationship in a satisfying manner.
- Enroll in an interpersonal skill-building class. Many of us do not have effective conflict management and communication skills. They can be learned. Your local college or any of a number of community service agencies may offer such programs.
- If you find that your marriage is in distress, admit to the possibility of needing the outside help of a counselor. Professional marriage counseling can be very effective if couples would just seek help before the relationship has broken down so far that it cannot be saved. Marriage counseling, however, does not work well if just one partner attends counseling sessions. Both the wife and the husband must attend if they hope to improve the marriage and reverse the disenchantment process that has begun (see Figure 13-5).

Figure 13-5

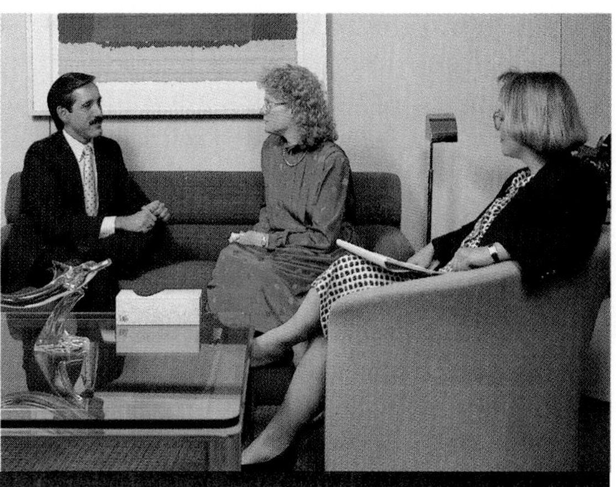

If marriage counseling is to be effective, both the husband and wife must be present.

ISSUES IN PARENTHOOD ACROSS THE FAMILY LIFE CYCLE

We have seen the potential rewards and challenges that children can bring into a family (Chapter 12). We have also seen the influences that children can have on the quality of the parents' marital relationship over the family life cycle. Now we will explore other issues of parenthood that add to its challenges in contemporary society.

The Problem of Infertility

Parenthood continues to be a popular choice for married adults in our society. Although we are seeing a slight increase in the number of married couples who voluntarily choose to remain childless, the vast majority of married adults will have at least one child.

But what about those who are *involuntarily* childless? What if a couple desires to bear children but finds it physically difficult or impossible? What steps can be taken, if any, to help these couples realize their parenthood goals?

Approximately 10 percent of American married couples are classified as having **impaired fertility**. That is, they are able to conceive a child, but find it difficult to do so. Another 13 percent are **sterile**. That is, they are unable to conceive at all.

The causes of infertility are physical in nature and can be associated with either the male or female. Causes of infertility in the male include low sperm count or defective sperm cells which do not result in a viable conception. Certain diseases among men, such as diabetes, mumps, certain sexually transmitted diseases, and endocrine (gland) disorders can lead to sperm production problems.

For females, fertility problems may be related to tumors or cysts in the ovaries that prevent ovulation, either regularly or at all. Infections which create scar tissue in the female's reproductive system can prevent the sperm cells from reaching the egg. Sexually transmitted diseases that are not cured in time are the most common causes of such problems. Hormone problems or disorders of the uterus can also prevent fertilized eggs from implanting properly in the uterus.

Infertility problems can be a source of great stress in marriages. Some couples try unsuccessfully for years to conceive a child, until their frustration at not being able to do so results in conflict. One spouse might blame the other for their fertility difficulties. The partner with the fertility problem may feel guilty for not being able to fulfill an important social role: parenthood.

Recent developments in medical technology have opened the door to fertility to many couples who, in past years, would have been unable to bear children. Some of these developments are controversial and involve serious moral dilemmas that have yet to be resolved.

FERTILITY DRUGS • Certain drugs can be prescribed by a doctor which promote ovulation in the woman by regulating hormone levels. Such drugs are quite effective in restoring the woman's fertility. However, these drugs can also lead to the release of many eggs, which can result in multiple births (twins, triplets, etc.). Use of these drugs has even resulted in a number of women bearing five or six babies (quintuplets and sextuplets) with one pregnancy.

SURGICAL TREATMENTS • Some cases of infertility in women can be corrected by surgery. However, many problems in the woman's reproductive system cannot be corrected. This has resulted in a number of other procedures that doctors can employ.

IN VITRO FERTILIZATION • In vitro fertilization (sometimes referred to as *test tube pregnancies*) is one such procedure used when surgery cannot help. This technique came to light in 1978 with the birth of Louise Brown in England. She was conceived in the laboratory of Drs. Robert Edwards and Patrick Steptoe. These doctors developed a way to combine a male sperm cell with a female egg in a specially prepared nutrient solution, so that fertilization would take place. Louise's mother could not bear children because of a blockage in her reproductive system that prevented her from getting pregnant. Drs. Edwards and Steptoe extracted the egg cell from Mrs. Brown and combined it with sperm cells from Mr. Brown. They then implanted the fertilized egg into the uterus of Louise's mother a few days following fertilization. The result was a healthy, normal 5 lb. 12 oz. baby girl born on July 25, 1978.

Since this pioneering effort, many couples around the world have been able to have children when they otherwise could not have had them. The method is safe and, in most instances, quite effective. However, one ethical concern with this procedure is the fact that it is a deviation from the *natural* method of fertilization—sexual relations between wife and husband. Some religions question whether or not we have the right to alter the course of nature by using the scientist's laboratory to "create life." Others say it is a matter of personal values and choice. If a couple chooses to overcome a fertility problem with in vitro fertilization and if it is allowable within their personal value system, then should they be free to do so? What do you think?

ARTIFICIAL INSEMINATION • This technique has resulted in millions of successful pregnancies world-wide. If the husband has a low sperm count, doctors are able to gather an adequate number to inject them into the uterus of the wife with a syringe. Sometimes the sperm are kept frozen at ultra-cold temperatures (−320° Fahrenheit) to preserve them until the couple is ready to have the child.

This method of overcoming infertility due to a husband's physical problem is quite safe and highly effective. Ethical questions have arisen, however, in terms of altering the *natural* course of fertilization. Also, questions of inheritance rights and legal status of the child have been raised when the wife is impregnated with the sperm of an anonymous sperm donor (if her husband was unable to produce any viable sperm cells of his own). Is the child born legitimate or illegitimate? Should the child be told of his or her anonymous natural father? As with in vitro fertilization, some say it is a matter of personal values and choice of the couple involved. What do you think?

SURROGATE PARENTHOOD • Perhaps the most controversial method of solving the infertility problem has been the use of surrogate mothers. Surrogates have been used by some married couples who find that the wife is physically incapable of getting pregnant or carrying a baby full-term. The couple hires a woman who is artificially inseminated with the husband's sperm. She is paid a sizeable fee to carry the baby through a full-term pregnancy, to deliver the infant, and then to hand the infant over to the couple who hired her.

Already this procedure has encountered serious legal and ethical complications. On the one hand, it has allowed some couples to have a child when other techniques were not available or would not work. However, actual cases have occurred where the surrogate mother wants to keep the baby after delivery. Court battles have raged over who has what rights in keeping the child. What if the surrogate mother desired to see the baby while it was growing up? Should the child be told how he or she was conceived and born? Should the identity of the surrogate mother be told to the child? If so, at what age? What if the baby is born with medical problems or physical handicaps and the couple refuses to take it? Some claim that this is a form of baby selling, which is questionable on legal and ethical grounds. Others question the morality of altering the course of nature in producing a child in such a manner. Because of these unresolved issues, some states have laws which prevent the practice of surrogate parenthood.

The issue of surrogate mothers has been hotly debated within the medical community, the legal community, and by many religious groups. What do you think? Are the benefits of any of these means of overcoming fertility problems—fertility drugs, in vitro fertilization, artificial insemination, and surrogate motherhood—enough to warrant their practice? Which do you find acceptable in your own value system?

ADOPTION • If a couple chooses not to use any of these means of overcoming fertility problems, another option is open: adoption. Most communities have adoption agencies that allow couples to legally gain custody of a child. Children are made available for adoption for any number of reasons: they may have been orphaned, abandoned or abused, or born to underage (teenage) parents who give them up. With adoption, parents are able to have more of a say in the age, sex, and physical characteristics of their child.

One problem with adoption concerns the availability of children with just the characteristics that the parents desire. A long period of waiting for an available child may follow. Adoptive parents are carefully screened by social workers to assure that they are sufficiently responsible and capable of caring for the adopted child. Adoption agencies want to make sure that adoptive parents are emotionally and financially stable enough to support the child. Such screening is a positive step toward assuring the welfare of the child. (It is interesting to note that society requires absolutely no such screening or proof of competence among people who bear their own children!)

Blended Families

When one considers the relatively high levels of divorce and remarriage in our society today, it is not surprising to see a rapid growth of a new family pattern: blended families. Sometimes these families formed after remarriage are called stepfamilies or remade families. In 1983, approximately 15 percent of all American children lived with one natural parent and one stepparent (amounting to 9.3 million children). Undoubtedly, this number will grow in the future if the divorce and remarriage rates remain at or about their current levels.

Many children of divorced natural parents will be part of two stepfamilies—the newly formed family of their natural mother and the newly formed family of their natural father. Stepfamilies may have children from previous marriages of both parents. All of the children may reside together, or some may live with the other natural parent. There may be children from both previous marriages and new children from the remade family.

It has been predicted that 60 percent of all children born in the 1980s will live in single-parent families for part of their childhood. The majority of these single-parent families will become two-parent families as the single parents remarry. Stepfamilies may provide a source of personal and family growth for those living in single-family homes. But, stepfamilies also introduce some special concerns which must be confronted and overcome if the new arrangement is to be a success.

Stepfamilies usually face more adjustment problems than intact families. This situation arises primarily because the newly formed family is a blend of two sets of rules, values, and family styles. Expectations and differences must be clarified and then resolved to ease the period of transition. Also, the "wicked stepmother" and "wicked stepfather" of fairy tales have created a stereotyped image of stepparents. Thus, some stepparents may have a strike against them before they even begin. The following are examples of issues facing newly formed stepfamilies.

NEW PLACEMENT OF SIBLINGS • The youngest child or baby of the family may suddenly gain several younger stepsiblings. Likewise, the oldest child in the formerly single-parent family may become the middle child in the new stepfamily. An only child who has enjoyed all of the family's attention may have to share some of this attention with stepsiblings.

NEW ROLE RESPONSIBILITIES • Children who had taken on many household chores and responsibilities in the single-parent family may find the new stepparent taking over their turf. They may be unsure of their new role or even feel that they have no role anymore. Similarly, a new stepparent without natural children may find their new parent role overwhelming.

LACK OF CLEARLY DEFINED ROLE RELATIONSHIPS • There is usually some uncertainty about how stepfamily members will interact. Do the children expect a warm, highly involved stepparent or do they prefer kind but reserved attention? Does the stepparent want to be involved in the stepchild's activities or prefer instead to have very little involvement?

NAMES FOR NEW FAMILY MEMBERS • Stepfamily members usually experience a period of discomfort as they determine what names they will use for each other. Some of the issues to be resolved in the early stages of stepfamilies include whether to use "Father/Mother" instead of a first name and whether to refer to a stepchild as my "son/daughter" instead of "stepson/stepdaughter."

NEW EXTENDED FAMILY MEMBERS • Siblings, parents, and other family members in the new stepparent's family may or may not wish to become involved with stepchildren. What is expected of the stepchild if these extended family members visit and interact with a stepparent or stepsibling?

DISCIPLINE • Discipline of stepchildren by a stepparent is a major issue for many stepfamilies. Does the stepparent act as the disciplinarian only when the natural parent is temporarily absent? Is the stepparent involved in determining rules and guidelines or does only the natural parent set these rules? Are rules equal among all stepchildren?

THE END OF FANTASY • For many young people the marriage of a parent marks the end of the fantasy that the natural parents will reunite. Coping with the realization that this will not happen is sometimes difficult for young people.

RESENTING ATTENTION GIVEN TO NEW FAMILY MEMBERS • Stepchildren often resent the attention the natural parent gives to the new stepparent. The children may have been the major focus of the parent's attention during the single-parent stage and may begin to feel left out. Stepbrothers and stepsisters may seem to be getting more than their share of attention.

CHANGES IN PHYSICAL SPACE • A move to a new home or to the home of a stepparent may bring additional concern to members of the newly formed family. Familiar surroundings may be left behind. Personal space may have to be shared with stepsiblings.

Stepfamilies, like single-parent families, need time for adjustment. Communication, increased understanding, and routine all help in the adjustment process.

Many stepfamilies that consider themselves successful have similar characteristics. These families exhibit the following behavior:

- They recognize that family members have different perceptions of what a family should be and they make attempts to identify and share these perceptions.
- They try to be realistic about the past. They neither hide nor dwell excessively on past happenings.
- They have learned to respect attitudes and feelings of other family members.
- They did not feel guilty when they did not immediately feel love for all new stepfamily members.
- They allowed time for stepparent(s) and stepchild(ren) to become well-acquainted before the marriage.
- They realized that stepparents cannot replace the missing parent. Rather, they understand that a stepparent can be an extension of affection, friendship, and deep caring.
- They refrained from comparing the stepparent with the natural parent who is not part of the new family.
- They welcomed the extended family of the stepparent/stepsibling as a positive factor in their lives.
- They established open lines of communication, allowing all members an opportunity to participate in family goal setting and decision making.

SPECIAL CONCERNS IN MARRIAGE AND PARENTHOOD

Marriages and families today face a number of special concerns. Two concerns, in particular, threaten the psychological and physical well-being of millions of American families each year: sexually transmitted diseases and violent behavior in the home.

Sexually Transmitted Diseases (STDs)

A number of relatively common diseases are spread from one person to the next by means of sexual contact. These diseases are known as **sexually transmitted diseases**, or **STDs**. A common belief is that STDs afflict only unmarried people, especially those who are sexually promiscuous. However, this belief is false. Anyone who engages in sexual intercourse and certain other types of sexual activity can be infected by an STD. This includes married, as well as unmarried, individuals. Also, pregnant women with an STD can transmit the disease to the unborn child either before or during childbirth, causing physical deformity, blindness, and possibly death to the young victim.

STDs can be caused by any of a number of microorganisms, including bacteria, fungi, and certain viruses. Most STDs have a medical cure, but some do not. If not treated promptly, most STDs can cause great damage to the person's health. Some will infect and damage the male and female reproductive systems, causing fertility problems later on (inability to conceive and/or bear children). Most STDs have painful symptoms. The infected person will know relatively early in the progression of the disease that he or she is sick. Others, however, show few symptoms, and the STD can cause significant physical harm before the person feels sick enough to seek medical treatment. Thus, one person may transmit an STD to another person with neither person being aware that one partner is infected.

The number of people afflicted with STDs is staggering. Each year, several million people in the United States alone acquire an STD. This number has increased greatly over the past 20 years in our society. The reasons for this increase in STDs are:

1. The rate of sexual activity among teenagers and adults (before marriage) with a number of different sexual partners has increased. More sexual contact with a greater number of people increases one's chances of getting an STD from someone who is infected.
2. Some of the most common STDs are difficult to detect early (such as gonorrhea and Herpes Simplex II). Thus, they are spread from one person to the next before medical treatment is even sought.
3. Many people are simply not aware of the prevalence of STDs today, their infectious nature, and how to prevent them. They therefore neglect to recognize the symptoms and to seek treatment before they have spread the disease to others.
4. Some people are unnecessarily ashamed or embarrassed to admit that they might have an STD. They delay seeking medical attention, hoping the STD will go away on its own. In the meantime, they are jeopardizing their own health and that of others with whom they are having sexual relationships.

One of the best means of preventing STDs is knowledge and safe sexual practices. Without accurate information, a person runs the risk of getting an STD regardless of whether or not she or he is married. Our goal here is to inform the reader of the more common types of STDs by identifying their symptoms and cures, if any. Be aware that there are other diseases that can be transmitted by sexual contact. Also, we recommend that you seek out additional information about these and other STDs from your parents, your doctor, and your local community health clinics. Anyone who suspects they might have an STD should consult a doctor or health clinic *immediately!*

ACQUIRED IMMUNE DEFICIENCY SYNDROME (AIDS) • Much concern has developed in the late 1980s over the STD known as AIDS. As of 1987, a total of 37,481 cases of AIDS had been reported in the United States. Males are victims of AIDS far more often than are females (34,741 cases in males, 2,740 cases in females). Approximately one-half of these cases have resulted in death.

AIDS is the most *deadly* of the STDs and it has no known cure. The number of reported cases is rising rapidly. One million or more cases of AIDS may occur in the United States by the year 2000.

AIDS is caused by a virus known as the **Human T Lymphocyte Virus III (HTLV-III)**. Other related viruses causing AIDS have also been recently discovered. The AIDS virus attacks and immobilizes the person's white blood cells, which normally function to fight off disease and infection. Without the protection of white blood cells, the AIDS victim's body is unable to defend itself against common infections and certain diseases. For many, death is caused by these "opportunistic" infections and diseases against which the body has no resistance.

AIDS is spread through body fluids, such as blood and male semen. AIDS has *not* been found to be transmitted through skin contact, saliva, or tears. It most commonly afflicts men involved in homosexual activities, but it has also afflicted intravenous drug users (those who inject drugs into the body with a syringe previously used by a person infected with the AIDS virus). Also afflicted by AIDS have been hemophiliacs (those lacking blood-clotting ability) and others who receive transfusions of blood that has been donated by a person infected with the AIDS virus. People involved in heterosexual (male-female) relations can also get AIDS if one of the partners is carrying the virus.

There is no known vaccine to prevent a person from getting AIDS, and there is no cure for AIDS victims. A person must have a blood test to determine if the AIDS virus is present. Also, blood donors today are tested for the AIDS virus before they are allowed to donate blood. However, this test may not detect the presence of the AIDS virus in a person's system for two to three months after they have been infected.

As with any STD, the best approach to dealing with the threat of AIDS is prevention through education and safe sexual practices. Of course, complete abstinence from sexual intercourse is the most effective prevention. Monogamous sexual relationships are also advisable (having sexual contact with only one partner who is known to be free of the virus). Use of the condom also helps to prevent the spread of AIDS, although no such method is 100 percent effective. For any person considering sexual activity, married or unmarried, consultation with your doctor or a health care professional is the best advice—before it is too late.

HERPES SIMPLEX II • This virus, also known as "genital herpes," has infected millions of Americans. It is one of the most common of all STDs. The herpes virus is most commonly spread through sexual contact of men and women. It produces painful symptoms in the woman's genital area in the form of open blisters and sores. Men, however, are less likely to even know that they have it. The problem here is that males can unknowingly transmit the disease before they realize that they are infectious.

The herpes virus has no known cure. Once a person has been infected, the virus stays in the central nervous system and can recur at a later time (often when the person is under stress). Certain ointments can be applied to the herpes rashes and sores, helping to relieve the pain and discomfort.

GONORRHEA • More than 1 million cases of gonorrhea are reported in the United States each year. It is caused by bacteria known as *gonococcus*. Its symptoms include painful discharge and a burning feeling during urination. Many females who have gonorrhea experience few symptoms and are unaware that they have it. This is seldom the case for males, who usually know right away if they are infected.

Gonorrhea can be cured by antibiotics, such as certain types of penicillin. However, through genetic mutation the disease is developing certain strains that are resistant to antibiotics currently in use. This is of major concern to scientists who are trying to discover new treatments as the old ones become obsolete. If left untreated, gonorrhea can cause sterility, blindness, and other harmful diseases. It can also cause blindness in newborns.

SYPHILIS • Syphilis is a less common STD than either herpes or gonorrhea. It infects approximately 25,000 in the United States each year. It is caused by a microorganism known as a spirochete. After a person is infected, syphilis develops in two stages. During the first stage, the person may notice an open sore in the genital area. As the disease enters the second stage, a rash and more sores develop on the body. The person may feel as if he or she has influenza, with swollen joints and nausea.

Antibiotics will cure syphilis. However, early treatment is essential. If left untreated, syphilis can lead to severe damage in the central nervous system, including brain and heart damage. Death can result. Pregnant women who have syphilis can transmit it to the unborn child, resulting in the same harmful consequences.

OTHER COMMON STDs • Other STDs that occur with high frequency are candidiasis (vaginal yeast infection), chlamydia (also known as one form of nongonococcal urethritis, or NGU), pediculosis pubis (pubic lice, or "crabs"), and trichomoniasis (vaginitis). For these and any of the other STDs, it is important that the infected person seek medical treatment immediately upon appearance of symptoms. More detailed information on all of these diseases can be obtained from your doctor or a community health care clinic.

Domestic Violence

Individual development is enhanced when families provide for the emotional and physical comfort of their members. Security and safety are major functions that families fulfill for both adults and children. Unfortunately, families can also inflict great emotional and physical pain on their members through violent behavior. Why is it that hurt replaces love in some families?

Family violence can occur in many forms. In Chapter 12, we discussed the dynamics underlying child abuse. Violence also occurs in marriage relationships (husband to wife and wife to husband). Reports of adolescents behaving in violent ways toward parents have also appeared. Elderly people in families can also experience abuse at the hands of younger members.

What constitutes abusive or violent behavior in families? Any behavior that is intended to cause physical or emotional pain or injury to another person is violent, or abusive, behavior. Such acts include hitting, slapping, punching, burning, biting, yelling, and the use of dangerous weapons (guns, knives, any hard objects). Parental neglect of a child by failing to adequately provide for the child's physical and emotional safety and comfort is also considered abusive behavior. Inappropriate sexual contact from one family member to another constitutes sexual abuse, another form of family violence.

The occurrence of family violence is far more common than most people think. In 1985 alone, it is estimated that more than 1 million children up to 17 years old were abused by one or both parents in the United States. More than 1.5 million cases of wife beating (husbands physically abusing their wives) took place. Hundreds of children die each year at the hands of their parents. These numbers do not even include the other types of family violence and abuse listed above. Clearly, domestic violence is a tragic issue of national concern.

CHILD ABUSE • In Chapter 12, we looked briefly at child abuse in the United States. A major issue in the case of child abuse is just what is and what is not abusive behavior. Most people would agree that beating up a child to cause physical injury is abusive. We would also agree that burning or hitting a child with a hard object is abusive. However, we begin to disagree when we speak of such parenting behaviors as yelling at the child or spanking the child. The line between abusive and nonabusive parenting behaviors begins to get blurry in many instances.

Many parents use some sort of physical punishment when disciplining their children. This can include grabbing, shoving, or slapping the child. Many people believe that such treatment does not constitute child abuse. What do you think? How much of this kind of punishment is too much? How hard should a parent be allowed to spank a child? How often? Is it all right to spank with a paddle or belt? What about verbal punishment of children in the form of yelling, screaming, and shouting? Just where does acceptable parental behavior end and child abuse begin?

Laws now exist making it a crime to brutalize, neglect, or otherwise inflict physical harm on children. Parents and others who are responsible for the care of children (day care workers, teachers, etc.) are legally obligated to provide for the physical safety of the child and to attend to the child's physical and emotional needs. Just because they are your own children does not grant parents the right to hurt or injure them. Moreover, teachers and child care workers, as well as doctors, nurses, and other health care providers, are legally obligated to report cases of suspected child abuse.

The trouble with child abuse laws is that they are difficult to enforce. This difficulty is caused, in part, by not having a precise definition of child abuse with which everyone agrees. Some people are afraid to report suspected child abuse to legal authorities. In many cases, it is hard to know for sure if a parent is abusing a child. Rather than run the risk of falsely accusing someone of child abuse, it is easier to say and do nothing. Others believe that what a parent does with his or her child is a private matter and that one should not meddle in another family's affairs. They cling to the mistaken belief that parents have the right to do whatever they want to their own children. Also, much of what goes on in families takes place "behind closed doors." Many children are severely beaten and battered in the privacy of the family's home, often injured or even killed before the child abuse is brought to the attention of the legal authorities. Unless it is detected and reported, the young victims of child abuse cannot be helped.

VIOLENCE IN MARRIAGE • Violence in families is not limited to abuse of children. Marriage partners also abuse each other by managing conflict in a physically violent manner. Hitting, pushing, slapping, throwing things, and using a dangerous weapon are the most common forms of marital violence.

Because of the superior strength of men, wife beating is the most injurious form of marital violence. Nearly one in three female murder victims in our society is killed by a husband or boyfriend. Wives, too, can behave in violent ways toward husbands, although often this violence is retaliation or self-defense from the attacks of husbands.

Many people believe that a marriage license is also a license to hit or hurt a spouse. They view the marriage partner as "their property," granting them the right to do whatever they wish. "What goes on behind closed doors is nobody's business but their own," they believe.

However, the laws of our society make it clear that these beliefs are not true. No one has the right to injure another person, regardless if he or she is your child, your spouse, or a nonfamily member. As with child abuse laws, however, family privacy makes it difficult to enforce laws against marital violence.

Many communities today provide shelters for battered women (married or single), and care for their children. The shelter's goal is to help the woman regain control over her life and to give her some time to consider alternatives to her present marriage relationship. Counseling services are also available in many communities to help both partners learn how to manage the relationship without violence. The availability of such services has raised the public's awareness of the marital violence problem.

However, shelters for battered women are only temporary. Often the woman re-enters the hostile home environment, only to experience retaliation by the husband or male partner for seeking help in the shelter. Recently, though, a growing number of wife-battering husbands have been arrested and convicted of the crimes they have committed. This is a clear sign that society will not tolerate abusive behavior inside the family.

PREVENTING DOMESTIC VIOLENCE • How can such tragic behavior in families be stopped? Is there any way to keep helpless children free from the abusive behavior of parents? What can be done to help violence-prone marriage partners discover alternative ways of handling conflict?

These questions have no easy answers. The key to prevention, however, lies in an understanding of the causes of domestic violence. Child abuse is related to a number of factors. These include:

- Parents' lack of education about normal patterns of child growth and development, resulting in unrealistic expectations of the child and of parenting
- Economic and other life stresses for the parent, such as illness or death in the family, unemployment, problems on the job, or marital conflict
- Bearing children that are unwanted and, therefore, unloved
- Parents having children before they are socially and emotionally mature enough to have them (as is true for many teenage parents)
- Having a child born with a mental deficiency or physical handicap, leading to frustration and disappointment on the part of the parent
- Social isolation of the parent, caused by the lack of a supportive network of friends, neighbors, and relatives
- Parents having alcohol or drug abuse problems
- Having children who are perceived as "problems," which include ill-tempered, highly active, aggressive, or otherwise difficult-to-get-along-with children

Prevention of child abuse depends upon our success in removing these conditions. Education for parenthood is one positive step that can be taken to help potential parents learn about normal patterns of child development. Parent education programs can also help to teach the skills of effective parenting (see Chapter 12), which can be used even in times of high stress. Some people may need help in deciding whether or not they are ready to bear children, financially and emotionally. Others need to be informed of the potential difficulties in parenthood, especially the high level of energy and commitment that effective parenting requires.

The problem with any preventive educational programs, however, is to motivate people to attend them. Even if they are made available free or at a low cost, many people who need them simply will not enroll. What do you think? How can we encourage potential parents to obtain parenting education? Should society require it of all people before they become parents? If so, how would this requirement be enforced?

Prevention of violence in marriage is also a complicated matter. Marital violence is related to a similar constellation of factors related to child abuse. Lack of interpersonal skills in the area of conflict management and problem solving, frustration, high levels of stress, and problems with work and career are just some of the reasons that marriage partners lash out at each other.

Education for marriage is one positive step that can be taken. Such programs help to identify whether or not a person is ready for marriage. They alert the person to the challenges and problems that marriage partners likely face in contemporary society. Premarital counseling can assist a couple in pointing out areas in which they are compatible and areas that might be potential sources of conflict. Getting a head start on solving such problems can prevent the frustration that may later result in violence. Also, many communities and colleges offer programs in interpersonal skill development. Learning how to communicate and how to more effectively make decisions and solve problems provides the marriage partners with positive alternatives to violence.

As with parent education, the problem with marriage education programs is motivating those who need them to enroll. What do you think? What can be done to promote marriage education in our society? Should we require it of all who plan to marry (that is, make it a requirement for getting a marriage license)? If so, how would this requirement be enforced?

WRAPPING IT UP

This chapter covered major life cycle issues that confront families today. The nature of the family life cycle is changing as a result of changing marriage and childbearing patterns, as well as the fact that we are living longer. Unless divorce terminates marriage, married partners today are spending a longer time alone together than ever before.

The *launching family* and *empty nest stages* of the life cycle provide new opportunities for enrichment in the marriage relationship. The return to the "couple relationship" without children often brings a renewed sense of satisfaction with the marriage. Without the responsibilities of parenthood to weigh them down, marriage partners typically find the middle years of life to be a positive experience through increased leisure and companionship activities together.

The aging family stage can also be a stimulating and enjoyable experience for many people. It remains a positive experience as long as the health of both marriage partners is good, and they are financially independent enough to live at the desired standard of living. Retirement brings with it added time to enjoy hobbies, traveling, and other companionship activities. Grandchildren provide strong and rewarding bonds for the aging person.

The end of the family life cycle is marked

by the death of one of the marriage partners. Death involves a predictable sequence of stages in the experience of grief and loss. Experiencing the death of a family member involves many emotions: grief, anger, hostility, guilt, and fear may be followed by a sense of joy, relief, and pleasure taken in the memory of the dead person.

Many people, particularly children, are unprepared to handle the stress associated with the death of a loved one. The topic of death and its inevitability must be confronted openly and honestly if healthy attitudes are to be formed. Death should be viewed as another normal part of life.

Successful marriage across all stages of the family life cycle is a difficult task to achieve in contemporary society. Not all marriages that stay together (that is, are stable) are defined as successful. Successful marriages are those that continue to meet the goals and expectations of both marriage partners over time.

The *process of disenchantment* can only be avoided if marriage partners consciously strive to maintain a satisfying marriage relationship. Disenchantment in marriage involves a growing apart in interests; increased conflict and role strain; and a decline in the love, affection, and experience of enjoyable companionship activities as time goes by. To prevent disenchantment, partners in marriage should seek out ways to maintain the feeling of love and mutual respect that brought them together in the first place.

Special concerns related to the family life cycle include infertility, blended families, *sexually transmitted diseases (STDs)*, and domestic violence. These four areas represent difficult challenges for marriages and families of today's society. To address any of them, family members need accurate information. They also need access to community services which exist to assist families in solving these or other special problems that might arise. Seeking help is a sign of strength in the family; it is not a sign of weakness. When it comes to meeting special problems, families today need, and deserve, all of the resources they can muster to create an environment that is most conducive to the individual growth and development of all family members—young and old alike.

Exploring Dimensions of Chapter Thirteen

For Review

1. Explain why the launching stage may be difficult for some parents and young people.
2. Explain the five basic stages of acceptance of death.

3• Identify the steps to maintaining a successful marriage relationship that lasts over the years.
4• What are the special challenges faced by blended families? How can blended families meet these challenges most effectively?
5• Identify the major causes of domestic violence.

For Consideration

1• Describe a positive way for a family to handle the launching of their three children.
2• Write a brief essay on why or why not you believe that marriage education courses should be mandatory (that is, required of all people who apply for a marriage license).
3• Describe how you feel about methods available today to help couples overcome infertility problems (surrogate motherhood, artificial insemination, adoption, etc.).
4• What should be done to help people become more educated about sexually transmitted diseases? Explain what you would do to slow down the rising rate of STD in our society.

For Application

1• Assess yourself and your own family to determine how easily the launching stage will be for you, your parents, and your siblings. Consider what progress has already been made in slowly growing toward independence from your family. Consider steps you will be taking to help move toward the launching stage. Discuss with your parents how you both feel about this stage.
2• Your friend Phil is having problems in school. His older sister was killed in a car accident five weeks ago. Phil seems unable to concentrate in school. Sometimes he appears to be daydreaming. At other times he is angry and irritable. How can you explain Phil's behavior? As Phil's friend, what can you do to help?
3• Invite a panel of experts to visit your classroom to discuss their work with victims of domestic violence (child abuse, marital violence, etc.). Consider including a local police officer, a worker at a shelter for battered women, a social worker who works with child abuse cases, and a family

counselor or therapist. Have them discuss their specific roles in dealing with the problem of domestic violence. Have them also discuss their views on how to best prevent domestic violence from happening, and what to do once it has occurred.

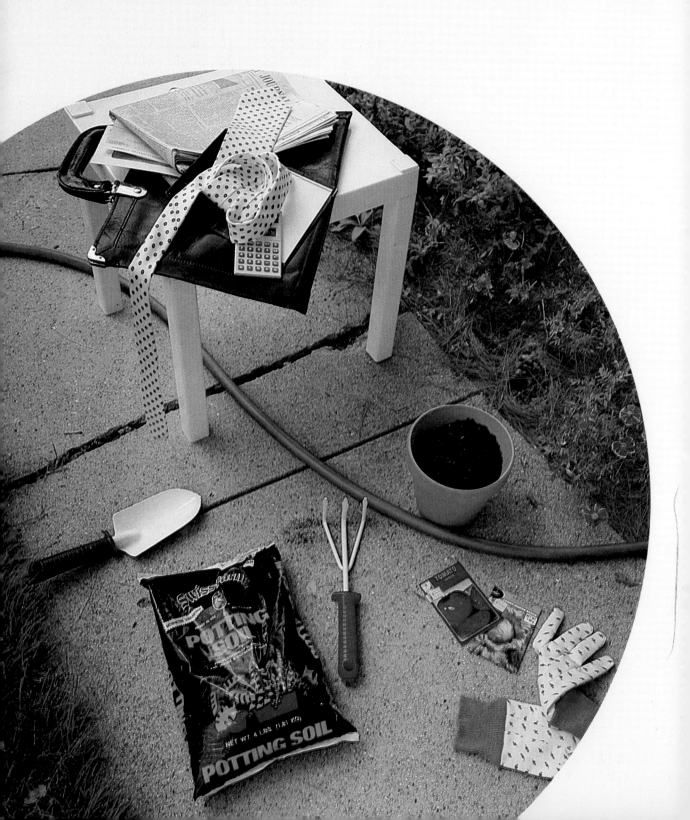
POTTING SOIL
NET WT. 4 LBS. (1.81 KG)
POTTING SOIL
TOMATO

part five

Combining Work and Family

The interrelationship of work life and family life is made stronger by more fully understanding our career/work goals and our family values and goals. Improved management in the home and in the work place can help balance the work-family relationship. Occupational and career decisions are made more realistic when family factors are included in the decision-making process.

Increasing numbers of individuals, by choice or necessity, are faced with balancing work and family roles. These two main areas of adult life—work and family—must fit together. This part provides materials and activities that will help you fit these two areas together and thus increase benefits for your family life and your productive work life.

Individuals and families do not exist in a vacuum. Individual family members and the family as a whole interact with society in many ways. One of the most influential of these interactions is with the work world. Direct results of employment such as income, economic benefits, and job satisfaction, clearly affect family life. More indirect effects of employment on families are related to the type of work schedule, the degree of work involvement, and the number of employed family members.

Likewise, the work world does not exist in a vacuum. It is affected by the workers' home and family situations. Workers who experience basically stable home environments with minimal frustrations are generally more dependable, productive workers. Basic skills and abilities learned in the home are carried over to the work world.

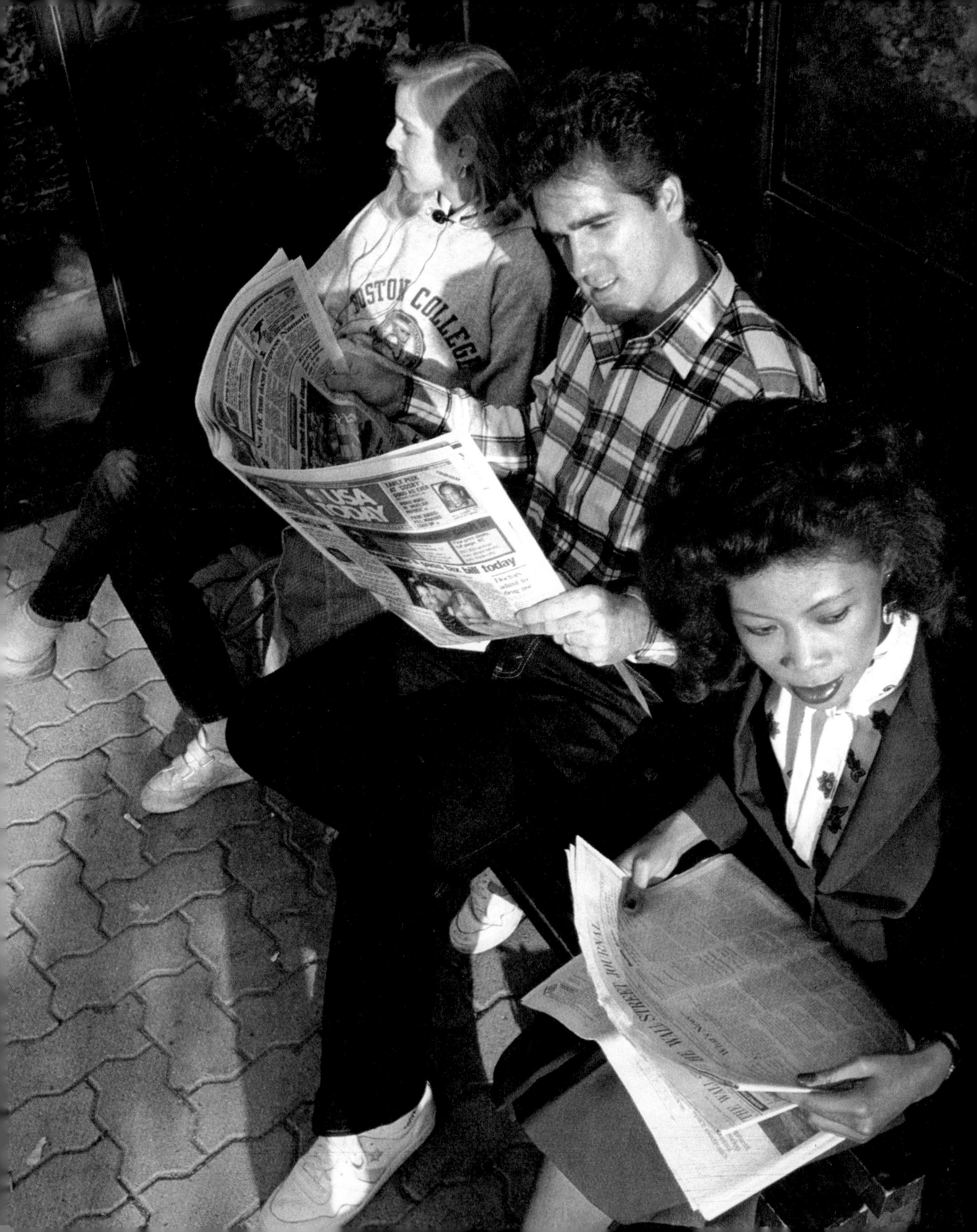
USA TODAY
bill today

fourteen

ACCEPTING WORK ROLES IN OUR SOCIETY

This chapter provides information that will help you to:

- Understand the meaning of work in our society.
- Identify reasons why people work.
- Understand changes in male-female work roles in our society.
- Consider multiple work roles for self and society.
- Realize the ways that nonworkers fit into the work ethic in our society.
- Understand what it means in our society if you are unemployed.

THE MEANING OF WORK

Work clearly has different meanings for different people. These meanings vary depending on motivation, individual needs, life stage, and general attitudes toward work.

Work need not result in pay. Many people work in the home and other places for no salary (Figure 14-1). However, in this chapter, the term **work** is used to refer to paid employment for a specific set of tasks. The work leads to the production of a specific set of goods or services.

Figure 14-1

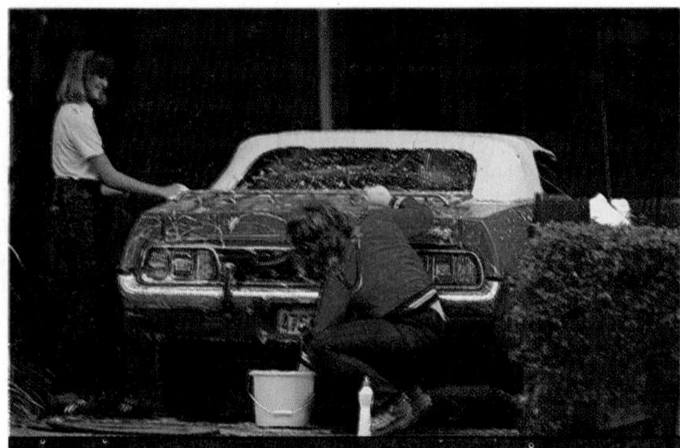

Is this work in your opinion?

Motivation

If you had sufficient money to live without working, would you work? At first this sounds like a silly question. Who would work when a person could spend time at the beach, travel, or do any other form of leisure activity? However, when people consider this question carefully, most indicate they would work. In one study, nearly 67 percent stated they would do some type of work even if they were not required to work for the income.

What is the motivation to work? What encourages people to obtain and keep jobs? In a government task force study, three basic reasons were found to motivate workers.

Economic need is the major reason most people work. The income gained from work allows people to pay their living expenses, save for major needs, and set aside savings for the future (Figure 14-2).

Figure 14-2

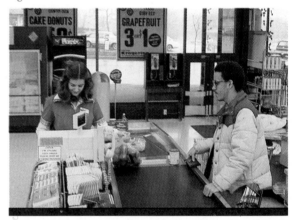

Economic needs and wants are the main reasons most people work.

Social reasons for working include establishing friendships. Many social relationships for young people and adults stem from work situations. In addition, social status is gained from work in general (having a job) and specific work (having a particular job). Social gains go beyond the status of the employee; they reflect on the employee's family members. Examples of this reflection are found in our society. Families in which adult members have prominent, influential jobs have a high social status, while those holding less prominent jobs have a lower social status. This status is not necessarily related to income. In some communities, trash collectors earn more money than college professors. Yet, a professor's family enjoys a higher status. Other social consequences of work may include location of residence, schools attended, and types of people with whom a person associates.

Personal reasons for working focus on the development of a personal identity and a positive self-concept. Work can build self-esteem and self-expression. It gives a purpose to life (Figure 14-3). As job success is built, an employee's personal worth grows and develops. People are pleased when they can provide a product or service valued by others. The work produced adds a purpose to our lives by allowing us to contribute to society in a much broader sense. Work organizes our lives and provides a framework for our lifestyle.

Figure 14-3

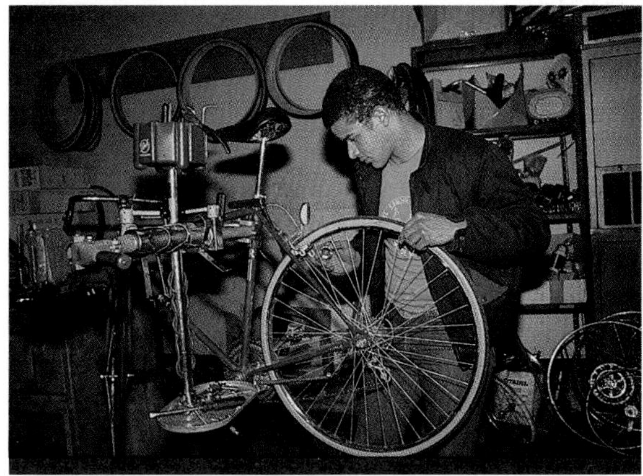

Work can provide self-expression even for young people.
Audrey Gottlieb/Monkmeyer Press

The importance of people's work becomes clear when you listen to people introduce themselves:

> I'm Jim Tyson. I'm a filing clerk for Modal Tire Company.
>
> I'm Joyce Holway. I'm an electrician.

Jobs provide people with an identity! Some types of work seem to provide more personal reasons to work than other types of work. Work that enables the worker to see a completed product or service is usually more personally rewarding than work that includes only one step of a process. Completing a total unit (a bookshelf, a sandwich, a potted house plant) seems to give people more of a sense of accomplishment than doing only a piece of the unit (assembling the boards for a bookshelf, adding the tomatoes to a sandwich, putting soil in a flower pot). The assembly line work in many American factories can cause feelings of frustration and lack of purpose to work. Many factories have changed from the original assembly line process to having each worker or team of workers create an item or portion of an item. For example, being able to see food items, car doors, or picture frames that you have produced can provide a greater personal identity. In turn, increased personal identity can lead to greater productivity.

CASE IN POINT

School Is Your World of Work

Whether or not you have a job, you are a worker. School life and all the extra-curricular activities surrounding it make up your work. The responsibilities, the time commitment, the possible conflicts with personal and family life, and the importance of attitude are easily equated to employment, even though going to school is an unpaid occupation. As you proceed through this chapter, consider your current work life (school and any additional paid employment) as well as your future work life.

Hierarchy of Needs

Maslow's Hierarchy of personal needs (discussed in Chapter 2) corresponds with motivation to work. In the lower stages when a person is striving to gain physiological and safety needs, a person is motivated by economic reasons. As movement progresses to higher levels, more personal and social reasons for work emerge. A job change affording greater dollar income but less personal gratification may be turned down at the higher levels of need fulfillment. The same job offer is likely to be accepted at lower levels of the needs hierarchy when income is more necessary to meet primary needs.

We often consider movement up the hierarchy to be a one-directional process. In reality, movement may be in both directions. As the work fluctuates, hierarchical movement also varies. For example, an individual may be succeeding on the job and functioning at the esteem of love and acceptance levels of the hierarchy. The loss of that job, failure to get the expected promotion, or increased job dissatisfaction can cause a return to the lower levels where primary needs reappear as a major concern.

CASE IN POINT

Andy has worked for the same company for four years. His wife is also employed. Together their incomes provide a stable means to gain food, clothing, and shelter. Andy is at the esteem level on the hierarchy of personal needs. He feels good about his life, his family, and his job. He enjoys achieving for the good personal feeling he gains from the achievements.

One day on entering work, Andy learns of a proposed plant shutdown. The plant may relocate, it may continue to operate with a quarter of the current work force, or it may close for a four-month period and reopen later. Whichever actually happens, Andy is concerned about his ability to provide for himself and his family. He drops from the esteem level on the hierarchy to the physical needs level. Paying the rent and providing food and clothing are now Andy's primary concerns.

If the plant stabilizes and Andy's job is again secure, he will be able to move up the hierarchy of needs again.

Life Stages

Reasons for working change as an individual moves through the life cycle. As a young adult, first jobs are often obtained to satisfy economic needs. Though experience and personal development may be gained, the dollar income and the independence it brings are the primary motivators for work. Dollar values may re-emerge as motivators for work at times of major expense such as when children are in college or during periods of prolonged illness of family members.

Later periods in life—particularly during retirement or semi-retirement—may allow people to place less emphasis on economic motivators. People may even work at self-fulfilling jobs for minimal or no money reward, provided that they have an adequate level of retirement income. The economic motivation to work is likely to remain strong for older people whose Social Security benefits and other sources of retirement income are inadequate to meet their needs.

Work Ethic

Motivation to work is affected by a person's attitude toward employment in general. **Work ethic** is the term used to explain an individual's or a society's attitude and philosophy about work. The American work ethic suggests that all able-bodied people should work and that work should be a major part of a person's existence. Efficiency and productivity are regarded as virtues, idleness and laziness are equated with weakness.

The statements below are responses to a national survey on work and the family conducted by the editors of *Better Homes & Gardens*. How do you agree or disagree with these statements?

> Hard work is still rewarded when the proper goals are set and strived for.
>
> I would like to believe that most people like their jobs, but I'm afraid that not many people I know really enjoy their jobs.
>
> Hard work and self-sacrifice may not always lead to success, but they surely bring self-satisfaction.
>
> I truly feel that the average American has lost the feeling of giving a good day's work for a good day's pay.
>
> Work for most people I know is on a survival level. Maybe the unrest comes from an inner prompting that tells us there is more to life than time, hurry, worry, and anger.

Americans have a strong work ethic, but not all Americans follow it. Individuals develop their own work ethic by observing their environment and learning from others. An individual who has observed lazy work behavior, poor work habits, and little incentive to seek or keep employment may develop a negative attitude about work. Likewise, people who have observed good work habits that have been rewarded are more likely to develop a positive work attitude.

CASE IN POINT

Horatio Alger wrote stories for young people. He wrote about poor boys who rose from rags to riches in America in the 1860s and 1870s. Luck, decency, and hard work were the virtues of his young heroes. These short novels, numbering well over 100 at Alger's death in 1899, brought about the phrase "Horatio Alger success stories." This phrase today represents the early American work ethic wherein the poorest individuals can become successful.

A strong work ethic encourages individuals to arrive at work on time, be responsible and loyal to the business, and strive for success at a particular job. The work ethic operating in our society includes rewards such as pay increases, fringe benefits, and promotions for such behaviors.

Some people expand the work ethic to extreme levels while giving only minimal attention to other aspects of life, such as family, personal needs, and leisure. These people are called **workaholics**. Like alcoholics who cannot control their excessive drinking, workaholics have difficulty controlling their work level. The stress caused by excessive work is harmful physically and psychologically. Heart disease and digestion problems often result from over-emphasis and over-exertion in the work world. Worry and frustration (sometimes to the point of nervous breakdown) are psychological results of workaholic behavior. A healthy approach to work includes a balance of a desire to work along with a realization that the stress caused by overwork is harmful.

Here are some points that will help you develop a healthy work attitude.

- Observe people who are successful at their jobs.
- Consider the social, economic, and personal gains from your work.
- Realize the need for everyone to develop a work skill.
- Consider how work gives meaning to your life and provides relationships and social structure.
- Contemplate the feeling of pride when achieving on the job.
- Realize the benefits of your work to society.

CHANGING MALE-FEMALE WORK ROLES

Almost any daily newspaper has articles discussing the changes in male-female roles. It is almost certain that such articles will include information on the changing work roles of men and women. Some sources may say that the new work roles of males and females have caused social role changes. Other sources will say the reverse. Whichever of these situations is more accurate, it is clear that a greater understanding of the role changes in our society will be beneficial in accepting the varying work roles.

Roles

A **role** is a set of expectations or behavioral standards applied to an individual in a certain position. A person's position as a student council member, a teacher, an athlete, or a police officer establishes expectations or standards of behavior. Roles exist based on sex, work, and position in families or other organizations. Though some expectations remain stable, most roles change over time and by situations.

History of Work Roles

In early tribal periods, men and women shared work roles and each provided food and shelter for families. Though the tasks were divided in order to allow the female to bear and raise children, most tribes functioned with females carrying out the roles of producers of goods along with the males.

In later agricultural periods in Europe and America, the family formed the typical unit of production. All members of the family capable of working were producers. Men did the more physically strenuous jobs such as heavy plowing and major construction. Women often milked cows, managed the farm produce, and did light plowing and household tasks. A grandparent was usually present to assist in home care, food preservation, and child care.

As work moved from farm to urban factory, the situation changed. It was difficult to deal with children at the factory site. Women were expected to remain at home with their children. Fewer extended family members, like grandparents, were nearby to assist with home and child care. Men were expected to shoulder the total responsibility of being the wage earner. Women were to manage the home and raise the children. Thus, two major roles—wage earner and homemaker—were established on the basis of sex.

The strict sex role division of work began about the time of the industrial period of our country in the 1900s. This distinction grew even stronger after World War II when returning soldiers needed factory and office jobs held by women during the war.

Figure 14-4

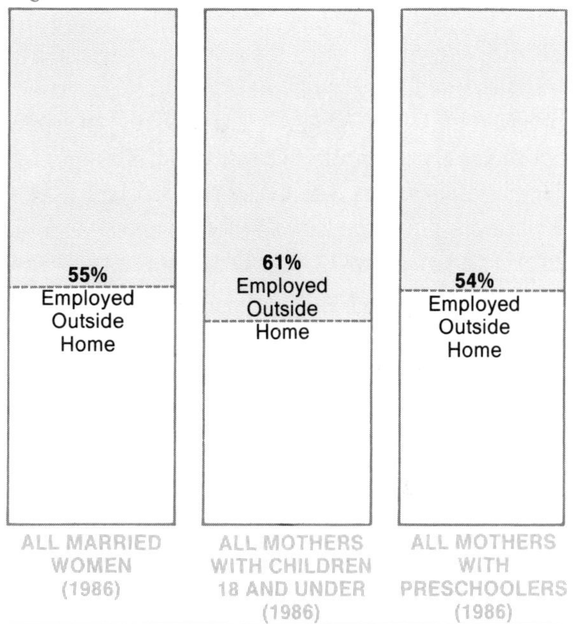

Employment of women outside the home is a major factor affecting current male-female roles. *Source:* U.S. Bureau of Census, Statistical Abstract of the United States, 1987, *Washington, D.C., p. 383.*

Current Male-Female Roles

We currently see a change from the distinct male-female work roles. No longer do many men and women feel they must respond to the rigid division of labor by sex. Multiple work roles—work on the job and at home—are becoming common to everyone, regardless of sex. Less frequently are these roles only for men or only for women.

A major factor in this shift in work roles is the number of employed women. The proportion of women in the work force is increasing dramatically. As of 1986, more than half of all married women and mothers worked outside the home (Figure 14-4). Of mothers with children of school age, 61 percent were employed. Of those mothers with preschoolers, 54 percent were employed. It is clear that now most women are combining the homemaker and employment roles, regardless of whether or not they have children.

With 55 percent of all married women employed, married men obviously no longer have sole responsibility for the wage-earner role. Also, there is a growing expectation that men will accept more household tasks as a shared responsibility (Figure 14-5).

As one man said, "With my wife working full-time, it's only fair that I share the work at home. If all the household work is to get done, I have to help." Generally, however, men have been slower to accept the household-family role than women have been to accept the employment role. In some families, the husband's involvement in the household work has been very limited despite the wife's involvement in the work force. There are

Figure 14-5

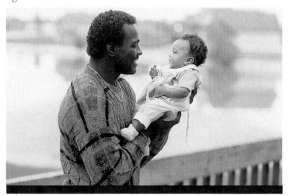

Males share household chores and childcare responsibilities. Multiple work roles for both men and women are common at work as well as at home.

Bill Smith/NFL Photos

several reasons for this, including the following:

- The general difficulty in changing from accepted social behaviors.
- Concern over others' perceptions if they do household chores.
- Lack of a male role model or example for role sharing. Men who had a father who assisted in household chores find it easier to accept shared work roles.
- Hesitancy on the part of some women to have their husbands enter a traditionally female household domain.
- Time involved for the husband to learn many of the household tasks.
- Hesitancy of both females and males to give up a comfortable position.

Spotlight on issues

Dual-Career Families

The terms dual-worker and dual-career both refer to situations in which the husband and wife are employed. The difference is that the dual-career family is one in which both partners are involved in employment that requires more than the standard work time. The work involvement often includes take-home work, weekend work, and business travel. Examples of such careers include doctors, lawyers, teachers, business executives, executive secretaries, accountants, and managers. In dual-career situations it is common for individuals as well as for the family as a whole to experience work overload.

Competing demands of career and family life present many challenges to dual-career couples. When each individual is involved in active work and family roles, total family activity is more than it is for families with less active roles.

Concern over fulfilling family roles is common in dual-career families. Many couples who choose dual-careers have not had family role models for this lifestyle. Consequently, their expectations may not be realistic. The occupational structures of their careers may involve social responsibilities and geographic mobility (having to move to a different city or state) that place additional stress on the family.

Some dual-career couples try to strike a balance between their work and family commitments by shifting their attention from one to the other at different times. At certain periods in their careers and in their family development cycle, they need to negotiate emphasis on career growth or on maximum family time. For example, some couples de-emphasize career commitments when their children are very young. Dual-career commitment is frequently a factor in postponing parenthood or deciding not to have children. Quality child care is often a concern of dual-career families both during the infancy stage as well as in later childhood.

Yet, studies reveal that children in dual-career families do not seem to be under more stress than children in families with only one working parent or with both working in noncareer jobs. However, dual-career parents seem to place increased strain on themselves to prevent stress on their children.

Despite these added concerns of dual-career families, studies show that most dual-career couples consider their lifestyle to be positive. Dual-career families seem to enjoy the benefits of two careers and seem to find ways to cope with the increased stress and strain. These families may use some of the following means to adapt to their lifestyle:

Scheduling: Families create work/home schedules that reduce or remove stress situations. Individuals negotiate work arrangements such as flexible scheduling, job-sharing, and other alternative work plans.

Role Priorities: Family members clarify their roles, deciding which ones are of greatest importance. This may involve decisions about their roles as employees, spouses, parents, and friends. It may also include decision making within the context of individual roles, such as setting priorities for being a good spouse.

Outside Support: Families may choose to pay someone to help with child care and household work. They also frequently welcome unpaid cooperative assistance from friends and relatives for child and home care. Informal networks of shared support are also common, where dual-career couples help each other with child care and home care.

Friendships: Families frequently make efforts to promote friendship activities with other dual-career families. Interacting with families that have similar concerns and goals seems to provide support for their chosen lifestyle. It also provides a shared support structure.

Compromising: Dual-career families may make adjustments by compromising, or agreeing to give up one aspect of a role in favor of another which may help the other partner. This coping strategy seems to work if compromises are shared among family members and among roles.

Personal fulfillment, increased standards of living, and pride in each other's accomplishments outweigh the strains of dual-careers for many couples. If you are considering this type of lifestyle you may find it helpful to talk to members of dual-career families to learn more about both the pros and cons of this arrangement.

Factors Involving Change

There are many factors involved in the changing work roles of men and women. Usually it is a combination of these factors that causes people to alter their roles.

ECONOMIC FACTORS • Numerous articles and discussions focus on why women go to work. The primary reason is related to economic necessity. Only a minority of women work for extra money. Most women use their income on daily necessities of life as well as saving for necessary goods and services for family and household. The importance of the dollar earned by women is obvious for those 19.3 percent of families in this country which are headed by single-parent mothers with one or more dependent children. It is also of major importance for women whose husbands are the major wage earners. It is frequently the wife's earnings which raise a family above the poverty level.

The economic reasons for women being employed seem to remain through the life cycle, though the particular needs may change. Consider the statements from the following women:

Young Couple Stage: "We've been married a year and a half. My income is necessary to help us buy the home we hope to have. We're also thinking of the money we'll need when we start a family."

Young Children Stage: "Perhaps we could survive on my husband's salary but not very easily. With the house payments and the car payments, my income is needed. Besides, I really like my work."

Older Children Stage: "With two children in college and another going to a technical school, I have to work. My income is important to their education."

Children Fully Launched: "We could manage now with one income, but with retirement ahead, we want to be sure to have enough set aside. Besides, I have three more years to reach retirement eligibility. I like my job, too. I'd miss it if I quit now."

CHANGING GENDER ROLES • As stated in the previous section, "History of Work Roles," the self-concepts of women have been traditionally tied to their roles as homemakers and mothers. Men found their identity through work outside the home, while women found their identity through work inside the home.

During the 1960s in America, this pattern began to change in a big way. Many women rejected the idea that their identity depended solely on housework and child care, due in part to a massive social movement, referred to as the "feminist" or "Women's Liberation" movement. Rigid role definitions for females were found to be stifling. Why couldn't women assume important jobs outside of the home, perform jobs traditionally held by men, earn money and social status, and then count on their husbands to help with housework and child care (Figure 14-6)?

Women began entering college in large numbers in pursuit of an education that would lead to well-paying careers. More women than ever before in our society counted on their work outside of the home to contribute to their self-concepts. Women's involvement in the occupational world became an important avenue for personal fulfillment, as it has always been for men. These changing role definitions for women, then, created an additional incentive: to seek paid employment as well as to be married and have children. Not only economic need, but the search for personal fulfillment through paid employment, have created a sharp increase in the percentage of women who work outside the home.

Figure 14-6

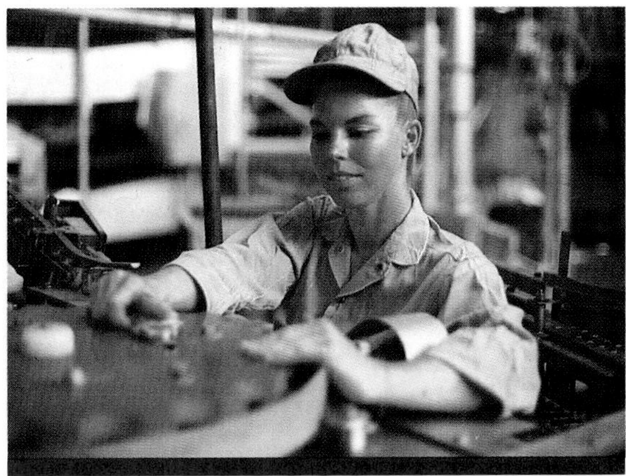

Women, today, often perform jobs that were traditionally held by men.
Campbell Soup Company

FAMILY LIFE CYCLE CHANGES • As recently as the 1920s, women spent most of their married lives raising their children. Families with five, six, or more children were desired, and many women spent 10–15 years of their lives in the childbearing stage. The life expectancy (the age when the average person dies) was much lower (Figure 14-7). In early America, the difficulties of childbirth and the large number of children born to most women allowed few women to see all of their children fully grown. The longer childrearing period and the lower average age of death left few years to be employed after children were grown. Today, women have longer spans of lifetime to devote to employment. For those women who choose to remain home while their children are young, there remains an average of 25 years for employment outside the home. Young people are often unaware of the length of time in a typical life span after the birth and early years of children. This lack of awareness is

Figure 14-7

Years of Life Expectancy at Birth

The life expectancy for people born in the year at the left is indicated by total population. Male and female differences are indicated.

Year	Total Population	Male	Female
1985	74.7	71.2	78.2
1980	73.7	70.0	77.4
1960	69.7	66.6	73.1
1940	62.9	60.8	65.2
1920	54.1	53.6	54.6
1900	47.3	46.3	48.3

SOURCE: U.S. Bureau of the Census, ***Statistical Abstracts of the United States***, 1987, Washington D.C., p. 69.

especially harmful for young women who make no plans for training and education toward employment. Throughout the country today, groups of people (primarily women) are gearing themselves for the work force after many years of caring for children and home. These **displaced homemakers** provide interesting advice to young adults.

CASE IN POINT

Cindy, 32 years old, with four children:

"I quit high school to get married when I was 17. I had four children pretty close together, and now the youngest is nine. I've tried being busy with community things, but I need to do more. My husband's income is fair, but it doesn't do much when you have four kids. I want to work, but there's not much available for someone without a diploma and no work experience. When I was 17, I thought I'd be ancient at 32. Now I see I've got lots of years left and need to be productive."

Regina, 29 years old with two children:

"I graduated from high school and went to a junior college for almost a year. I dropped out because it seemed like I had to study so much and my friends were out having fun. They had jobs and were earning money. I got a job as a cook's helper at a restaurant, and then I met Bill.

"We got married. He worked with a trucking company, and I got a different job with a candy company. The babies came, and I quit work to stay home. Two years ago Bill lost his job. Things got really bad and we did a lot of fighting. He left me, and I've been alone for almost one year. I'm able to get public assistance money, but that's no way to live forever. I want a good life for my kids and for me. I have a long life ahead. I'm starting a job training course in welding. I've found I'm very good at this and my instructor is helpful. Hopefully, I'll be a paid welder next year."

Reba, 45 years old with three children:

"My youngest child is a senior in high school. I've spent a lot of good years with my family, and I enjoyed it. Now I want to do something in addition to my home and family. Before I got married, I wanted to be a teacher and I had finished two and a half years of college. Though I no longer want to teach, I do want to go back to college. I'd like a degree in library science. I've done lots of volunteer work in the library and I love research work. I'm very excited about this whole new stage of my life."

These three women have very different experiences. Yet, their situations point out the large segment of the life cycle left for productive work years after the early child-rearing years. Consideration of these years is necessary in career and life planning.

The life-span changes also affect work roles for men and women in relation to mid-life career changes (Figure 14-8). The increased life expectancy allows many people to consider a new occupation at mid-life. Job dissatisfaction and opportunities in new fields may encourage people to enter a new career. Unique retirement systems and jobs that are more suitable for youth also urge people to make a job change at mid-life. These mid-life job changes often offer and/or require changes in sex roles. The following situations are examples of career and role change.

Figure 14-8

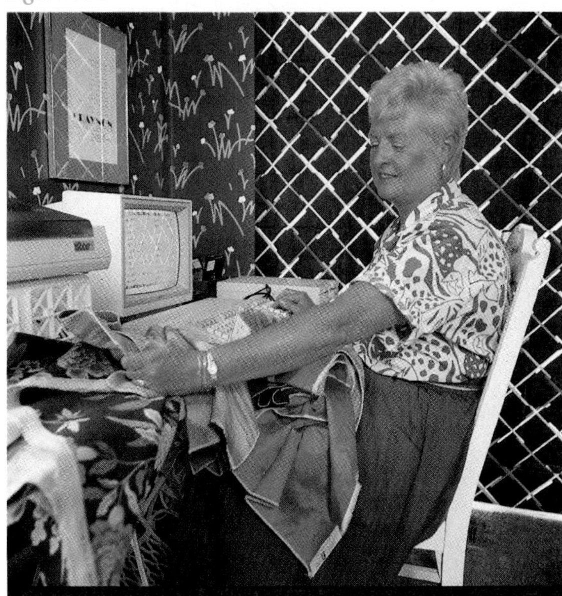

Increased life expectancy causes many people to consider a new occupation at mid-life.

CASE IN POINT

Winston joined the Army after graduating from college. He served 20 years and retired at age 42 as a Captain. Winston considered looking into jobs as a security specialist since his military work was in this area. However, he had achieved quite a skill in jewelry making, a hobby he began many years ago. He had sold several pieces at high prices and was beginning to realize he had some real artistic talent. Winston and his family decided to try this new career which required a role change for the entire family. Winston worked in a basement workshop creating the jewelry. Winston's wife was able to devote more of her time to her job as a legal secretary—a career that had been limited because of the many military relocations. Winston and the children often prepared the meals: general housekeeping tasks were shared. Summer weekends often found the family at craft and jewelry fairs where Winston began to gain a reputation for quality work. This career change provided altered work roles that blended satisfactorily into Winston's family.

Carmen is a single parent with two teenage children. She had worked as a salesperson and manager in a fabric store for seven years. She had received a few promotions, but she was not satisfied with her salary. She also felt the job offered little excitement or challenge. Carmen had often helped a friend in his bookstore. She enjoyed sales but had skills at managing, ordering, and bookkeeping. When her friend asked if she was interested in a partnership as half-owner and full-time operator of the store, she hesitated. She worried about her ability to support herself and two children if the business should fail. After much thought, Carmen entered into a partnership with her friend in the bookstore. She and her children have had to alter their schedules and roles in order to manage the bookstore operation. Her children often help in the store and they share more of the work at home.

The above situations are examples of mid-life career changes that caused work role alterations. Both Winston and Carmen had a need and desire to consider a new job that filled personal and economic needs in their remaining employment years.

Acceptance of Integrated Roles

Many individuals have no difficulty accepting multiple roles made necessary by a changing employment structure. They readily accept males and females sharing both employment and homemaking roles. These shared roles are sometimes referred to as **integrated roles**. Role integration is the lessening of the distinction of work roles for males and females. Role integration allows family members, regardless of sex, to do what needs to be done in order to maintain a stable, positive family life.

Sometimes individuals have difficulty accepting integrated roles. They are uncomfortable with roles other than the traditional male bread-winner and female homemaker roles. Such people have particular problems when circumstances force them to accept nontraditional roles. There are some factors that may hinder acceptance of female employment roles and male homemaker roles.

PARENTAL ROLE MODELS • When parents perform work roles and homemaking roles in an integrated fashion, young people are less likely to rebel against such role expectations. This is especially true if the parents enjoy the integrated roles (Figure 14-9).

Consider the following families. Which families exhibit integrated role behavior? How equal is the sharing of multiple roles? How do you think Pete, Jud, Rebecca, Harvie, Jodie, and Brent will handle integrated roles when they are adults?

Figure 14-9

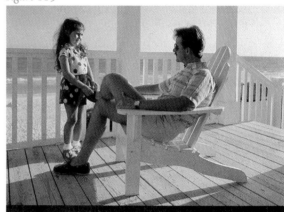

Fathers who enjoy nurturing their children's aspirations allow family members to seek emotional support from either parent.

Florida Department of Commerce/
Division of Tourism

CASE IN POINT •

Paul and Yolanda have stable jobs with full work schedules. Both enjoy their work and their home life with their son Pete, age 4. Both Paul and Yolanda realize the necessity of sharing work at home. Cleaning is a shared task, usually on Saturday mornings. Laundry is shared also and usually done on evenings throughout the week. Yolanda enjoys cooking and prepares most meals, although Pete helps with much of the kitchen work. Paul does most of the yard and garden work, which he enjoys.

Rose and Marvin are both employed. Rose does nearly all the household work plus her full-time job. She often does laundry and cleaning late at night and on weekends in order to get everything done. Marvin manages the car maintenance and sometimes will deliver Jud and Rebecca to their school activities.

Edna is a single parent with a young son, Harvie. Edna works full-time and has total responsibility for household care, car maintenance, yard work, and all work and family activities. She recently repainted and wallpapered the first floor of her home with the help of Harvie and her friend, Anne.

Kim and Frank are both employed. Frank's mother, their daughter, Jodie, and Brent, Kim's son by a former marriage, reside together in the country. Frank has an office at home and manages the majority of the household chores. Frank's mother works full-time in real estate and helps with some household work in the evening. Kim works outside the home plus operates a dog kennel. Kim does household cleanup periodically and manages most of the laundry. Food preparation is often done by Jodie, Brent, and Frank.

COMMUNITY ROLE MODEL • Young people residing in communities where integrated work roles are common are more likely to accept such role expectations. Young people living in communities where a male running a vacuum cleaner is an oddity tend to hesitate in accepting integrated roles. Communities where women who are employed full-time are rare will probably produce fewer people who readily accept integrated roles.

SELF-CONCEPT • People with positive self-concepts more readily accept integrated roles. When individuals have secure feelings about themselves and do not feel they must prove themselves to others, they can better accept new roles. People with a positive self-concept do not need to prove their masculinity or femininity by performing particular work roles.

NEED • Acceptance of integrated roles increases with the need to perform or fulfill the roles. If economic situations force women to join the work force, such roles are more readily accepted. This was evident in World War II when women entered factory work. If situations dictate that women are not able to carry out the traditional homemaker role, males are more likely to fulfill this role. Men may carry out the homemaker role in homes where there are disabled women, women who are pregnant or have just given birth, or there is no woman in the home. Even people who strongly dislike integrated roles will accept them under such conditions.

NONWORKERS IN OUR SOCIETY

The discussion of the meaning of work earlier in this chapter indicated the importance we place on work in our society. The work ethic emphasizes the virtues of efficiency and productivity and equates idleness with worthlessness. For many, work provides a place in the human community. Clearly, we live in a work-oriented society.

How, then, do nonworkers fit into the work ethic? How do jobless people gain a sense of worthiness? How can the unemployed deal with work roles that are so important in our society?

Retired People

People who have retired are usually faced with mixed feelings with respect to their work roles. In a climate that prizes work and productivity, retired persons may see themselves as individuals with second-class status. There are conflicts between the measures of success in the work force (affluence, power, productivity) and the typical outcomes of retirement (lowered income, powerlessness, lack of productivity).

Loss of the work role can affect the status and social image of the retiree and cause significant identity problems. Feelings of uselessness and lack of self-satisfaction are typical for people who have not prepared themselves for retirement.

Retired people can benefit from preparation for the retirement years. Establishing hobbies, interests, and activities that will play an important part in a person's retirement years can eliminate feelings that they have nothing to contribute (Figure 14-10). Developing an identity in addition to the work identity will help maintain a positive self-image in the retirement years. The retirement period can be more satisfying if there has been a balance between the work identity and personal identity. Some may be able to enter retirement more gradually through "partial retirement" programs, where the worker reduces the number of hours worked before leaving the job altogether. This plan helps to reduce the shock of moving from a full-time work role to one that involves no paid employment.

Realizing that work need not be paid work can also help the retiree. Work in the home, volunteer work, and helping relatives, neighbors, and the community provide work roles that are considered important in a retiree's

Figure 14-10

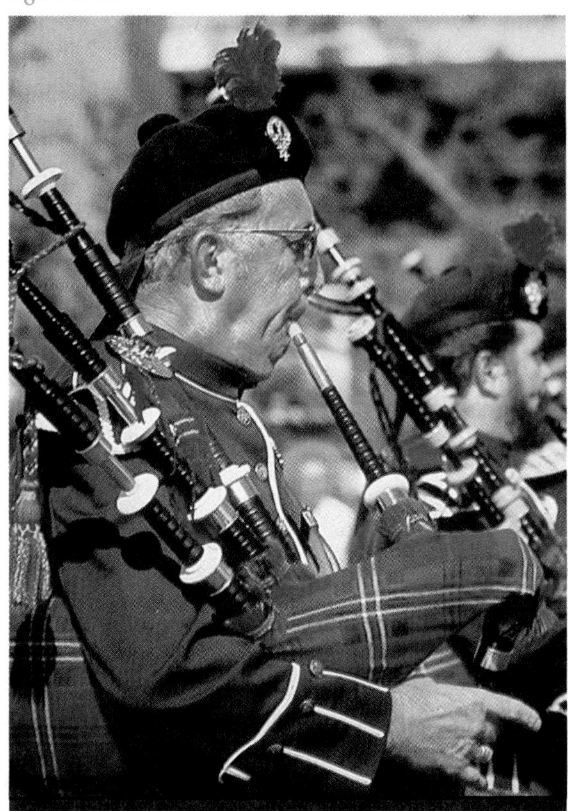

Sometimes retired people have difficulty accepting their nonworking roles. Establishing a hobby can eliminate feelings that retired people have nothing to contribute.

The Salt Lake Valley Convention and Visitors Bureau

life. Accepting the importance of these roles is necessary to satisfactory retirement life.

The Unemployed

Earlier in this chapter we discussed the importance of the work ethic in American society. A positive attitude toward work contributes to productive work activity and good work habits. However, not all who possess a work ethic and a desire to work are able to find employment. Lack of training opportunities, unequal access to education, discrimination, and prejudice are just some of the reasons that people find themselves unemployed. Also, as our society moves ever more rapidly into the computer age, more jobs require skills in advanced technology and information processing. For example, opportunities for computer programmers have grown recently while the need for railroad engineers and assembly-line workers has declined. A growing number of workers are thus finding that job skills in such areas as manufacturing and industry are obsolete. These skills are in less demand than they once were when our economy was based almost entirely on heavy industrial production. Consequently, a growing number of dislocated workers are joining the ranks of the unemployed because their job skills no longer meet the requirements for available jobs.

Unemployed people also include those who have recently been dismissed from a job because of plant closings, lack of work, or unsatisfactory performance. The unemployed include those who have been out of work for a period of time but are still avidly seeking a job. In addition, there are the young unemployed who have not been able to find jobs.

The unemployed suffer from loss of identity. Though joblessness is an economic event, it can cause severe psychological and physiological anguish. The unemployed often suffer from feelings of uselessness in a world that rewards the useful. They usually blame themselves for the loss of a job even in situations where the job loss was beyond their control. Outward behavior of humor, nonchalance, or blaming the system often mask feelings of loneliness and loss of place in society.

Spotlight on issues

Unemployment and the Family

Every year, thousands of Americans lose their jobs through plant closings, layoffs, and firings. In addition to providing an income, a job can also influence our self-concept to the point where our identity can become closely tied to our vocation and sense of productivity.

Many people lose more than their income when they lose their jobs; their feeling of self-worth may be shattered. Unemployment may bring on feelings of uselessness. Worry, anger, fear, and frustration are common reactions when a family member loses a job.

What can be done when someone in your family becomes unemployed? The most important thing is for that person to maintain emotional health. This can be fostered by using the following suggestions while an intensive job search is underway:

Avoid Idleness: Decide to be active. Watching too much television can hinder job hunting. Furthermore, television commercials showcase costly items which an unemployed person may not be able to buy. This may cause the person to become frustrated and depressed. Likewise, do not begin to depend on alcohol and drugs. An alert and attentive attitude is needed to find a new job.

Consider Job Hunting As Work: Make a plan or schedule for each day. Make a list of job openings and possible contacts who might be of help. Read newspaper classified advertisements and contact former employers.

Socialize: It is helpful to see friends and to share concerns with others. Nothing is accomplished by trying to hide the fact of unemployment. Don't be afraid to ask for help. Friends, neighbors, and former co-workers may know of job openings. Just talking about the situation may be helpful.

Get Physical Exercise and Maintain a Good Appearance: People with alert minds and bodies always function better. It is important to look well-groomed for job interviews; applicants who look like they're suffering—with sloppy clothes, bowed heads, messy hair, and sloped shoulders—aren't likely to get the job.

Take Available Work: Do not be too proud to accept certain jobs. Though it may not be the desired type of work, it can bring in money and may lead to other work. Consider volunteer work that may create job openings as well as provide good background skills.

Explore New Areas: Use this period to search out new areas of interest that may later lead to a job. People without work can visit public libraries and other facilities to broaden their knowledge base.

Relate to Family Members: Use this opportunity to strengthen family relations. Take advantage of a less rigid schedule to spend time with loved ones.

Brush up on Job Search Skills: Review job-interviewing techniques, write a new resume, and practice communication skills by using a tape recorder. Take advantage of job search classes or mini-courses offered at vocational schools or other community sites.

For many, the difficulties of unemployment are heightened by the need to seek unemployment benefits and/or public assistance. Personal and family pride may postpone the request for such assistance. When it is necessary to resort to the welfare system, the nonworker may feel rejected, saddened, and angry. It is important in times like these that family members try to support and encourage the unemployed member. This is *not* a time to blame or cast shame upon the nonworker. Becoming employed again will be much easier when family members maintain a loving and supportive atmosphere that bolsters the nonworker's self-concept.

Jobless people can help to maintain their sense of identity by working at finding a job. Continuous search of job ads, employment lists, and personnel offices may yield a job opening. Job retraining is a key to finding a job that is more in demand. In the future, workers will have to be willing to acquire skills that are suitable for more than just one type of occupation. Such transferable skills will provide some insurance that a worker will not become obsolete with advancing technology and a changing job market.

Nonworkers need to gain perspective of the current economic system. They must realize that they may be victims of economic stress periods or rapidly changing technology. Though this will not put bread on the table, it may help them see that they may not have been personally responsible for their situation.

The Unemployable

Another category of nonworkers is the unemployable. For various reasons, these people have been jobless for long periods of time. The unemployable may have had sporadic short-term periods of employment. Yet, they usually are not capable of long-term employment. The unemployable often suffer from a lack of education and experience. They also may be without employable skills, such as willingness to report to work on time on a daily basis, willingness to follow instructions, or awareness of responsible behavior on the job. Female heads of households with very young children may be part of this unemployable segment because they have no affordable child care services available to them.

The unemployable include severely handicapped people without job skills. People unable or unwilling to work for physical or psychological reasons are also included in this category.

These people generally rely on welfare for their income. Like the other types of nonworkers (retirees and unemployed), they suffer from the frustrations of existing in a world where the work role is rewarded by dollars and respect. The long-term unemployable often suffer from acceptance of their situation to the point of having no hope or thought of change.

Our society has difficulty dealing with the unemployable. Concern is heard about the rising welfare costs paid by tax dollars. It is frustrating for many workers who adhere to the work ethic to accept those who cannot or will not follow this philosophy. People cite those who misuse public assistance for personal gain and generalize this behavior to all of the unemployable. It is hoped that reform movements in the welfare system will help meet both economic and social needs of the unemployable. Such reform may focus on helping unemployable people locate an appropriate job. Other reform efforts include provisions of job skills, building self-confidence, and provision of goal setting and job hunting techniques. For example, with advances in medical technology and vocational training, many more handicapped people today are able to land jobs and become productive workers than ever before. Blindness, deafness, and crippling illnesses and injuries no longer imply that a person cannot lead a productive and satisfying life at work. However, despite these advances, provisions for those unable to maintain an income continues to be a concern to our society.

Work can mean many things to many people. It is important to consider how work and its motivation influence a person's work and family situation. The better family members can incorporate the motivation into group and individual goals, the better they will be able to reduce the likelihood of conflict between work and family.

WRAPPING IT UP

Family life and the world of work interact in many ways in our society. Work means different things to different people. In this book, *work* refers to the paid employment for specific tasks that are done in order to produce goods or services. People work for a number of reasons: economic need, to establish social ties and social status, and for personal fulfillment. As people grow older in the life cycle, reasons for working shift from economic need to personal fulfillment.

The *work ethic* in American society is strong. Being efficient and productive are regarded as virtues, while idleness and laziness are regarded as weaknesses. We expect able-bodied people to work, whether they are students in school or paid employees in the work force. People who take the work ethic to its extreme are *workaholics*. Their involvement in work activities is excessive, to the point of excluding other important life activities and causing health problems.

Role expectations for workers have changed significantly in our society. In particular, the work roles of males and females have changed to where the majority of married women are mothers and employees outside the home. Multiple work roles involving work both inside the home and on a paid job are now common for both males and females.

Growth in the number of women in the work force is due to life-cycle changes, where women today are living longer after their children are grown and leave home. Also, more women are working due to the need for additional money in the family to pay for such necessities as food, clothing, and housing. More women today are also employed outside of the home due to changes in self-concept. Productivity, sense of achievement, and earning income have become important parts of the personal identity of many women.

Added stress and strain can be found in dual-work and dual-career families. Husbands and wives in such families must cope with time management problems and shifting role priorities. Sharing of household duties and compromising in times of scheduling and role conflicts are necessary if the benefits are to outweigh the disadvantages in dual-career families. Couples who are able to adopt *integrated roles*, where employment and homemaking roles are shared by the husband and wife, are free to do what needs to be done to maintain a stable, positive family environment.

There are different types of nonworkers in our society. *Retired* individuals may suffer a loss of social status and develop a feeling of uselessness when they give up the work role. Developing an identity in ways other than just work role can help retired people cope with this transition in their lives. The *unemployed* and *unemployable* may also experience significant psychological stress. Lack of education, job skills, access to jobs, and knowledge of how to search for jobs all hurt the unemployable person's chances of finding employment. In a society that rewards productivity with paid employment, the unemployed must face a serious challenge to their personal identities and sense of self-worth. Support from family members is critical to the unemployed person's psychological health and motivation to search for employment.

Exploring Dimensions of Chapter Fourteen

For Review

1• Explain the basic motivators for people to work.

2• What are the basic factors that relate to the change in male-female work roles?

3. Define work ethic.
4. What are integrated work roles?
5. What are the major types of nonworkers in our society?
6. What are the major problems facing the unemployed? the unemployable? the retired?

For Consideration

1. Create your own definition of work.
2. Explain how the hierarchy of personal needs relates to motivation to work.
3. Consider two individuals: One who readily accepts integrated work roles and one who cannot accept them. Consider possible reasons for this acceptance and rejection.
4. In what ways does our society inflict problems on the nonworker? What can be done to prevent or solve these problems?

For Application

1. Explore the early stages of the American work ethic (late nineteenth century, early twentieth century). Read a Horatio Alger story emphasizing that hard work leads to success. Review political slogans, songs, magazine articles, and plays to learn of the work ethic concept in that time period. How did this philosophy affect the building of our country? In what ways does this ethic still apply? In what ways has the ethic weakened?
2. Explore agencies that assist nonworkers. Interview personnel. (For example, workers at retirement centers, retirement counselors, unemployment counselors, public assistance workers.) Learn how the nonworker affects the person's family members and society as a whole. Determine possible ways to assist both the nonworker and the nonworker's family.
3. The play *Death of a Salesman*, by Arthur Miller, depicts the psychological anguish experienced by a man who believes strongly in the work ethic, but who becomes unemployed. Read this play, and try to understand

how Willy Loman feels when his successful career as a salesman comes to an end. How do his wife and children react to his work experiences? What could Willy or his family members have done differently to prevent the tragic ending they experienced?

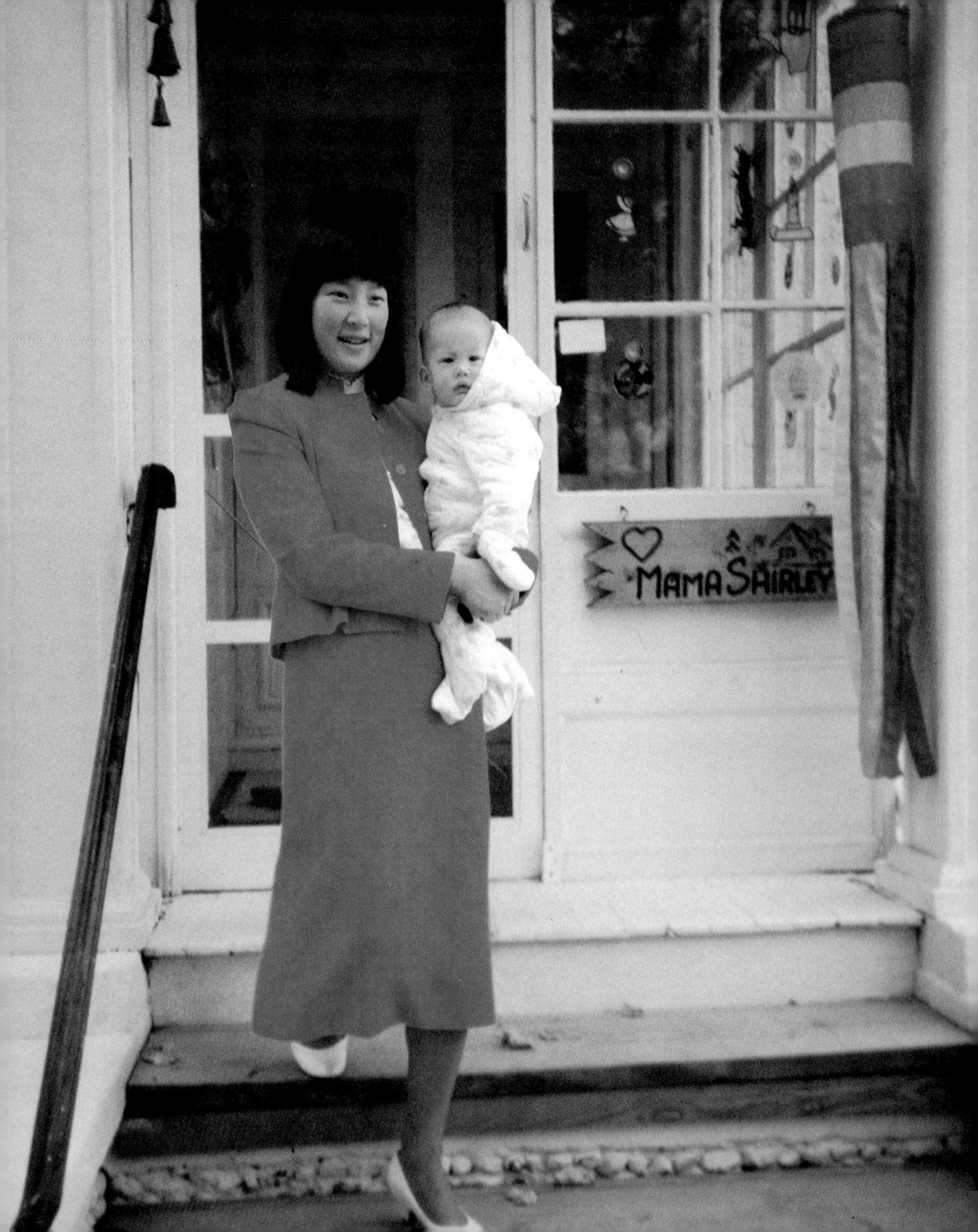
MAMA

fifteen

BALANCING WORK AND FAMILY

This chapter provides information that will help you to:

- Understand the interaction of work life and family life.
- Assess family values and goals related to work life and family life.
- Recognize basic techniques to assist in the management of work life and family life.
- Recognize support systems helpful to families in balancing work life and family life.

Work or school life and family life present many situations that require careful balancing of these two worlds. Requirements of the work world may conflict with goals and values of the family world, and vice versa. Likewise, school life and home life may conflict. Athletic practice each evening and weekend may limit family interaction. Responsibilities to family members may conflict with needed study time.

Statements such as, "Family comes first," or "My family knows this work I'm doing is all for them" are not helpful enough to counteract feelings of guilt or rejection. A more thorough understanding of the interaction of the work and family worlds is helpful in relating to work/family issues. Assessing family values and goals and gaining awareness of management techniques and support systems supply practical assistance.

THE INTERACTION OF WORK AND FAMILY

The Industrial Revolution was a milestone in the changing of male-female work roles. It was also a milestone in relation to the interaction of work and family. Prior to the Industrial Revolution, there was little or no separation of the work site and the family home. Work and family activities were bound together based on their same or close location. Families actually produced the food, clothing, and other goods that they consumed. The Industrial Revolution brought rapid changes. The development of industrial cities caused a separation of work and family. Thus, a separation in the roles of worker and family member was formed.

Because of these two distinct work-family spheres, the interaction of the work world and the family world is not easily recognized. Until recently, the worlds of work and family have appeared to be two distinct, unrelated worlds. The public world of work based on economic relationships and the private world of the home based on love relationships may be considered separate entities. It has been thought necessary that each world should act independently with its own functions and rules. Consider Sara's experiences when she began teaching high school 25 years ago.

CASE IN POINT

When I was in college, I remember my professors telling me that it was absolutely necessary to separate your teaching role and your family role. They said, "Never take your home concerns and problems to the classroom. Leave home things at home." I really took their advice seriously. I tried not to do much school work at home. I tried not to let my home and family life affect my classroom. It was very hard. I ended up feeling frustrated both at work and home, and I felt guilty if I did anything to let the worlds overlap.

As the years went by, I realized I was trying to do the impossible. My work life and home life are highly related. A busy time at school, a winning athletic season, or a teachers' strike does affect my family life. A concern or major family activity does cause frustration for me at school. I've now accepted this and seem to be able to function better. I really think that by sharing more work situations with my children and husband they can better understand my life at work. They see why I act as I do. I also find that my students see me as more human when I periodically mention a home situation that has affected my thinking and behavior.

Today people realize that the two aspects of life—our job and our family—are interrelated (Figure 15-1). Though the work site and the home are usually separate, what we do in one sphere affects what happens in the other. There is continual interaction between

Figure 15-1

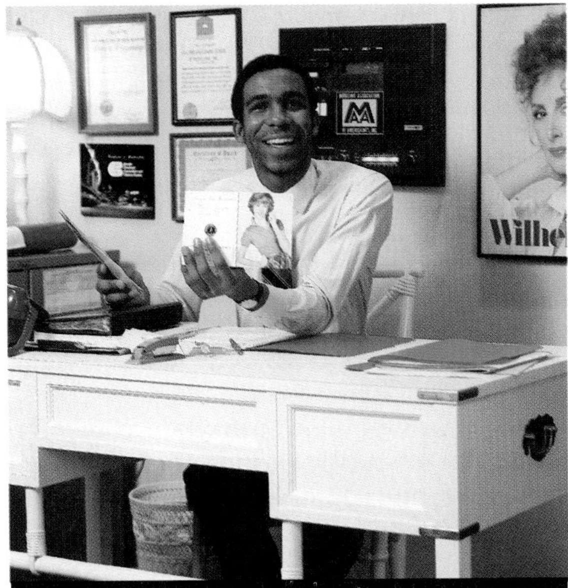

This employee appears happy, healthy, and energetic. These positive characteristics would not be possible without a rewarding home life. One's home life affects one's work life.

Figure 15-2a

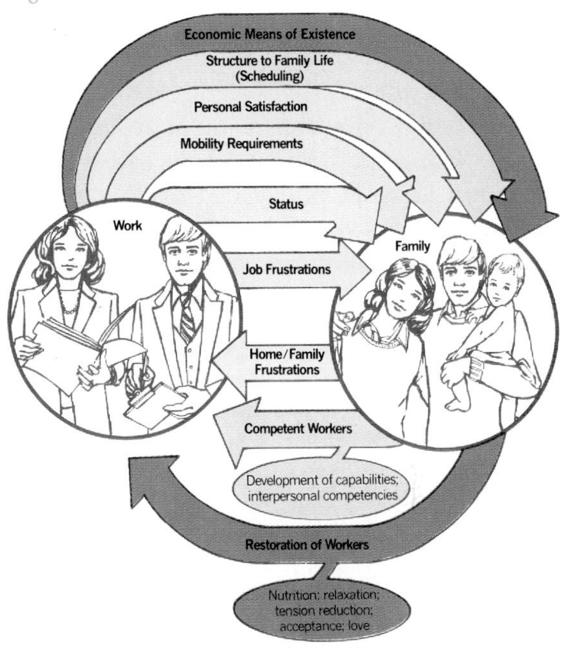

The worlds of work and family are not separate. They are strongly related.

Figure 15-2b

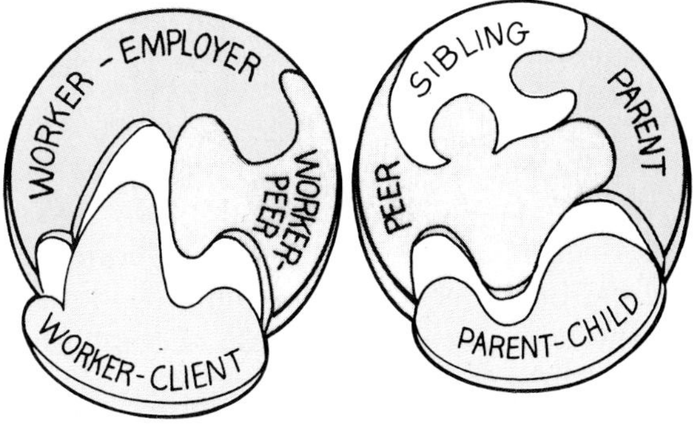

Within both the work world and the family world, there are various interactions.

these two aspects of our lives. The structure of the work system has a major influence on the kind and quality of family life. Likewise, the well-being and potential productivity of family members influence the work system. In both positive and negative ways, the two spheres impact on each other. Using Figure 15-2a and 15-2b as guides, consider these impacts.

The Effects of Work on the Family

There seems to be ready acceptance of the impact of work on the family. Most people understand, usually from first-hand experience, how the work world has both direct and indirect effects on the family and family members. A family's **economic means of**

existence is gained from work. The work world allows the family's economic function to take place. It is easy to understand how families are affected by a plant closing, a loss in sales, or a sudden expansion in productivity and profits. A new approach in sales or an alteration in work policy can make a direct and strongly felt impact on family members. Consider the following situations and the impacts they had on the economic means of existence for these families.

CASE IN POINT

The plant office decided to cut back its costs so now we have to wash our work uniforms. It's really expensive to have it done at a laundry, and our old washer can't manage those big uniforms. We have to make a special trip to the laundromat each week to wash my uniforms in a heavy-duty washer. It takes time away from home, and it's a bother.

We had budgeted to use some of the income from the corn crop to fix the front porch. Then we had a hail storm and the crop was nearly ruined. We'll have to hold off until next year to get the porch fixed.

My mother is doing really well at her job at the beauty parlor. More customers are asking for her. She can now set her own hours. Meals and evenings aren't as mixed-up as they were.

Personal satisfaction comes from the tasks performed in the work sphere. Self-concept evolves from the accomplishments at work and the rewards received for these accomplishments. The self-concept, in turn, affects our actions at home. People returning home after a successful and personally satisfying work day are likely to have positive family experiences. People returning home after an unfulfilling, frustrating work day are likely to have less positive family experiences.

Status is gained from the particular job as well as from work in general. This status is reflected on the worker and others in the family sphere. Whether or not the status received is satisfactory, it has an impact on the family.

The work sphere may require **relocation** to a different city or state in order to maintain jobs. This requirement varies with the type of employment. Positions with the military and large corporations require frequent moves. Some companies allow workers a choice of advancement with a relocation or of remaining in the current location without advancement. Whether a definite requirement or an option, relocation clearly affects the family sphere (Figure 15-3). Recently companies have required fewer relocations because of the high cost of such moves to the corporations involved. At the same time, there is an increase in relocation among blue-collar workers because of plant closings or plant relocation.

Figure 15-3

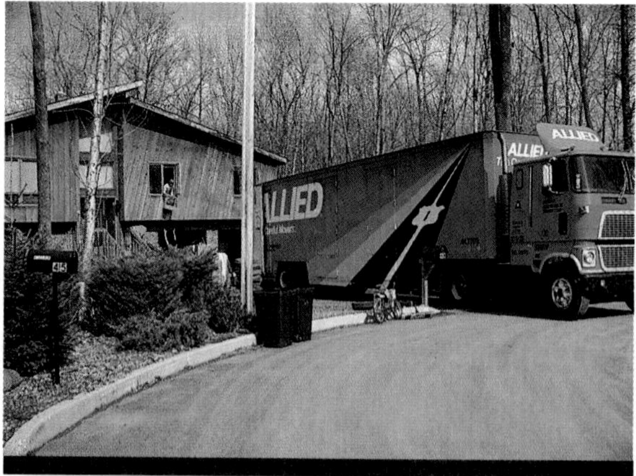

Relocations clearly affect the family—sometimes positively; other times negatively.
Renate Hiller/Monkmeyer Press

In such cases, workers are told they can maintain their job if they go with the company. When jobs are difficult to find, families will often accept an unwanted move in order to maintain an income.

Relocations are particularly difficult with multiple-worker families. Decisions need to be made, not only about the effect of the relocation on the family in general, but also about the impact on the careers and jobs of other family members.

Relocation can have both positive and negative aspects. Some families frequently relocate and seem to thrive on the experience. Other families can have a single relocation and find it a devastating experience. Consider these two situations and determine causes for the different responses to mobility.

CASE IN POINT

Sid and his wife, Robin, and their three children have moved eight times in the past 17 years. Sid is with the military, and relocating is part of the military life. The frequent moves have affected Sid's family in several ways. Robin has usually found some kind of part-time work often below her skills and abilities. Because of the family's frequent relocation, she has little chance for advancing in a job. The children dislike leaving friends they have made, but they have learned to adjust quickly. They make new friends and become acquainted with communities easily. Sid's family is very close, perhaps because they often rely on each other during resettlement. They all appreciate the opportunities these relocations have offered including meeting new people, seeing many places, and enjoying several foreign countries.

Muriel has worked at the plastics company for eight years. Rumors began circulating about the closing of the plant because of changes in management policy. Muriel looked for a job, but could not find one. When the plant closing was announced, workers were told they were guaranteed jobs at another division of the company in an adjacent state. Muriel and her two children moved in order to maintain a job. However, the move has been difficult. Finding a place to live, adjusting to new friends and new schools, and becoming familiar with new surroundings have been a major task for all three family members.

Spotlight on issues

The Work-at-Home Lifestyle

Most people don't think of the home as a place of employment. Instead, they consider the home as the place to return to after the day's work is finished. Yet, every year more Americans choose to work at home. In 1980 a national survey showed that 6 million people were employed within their homes. Recent surveys indicate that one out of three Americans would prefer to be employed at home.

The work-at-home lifestyle is often called the **electronic cottage**, in reference to the increasing use of electronic equipment and services that make possible new types of employment in the home. This term may be deceiving since many types of employment in the home do not involve electronics, computers, or telecommunications. But electronic materials have become an important factor in the creation of more work-at-home jobs. Telecommunication systems, home computers, word processors, and an increasing number of electronic devices have contributed to the transformation of the home into a workplace.

The impact of working at home is not yet clear, nor can anyone say for sure how widespread this lifestyle will become. Some of the advantages of at-home work include decreased transportation costs and time, increased work-time flexibility, easier management of work and family interaction, and increased family time together. In addition, children reach a better understanding of an involvement in their parents' work.

Not all those who have tried the work-at-home lifestyle have found it desirable or workable. Some workers find the disruptions by family members and the limited contact with co-workers harmful to their productivity. A high level of self-discipline is needed to resist the temptation to do household chores during work periods. Some at-home workers who are not self-employed find it difficult to regulate work time without a supervisor present.

Contrary to some current perceptions, working in the home does not necessarily eliminate the need for child care services. Work that requires high levels of concentration may make child care assistance necessary for part of the day.

People who have successfully managed employment in the home give the following suggestions for families considering the work-at-home lifestyle.

- Establish self-discipline appropriate for your own work style. Working in the home allows flexibility in timing of work and in taking breaks from work. Still, a general work pattern is usually necessary.
- Create a means for communicating with peers. Networks of people working in similar endeavors can be organized to meet informally. These networks provide both social and professional interaction necessary to stay aware of trends and stimulate new ideas. Electronic networks may be able to provide this communication.

- Maintain physical and psychological boundaries. Family members may infringe on a worker's time and space, especially at the start of this new work-at-home lifestyle. Guidelines as to when, how, and why workers are to be interrupted can lessen this problem.

There are positive and negative features of the work-at-home lifestyle. Families that have tried this way of working seem to find the positive aspects worthwhile and the negative ones controllable. How might your family function in a work-at-home lifestyle?

The work world adds a *structure* to the family life of the worker and the worker's family members. The structure differs with respect to the type of work. Some jobs do not require work beyond normal working hours. Other jobs require an absorption of the worker beyond the standard work hours (Figure 15-4). This absorption may involve family members as well as the worker. For example, consider farming, operating small shops or businesses, pastoral or ministry work, small town medical or other professional work. These occupations require involvement of the worker beyond the standard daily work time. They often absorb the worker's attention during nonworking hours. They also absorb time and attention of family members (Figure 15-5). Spouses of ministers are usually expected to fulfill a particular role related to the ministerial work. Farming and small business operations frequently involve most if not all family members. It seems clear that people involved in absorbing work can expect their work sphere to have a significant impact on their family sphere.

Scheduling a family activity is highly affected by work schedules. Mealtimes, bedtimes, social activities, vacations, leisure activities, and the amount of participation in community, religious, and social activities are affected by work schedules. The amount of flexibility allowed in particular jobs also affects the family sphere. For example, some jobs allow

Figure 15-4

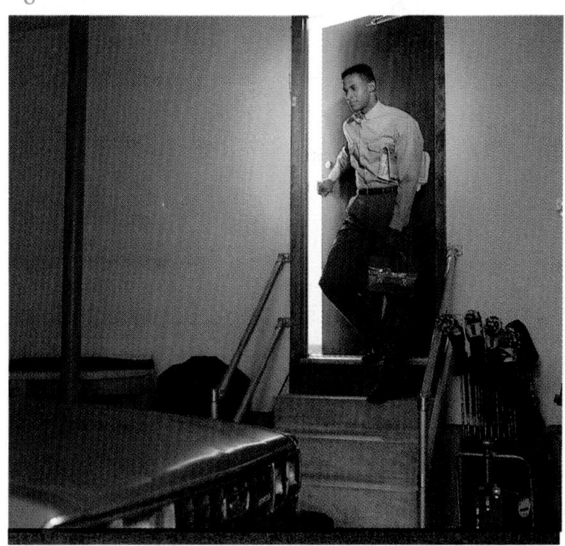

Some jobs require the worker to begin work at night. This work schedule affects family members as well as the worker.

Figure 15-5

Degree of Family Absorption in Work

HIGH ABSORPTION	MEDIUM ABSORPTION	LOW ABSORPTION
• occupation highly visible to family members • family members collaborate	• occupation has medium visibility to family members • family members provide some support	• occupation is physically exhaustive • home offers refuge and recuperation from work • family members play peripheral roles in occupation
Types of work: craft work; small business; some professional; farming	*Types of work:* bureaucratic; clerical; mid-management; technical	*Types of work:* mining; factory work; some clerical; highly technical and specialized

the worker to leave the work place at midday for a child's school program or other family-oriented reason, and to make up this time during off hours. Such flexibility has a positive impact on the family sphere.

Consider the following brief examples of work schedules structuring family life. Do you consider these positive or negative?

CASE IN POINT

Ellen could leave her home at 8:00 a.m. and be at work on time. However, because parking is limited, she must leave at 7:15 a.m. in order to get a parking space. She would start work when she arrived, but she is not able to count this as work time. Instead, she must waste 45 minutes each day away from her family without payment and without completing work.

Bill has to work the late shift every three weeks. During this time, his family has difficulty managing to keep the house quiet so Bill can sleep in the daytime.

Cara works the 9:00 p.m. hospital shift. She sleeps from 8:00 a.m. to 2:00 p.m. Then at 3 p.m. when her children come home from school, she can spend time with them.

Phil works at the City Recreation Department. His wife complains that when she has time off from her job—weekends and evenings—Phil is busy with his job.

Sue's mother is a doctor. Sue says that nearly every time there is a school activity that parents are to attend, her mother gets called away for an emergency.

Most employed people have some kind of **job frustrations**. Few people interact in their family sphere without sometimes letting these work frustrations affect their family life. Some individuals may communicate these frustrations openly while others keep silent about job concerns. However, most people are unable to prevent frustration of the work world from somehow affecting the family world. Being able to find a satisfactory way to handle frustration is an important task for most workers. Workers need to release some of the work-world frustration without dominating the family sphere with the frustration. An unpleasant attitude will affect work and family (Figure 15-6).

Figure 15-6

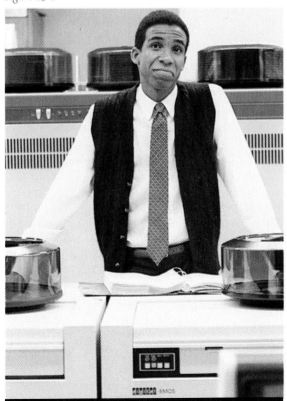

An unpleasant attitude, often caused by job frustrations, affects work and family life.

Effects of the Family on Work

It is clear to most people that the work world affects families. However, less thought has been given to how the family affects the work world.

Providing **competent workers** is a major way that the family sphere affects the work sphere. Employers are well aware of the need for competent workers in their businesses. Competence on the job entails skills that fit the needs of the particular work. These skills may be learned through education in a specific job training program or they may begin very early in life at the actual job site. Aside from these specific skills, many general capabilities and competencies are needed for most jobs. Many of these capabilities and competencies are gained in the home from family members. These include interpersonal communication, relating to fellow workers, accuracy in work, and attitudes toward work. Responsibility, promptness, and a positive attitude are also learned in the home. The family's provision of competent, capable workers affects the work world. Consider this storekeeper's situation.

CASE IN POINT

I hired a young man three months ago. His teachers told me he worked hard in his classes. His grades are good, and during the three weeks of training he seemed to catch on quickly. But he just can't seem to relate well to customers. I've tried to work with him, but he continues to have a surly, unpleasant attitude toward people. I don't think he means to be rude, but that's how he appears. Last night I met his father. He had the same unpleasantness about him. I'm just going to have to find somebody else for the job!

This young man may have gained his manner of relating to others from many sources. However, it appears that his home/family situation has fostered this way of reacting. The family sphere in this case has impacted negatively on the work sphere.

Restoring workers is another activity that takes place in the family world which impacts on the work world. The family sphere provides a psychological and physical restoration for workers. In the home, a worker can relax and reduce tensions (Figure 15-7). Proper nutrition and adequate sleep give the worker renewed strength for the job. Acceptance and love from family members restore the worker and give new perspectives to a person's life. Pleasant surroundings enhance this relaxation and acceptance. Single people find the same relaxation and tension reduction in their home surroundings. Friends and extended family members provide acceptance and love.

Figure 15-7

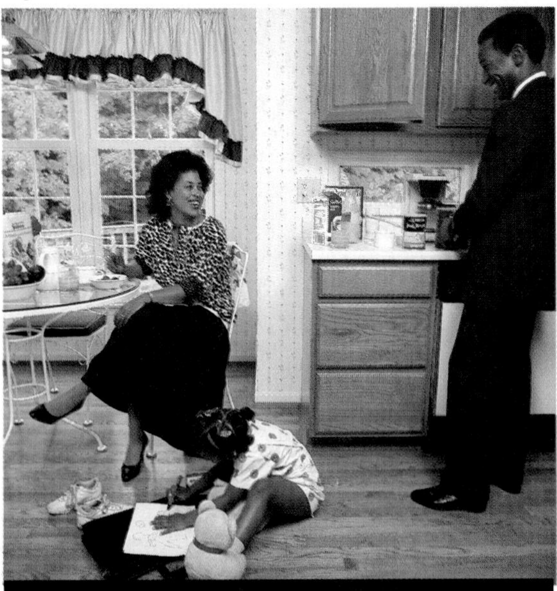

Workers are restored physically and emotionally by the interaction among family members within the home.

Clearly, not all family spheres provide the need for necessary restoration. When the home sphere repeatedly and severely fails to provide this restoration, it will adversely affect the work sphere. The repeated impact will likely produce dissatisfaction with the worker, which may result in lack of promotion or loss of the job.

Consider the following failures to restore the worker in the family sphere. Are these situations only temporary or long-term? How do they impact on the worker, the worker's family, and the employer?

CASE IN POINT

Joan and Frank had a baby daughter last month. Frank took two weeks of paternity leave. Now he is back at work. The baby has not yet managed to sleep through the night, and the last three nights were particularly difficult and tiring for all three family members. Frank is tired and has been irritable with his co-workers.

Shanna has never developed good nutritional habits. No one in her family eats breakfast, but each person usually has a rich pastry at mid-morning. Shanna's summer job in the park requires physical stamina. By 10:00 a.m., Shanna is dragging and can't seem to keep up with the rest of the work crew. Both yesterday and today, Shanna's supervisor complained about her slowness and her poor job of weeding the flower beds.

Both Dorothy and Paul like to return from their jobs and relax together in their living room or on their porch. Often their children join them. Though this relaxation is brief (they usually start dinner after about 20 minutes), they find it to be a good way to unwind. For the past week, Paul's brother, sister-in-law, and young son have been visiting. Not only must Paul and Dorothy entertain their guests, but they also must give up their relaxation period.

Andrea has lived alone for four years, except for her dog, Shelly. Shelly was killed by a car two months ago. Andrea had always looked forward to Shelly's greeting when she returned home from work. Shelly's evening walk provided Andrea with exercise, relaxation, and the opportunity to meet people in her neighborhood. Andrea feels foolish telling people how much she misses Shelly. Yet, Andrea realizes that the absence of her special friend is affecting her behavior at home and at work.

Just as people bring work frustrations to the family sphere, so do home/family frustrations enter and affect the work sphere (Figure 15-8). Breakdowns in the home and family cause major problems in the work sphere. Divorce, separation, loss of a pet, alcohol or drug abuse, major illness in the family, and confrontation with the law have a major impact on a person's performance in the work world. Common illnesses, daily school concerns, family disagreements, and scheduling conflicts are less severe but still affect the work world. Absenteeism from the job and lack of attention while on the job may result from these family/home frustrations. Workers who bring frustrations to the work world affect their own productivity and that of the company.

A more positive interaction of work and family is possible with greater effort on the part of both families and employers. Policies that reflect family needs and provide support systems to families can be provided by the corporate/business system. In turn, families can assess their goals and values, improve management skills, and provide their own support systems.

Figure 15-8

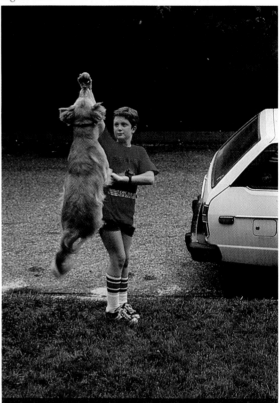

Losing a loving pet can affect the work sphere.

ASSESSING FAMILY VALUES AND GOALS

The balancing of work and family is improved when family members have a clear understanding of their values and goals related to employment. Assessing these values and goals both as an individual and as a family gives direction to dealing with work/family concerns.

Family-Work Values

As stated in Chapter 3, a value is a belief or feeling that something or someone has worth. What degree of worth do you and your family members place on work? Do you and other family members consider work a necessary evil that must be carried out in order to live? Is work an element in your life that provides meaning and feelings of achievement and success far beyond the dollar it may bring?

Family-Work Goals

A goal is an end toward which effort is directed. Values not only influence the types of goals we set, they also influence the amount of time, energy, and effort we are willing to put forth to see our goals accomplished. Work values that are based only on economic benefits produce different short- and long-term work goals than do work values that emphasize self-fulfillment.

Using the Family-Work Value/Goal chart that follows (Figure 15-9), determine if your family values and goals are oriented primarily toward income or primarily toward career. Does your family's orientation lie somewhere between these values? What value/goal orientation would you prefer your current family to have? What value/goal orientation would you like your future family to have?

Consider the following situations. Ask yourself if the interaction represented in these examples flows from the work sphere to the family sphere. In which situations does the work sphere positively or negatively affect the family sphere? How? Why? In which situations is it possible to see the family sphere having a positive effect on the work sphere negative effect? Explain.

1. The autumn sales meeting in Carl's company requires a lot of take-home work for Carl.
2. Ms. Lane, the school principal, enjoys knowing students and seeing them grow up to take their places in the community.
3. Greg does well at his part-time job in the clothing store. He has a real ability to relate well to people.
4. Mr. Carson's recent divorce has been very upsetting for him. He has trouble concentrating on his job.
5. Eva feels good when she returns home from work, hugs her husband, and gets kisses from her two children.
6. Jane's difficult semester at college was helped by the love, affection, and acceptance shown by her parents and sister.
7. The plastics company closed. The workers were told they could keep their jobs if they moved to the new plant.
8. Paul's mother is a minister. Her schedule during evenings and weekends is very busy.
9. Sid was so disgusted with his boss that he came home, slammed the door, slumped in his chair, and drank three beers.
10. Doris got the job at the greenhouse because her father had taught her about plant care and plant identification.
11. Sonia's mother is the school superintendent. All of the teachers know Sonia and expect the best grades and behavior from her at all times.

The goals and values related to work and family might be better understood by consid-

Figure 15-9

Family-Work Value/Goal

	Primarily Income-Oriented	Integrated	Primarily Career-Oriented
Value of Work for the Family	Work brings only financial means of existence: necessary evil	Work is highly valued yet other aspects of life are equally valued.	Work provides major meaning and fulfillment for family members.
Identifying Behaviors	• Family finds major pleasures in outlets other than work.	• Pleasures received from both work world and other aspects of life.	• Pleasure is gained mainly from work world.
	• Family activities are totally apart from work world.	• Family activities contain a mixture or balance with the work world.	• Many or most family activities revolve around the work world.
	• Family members only vaguely aware of actual work of other family members.	• Awareness of actual work activities of other family members.	• Family members are strongly aware of and may be involved in some aspect of each other's work world.
Goals	• Short range: continue to maintain job in order to have income.	• Short range: seek career/work challenges tempered with meaningful personal and home life.	• Short term: continually improve work position in order to gain new challenges and personal growth in the work world.
	• Long range: discontinue work as soon as financially possible in order to seek pleasure elsewhere.	• Long range: retire at typical stage; maintain interest in work world yet develop new interests and capabilities.	• Long term: extend work life as long as possible; retire late or not at all; work interest continues into later years.

ering three families: The Moneysmiths who are primarily income-oriented; the Fulfillers who are primarily career-oriented; and the Middlers who have an integrated orientation. Consider these families and how their work values affect their long- and short-term goals.

CASE IN POINT

The **Moneysmiths** are primarily income-oriented. Mr. Moneysmith works with a large corporation where he makes all arrangements for the business trips for the top executives. Mr. Moneysmith's desk job keeps him busy from 9:00 a.m. to 5:00 p.m. but seldom requires time during evenings or weekends. Mrs. Moneysmith is a temporary office worker employed at various places each week. She also does some typing from her home. The Moneysmith's main interest is in a horse farm outside the city which they purchased five years ago. They spend nearly every weekend there, and their lives and the lives of their three children center around horses and horse farm activities. Mr. Moneysmith plans to retire as soon as possible and move to the farm.

Mr. **Fulfiller** is a landscape architect who previously worked for a large company. He now owns his own business where he plans and implements landscaping for both businesses and residences. Ms. Fulfiller is a kindergarten teacher, very devoted to her profession. She has received various awards for excellence in teaching and is highly respected. She also has a hobby of photography which she applies to both her schoolwork and to landscaping work. She has a photo diary of all the landscaping architecture projects completed by Mr. Fulfiller. Both Mr. and Ms. Fulfiller bring work home with them in the evenings and on many weekends. Bob Fulfiller, their son, just entered college where he plans to take small business management classes and later assist his father. Sue Fulfiller is still in high school, but she has an avid interest in horticulture and plans to study this further beyond high school. Both children have accompanied their father on many of his jobs. Many family vacations are centered around visiting outstanding landscaping sites. Family communication often centers on this topic. Mr. and Ms. Fulfiller both plan to continue their careers: they probably will choose late retirements. Mr. Fulfiller feels that even after officially retiring, he will probably continue with a job here or there.

Mr. and Mrs. **Middler** are X-ray technicians who met while in school. They work at different sites—Mrs. Middler at a hospital and Mr. Middler at a large X-ray laboratory. Both enjoy their work and discuss it often at home. Their daughter seems to have some interest in the medical technology field, but their sons have other interests. Though the Middlers are very involved in their work, it does not enter their home lives to a great extent. Family activities center primarily around sports. The Middlers both plan to retire at the usual retirement age. They may then pursue their hobbies of gardening and china collecting.

It should be clear that none of these models is best. All three families contain members who are good workers, who do their best for their employers in their specific jobs, and who are concerned with society as a whole. All three models can function positively if family members are aware of and accept family-work values and goals.

MANAGING TIME

It takes wise use of time to balance work and family. Hectic schedules of family members, coupled with the required time and energy of multiple worker families, can cause frustration. Wise management of time is vital to successful families.

Often the lack of time seems to become a monster or a villain in the work/family interchange. This monster can be tamed by several techniques. You may already use some of these techniques without considering them a method of improved management.

Scheduling Systems

Active families need some type of system for scheduling activities. Mechanisms as simple as a chart, calendar, task list, or memo board can help organize family members and keep activities running smoothly.

Even activities that seem to affect only one individual can have an impact on other family members. This is especially true when transportation and care of other family members are involved. A large calendar taped to the refrigerator or other prominent spot can be helpful in coordinating work and family activities. A chart or list can be created by family members to meet special needs of their own family.

School systems and social organizations that schedule their activities in advance are helpful to families in their planning. Arrangements often can be made to deal with complex schedules if advance notice is given.

Some families have established a coordinator's job which rotates from member to member. The coordinator has the responsibility of seeing who will be home on what evenings to stay with younger children. The coordinator also makes connections between members to cover transportation needs. In general, the person knows where people are, how they get there and get back, and who will be at home. Though this task traditionally belonged to a parent, children in many homes are able to play the role of coordinator.

Communication Systems

The best calendar or chart and the most highly developed communication skills will not be helpful unless family members have some system or plan for communication. For many families communication is based around mealtime—specifically the evening meal. This is usually the time for relating happenings, feelings, ideas, and present and future activities. Other families may have other communication points—in the evening before bedtime, during the after-dinner clean-up, or in the morning before work and school.

A time set aside for communication of various family and work issues and for sharing a family time is helpful. Planned family sessions, to be discussed in Chapter 18, are helpful organizational tools.

Quality vs. Quantity Time

In Chapter 5, we discussed that people can talk and really not communicate. Likewise, people can spend many hours together without gaining or giving any benefits from the togetherness. The quantity or amount of time together is not necessarily related to quality or degree of good received from the time. A parent may insist on spending the majority of the day in the presence of his or her child. Yet, this time together may provide little quality-interaction. Being engrossed in work of the home, watching television, or otherwise being preoccupied can provide quantity time but not necessarily quality time. Being busy with chores, acting as chauffeur, observing family members in sports activities, reading the newspaper, and watching television are some of the activities that may amount to high quantity but low quality family time. Efforts can be made to transform quantity time to quality time.

- Turn off the television after the presentation and discuss the program.
- Make a deliberate effort to discuss situations at mealtime.

- Use the family interest in sports or other activities (whether participant or spectator) as a building block to discussions.
- Turn a wasted few minutes into a meaningful exchange by going for a short walk. Jog together and walk home.
- Make an attempt to listen to what other family members are saying.

Of course, if you can't get *any* time together as a family, it is difficult to have quality time. But most families do have time which they poorly manage or misuse. By taking a critical look at how we spend our time within families, we can see some wedges in which we can place some valuable family interaction. Consider Bill, Sandra, and their six-year-old son, Charlie. After considering their daily schedules, they found three spots in which they wasted valuable time together:

20 to 30 minutes before the evening meal: At this time, Sandra usually cooked, Bill checked the mail or vice versa, and Charlie watched television.

Change: Now Sandra and Bill alternate meal preparation while the other reads aloud a chapter in a book to Charlie. All three share the kitchen and the story. Bill and Sandra enjoy some of the classics such as *Swiss Family Robinson.* Discussion of the story usually carries over into the meal. Charlie's interest in books has increased, and this action has provided a good break from work-world activities.

30 to 45 minutes after mealtime but before Charlie's bedtime: Bill read the newspaper each evening after the meal was cleared away. This took most of the available parent/child time.

Change: Bill has decided to hold off his newspaper reading until after Charlie's bedtime, allowing more family time to be shared among the three.

30 minutes before the 11:00 p.m. news: Sandra and Bill always watched the 11:00 p.m. news before bed. They used this as their major means of catching up on the happenings of the day. They usually sat before the television, half watching something uninteresting and waiting for the 11:00 p.m. time slot. Bill often dozed in the chair.

Change: They decided this was a time waster. They now deliberately turn off the television until the 11:00 p.m. hour. They can share many things in these few minutes.

Though none of these time slots is large, they total approximately 90 minutes of quality interaction during the day. This method of assessing family times can assist families with heavy work commitments. Families can find time or make more time to share together.

Setting Priorities

Giving a rating or a ranking is called setting a priority. When a group of active people have their work and family goals coupled with household tasks and activities, setting priorities is usually necessary. From time to time, an individual or family activity will have to be given a low ranking or rating or possibly eliminated. Some household tasks may have to be set aside temporarily or permanently. (Not every task and chore carried out in the home is necessary.)

CASE IN POINT

Sandy's family reached a mutual decision that they were involved in too many activities. Their schedules were so busy, it seemed they seldom had time to see each other. Sandy's mother, her brothers, and Sandy made lists of each activity or club in which they were involved. Then they ranked each one for the amount of enjoyment gained personally and the amount of good this activity did for others. Sandy found that there were three clubs she was a member of in which she had no interest. The activities were neither enjoyable nor of much aid to others.

Sometimes setting priorities and saying no to requests for your services can be difficult. Limited time requires such ranking if a group of people is to function successfully.

Lowering Standards for Low Priority Items

Chores can be ranked just as other aspects of family life. Standards need not be as high for the low priority items. For example, if your family puts a low priority on the value of sparkling windows, less than perfect standards can be applied for window washing in your home.

If your family does not value sweets, is weight conscious, and seldom has time for dessert, then you could clearly rank dessert preparation as a low priority item. Lower standards in dessert preparation and selection would be in order. The lowering of standards on low priority items allows time and effort to be placed on the high priority items as well as on the family interaction itself.

Delegating Responsibilities

Many times household activities remain with one or two people when others in the family are capable of handling these tasks. Working mothers, particularly mothers who have returned to the work force, may be hesitant to ask family members to take over household chores. This "Super Mom Complex" eventually causes frustration and conflict in many situations.

Delegating responsibility to all family members is a learning experience that is relatively painless if several precautions are taken.

Teach the task or skill to the family member. For example:

- Show the best way to safely load the dishwasher.
- Explain exactly what to ask when having the automobile oil changed.
- Make reminder cards to help people remember how to set the washing machine and dryer.

Make the expectation clear. For example:

- Make lists of jobs to be rotated, and put the job lists in a prominent place.
- Have clear statements of what is expected: "Scrub bathtub with cleanser and sponge. Rinse thoroughly." This cannot be interpreted as a quick rinse job.
- Make clear who does what and how often and for how long.

Show consideration and appreciation for tasks even if not done to the level at which others had done them in the past. Comment on originality, creativity, or a different or more efficient way of achieving the same goal (Figure 15-10).

Figure 15-10

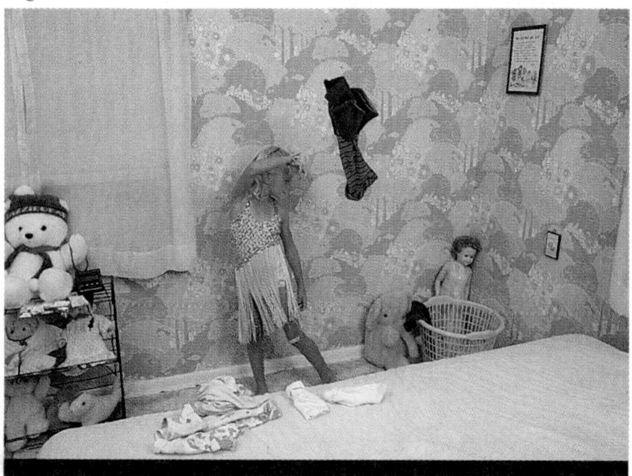

Dirty socks reaching the clothes basket by means of a book shot from across the room may get to the laundry faster than otherwise.

It is not only children who must encounter new tasks. Adults who have not done a particular task must learn new skills just as children must.

DEVELOPING SUPPORT SYSTEMS

One of the greatest aids to families in balancing work and family is a system of supports. A support system is a collection of people and services who directly help with managing the family or can serve as a backup in particularly difficult times. In past generations, extended families provided such services. Family and neighbors often functioned as support systems without considering themselves as such.

Family and neighborhood ties still exist for many people. However, increasing mobility leaves many families without the help of extended family and close friends. Another change from past generations is that grandmothers who once played major child care roles may now be employed full-time. The grandmother may not be able to assist even if living close by.

Multiple-worker families (families in which more than one adult is employed) and single-parent families have particular needs for support systems. The time conflict and compounded responsibilities of these families usually require extra support to keep things running smoothly. People in such families need to take action to develop systems of assistance and support. Families need to reach out to establish or construct a support system.

Individual and Family-Developed Systems of Support

Reaching out to local friends and acquaintances is often necessary in order to initiate a support group. A willingness to pool activities and participate with others is a part of most support systems.

PERSONAL SUPPORT SYSTEMS • Consider the following examples of support systems and determine how many your family uses or might use. How do you assume such systems developed? What action was taken to establish the support?

CASE IN POINT

Claudia Gray is a single parent with two preschoolers. Claudia has joined with three other parents to share child care. On Tuesday evenings, Claudia will care for any of the other families. On Thursday, Claudia can leave her children with the family on duty and have an evening to herself for shopping or relaxation. These four families all serve as emergency helpers. A sick child sent home from school or from day care can use the backup aid of one of the families.

Andrew and Shelly Kovaks both work full-time jobs. Their three children—ages 7, 10, and 11—are cared for after school by a neighborhood mother who does not work outside her home. Andrew's aunt living in the same town helps with child care occasionally in emergency situations. This happened when their young son had a case of chicken pox and could not go to the neighbor's house. In addition, Andrew and Shelly have had a college student stay overnight with the children when both parents have to be out of town. This support system of child care allows Andrew and Shelly to handle their workload without undue worry about the children.

Phil Jiminez has never married. In his apartment building he has found four other single people: Jane, a retired widow; Pete, a divorced insurance agent; Ellen, a middle-aged accountant; and Carlos, a young social worker. These five people have established a rotating Wednesday supper at their homes. This has provided a system of friendship, shared interests, and neighborhood concern for one another.

Kelly, 15, and Kevin, 13, are responsible young people who live with their father, Frank Hogan. They no longer need child care services after school. Yet, the assistance from retired neighbors, Don and Gladys Powell, supplies a support system that is helpful to Frank and the children. If Kevin or Kelly need help or assistance, they can always go to the Powells. They often stop in to chat or sample Mrs. Powell's baking. In turn, Frank and his children often help the Powells with tree trimming, furniture moving, or other physical work.

Sheila McMullen does not get home from work until 5:45 p.m. Soccer practice for her daughter, Carmen, starts at 4:30 p.m. and ends at 6:00. Sheila contacted several parents of Carmen's teammates who could deliver the children to the soccer field. Sheila picks up the children at 6:00 p.m.

COMMUNITY SUPPORT SYSTEMS • The above examples reflect small neighborhood or cluster groups of support services. Families must often work to establish wider, more general community support to assist working families. Community services to assist people in particular circumstances may never come about unless action is taken to create such services. This action is usually sparked by one or two people who can relay their concerns to others and generate a wider circle of interest and concern. Consider the following action by Marion and Sid.

CASE IN POINT

When Marion Goldstein began working after seven years of being a full-time homemaker, she and her husband, Sid, realized that many of the school and community activities conflicted with working parents. Marion, Sid, and a group of other working parents met with the school superintendent to point out several concerns:

1. Activities (choir groups, drama presentations, etc.) held during work hours and requesting parent attendance

2. Parent-teacher conferences held during the school/work day with little advance notice to schedule arrangements
3. School emergency records reflecting only "father's place of employment"
4. Community center offering classes for parents and children only on weekday afternoons rather than including Saturday afternoon
5. No bus service after school hours for junior high and high school students involved in extracurricular activities
6. No provision for after school child care of elementary grade students

The school and community system has begun to react to the situations highlighted by this parent group. As more working parents request assistance and support from the school and community, changes may occur. These parents will need to assist in the process by volunteering time and providing extra payment for services.

A personal/family need shared by many people motivated the above action. Community action that assists individuals and families has been responsible for an array of support services. Day care for both children and adults, group-sponsored "parents night out," organized groups to assist in car care or household maintenance, and structured organizations of carpools serve as examples. Such group action assists families in balancing the work world and family world.

What structured support services are available in your community? How were they started? What support services are needed?

Employment-Oriented Support Systems

As employers see the relationship between well-organized, stable families and work productivity, they are more likely to provide family supportive benefits for employees. Many businesses have employment policies that can assist individuals and families in dealing with their home and family life. Many of thc policies help to reduce the stress employees feel when the demands of the job conflict with the demands of the employee's family. In addition, there are benefits and services that can be supplied by the employers. Employee benefits, policies, and services which provide a network of support are discussed below.

REARRANGED WORKWEEK • A variety of schedules are included within the term rearranged workweek. Any schedule different from the standard five-day, 40-hour, Monday-through-Friday arrangement is considered a rearranged workweek. New types of work schedules are being used increasingly throughout the United States work force. Such alternatives to the standard, structured work schedule have the potential to meet the needs of both families and employers.

These rearranged or alternative work schedules can be applied to nearly all types of work but are particularly suitable to certain types of employment. Services that cater to public needs such as libraries, department stores, auto sales, and transportation services usually use rearranged work hours. Services that are provided round-the-clock (hospitals, police departments, food production, data processing) must have rearranged work schedules.

Of the various types of rearranged schedules responsive to worker needs, the most common are flexible worktime, job sharing, and compressed workweek.

FLEXIBLE WORKING HOURS (FLEXTIME) • This allows a worker to work a determined number of hours within a particular time period. In most situations, there is a common core time when all workers must be on the job. The flexible period is at the beginning and end of the day when workers decide their own arrival and departure times (Figure 15-11). For example, people in the Fanco Corporation are required to work eight hours a day anytime between 7:00 a.m. and 8:00 p.m. There is a common midday time (core time) for all workers to be present. One employee may come to work at 11:00 a.m., take a lunch break from 3:00 to 4:00 p.m., and then work until 8:00 p.m. Another employee can arrive at 8:00 a.m. and leave at 5:00 p.m. Both employees chose their work hours to meet their personal and family needs.

There are many advantages to flexible working hours. Work can be planned around children's school hours; heavy traffic times can be avoided; and workers can participate in more community and service activities. Flexible schedules tend to reduce absenteeism. Employees on flexible schedules appear to be more satisfied with their jobs. Many companies have found greater work productivity with flextime.

Employers have some concern related to flexible hours because of time and effort involved in managing the workers' schedules. In some cases, flextime may increase building operation costs because of the longer time period involved each day. Most problems or concerns related to flextime, however, seem to be at the initiation stage. As workers and employers grow accustomed to the structure, they usually find that it is beneficial to all.

JOB SHARING • When two people voluntarily divide the tasks and responsibilities of one full-time job, they are **job sharing**. Salaries and fringe benefits are calculated by the amount of time each person works. For example, Paula and Charles share a computer operator job for an insurance company. Each works a half day (four hours). This situation allows both Paula and Charles to have a source of income, keep their skills updated, and yet have time for other pursuits. (Paula is busy

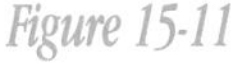
Figure 15-11

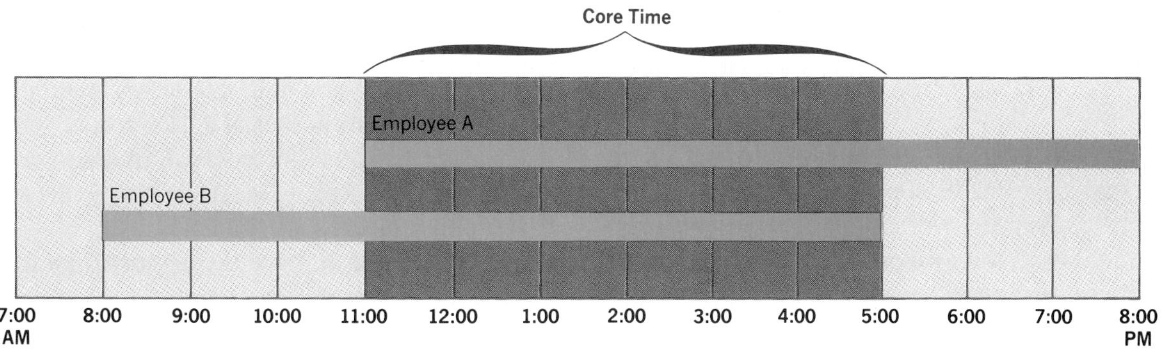

caring for two small children; Charles is taking advanced courses at the university.)

Their employer welcomed this job sharing for Paula and Charles. Both are good workers and may wish to work fulltime later on. Many employers have found increased productivity and low absenteeism with job sharing. There are minor increases in record keeping and taxes for the employer. But once established, job sharing seems beneficial to both worker and employer.

COMPRESSED WORKWEEK • This allows a worker to be on the job less than five days a week but with concentrated hours of work each day. Usually a compressed workweek consists of a four-day, 40-hour work schedule with 10 hours of work each day. Such scheduling allows the worker more compressed family and personal time as well as more compressed work time. Three-day weekends are an advantage of this scheduling. The disadvantage is a long, ten-hour work day which can be very tiring for some people. For people who tire easily, this schedule could be negative to both work productivity and home life.

Employers can save money with compressed work hours. Plant start-up and shut-down costs can be cut significantly. However, some types of work and some types of employees do not fit the compressed workweek.

SUPPORTIVE BENEFITS • Employers have begun to provide supportive benefits other than rearranged workweek to workers. Such benefits are slowly becoming part of employee benefit packages to assist family life of the workers. These include health insurance and life insurance programs which assist the worker and his/her family in the event of illness, accident, or death. Disability and worker compensation programs provide a continuous flow of income to the family when the worker is unable to work due to illness or injury. Without such supportive benefits, workers and their families are vulnerable to catastrophic losses in income in the face of crisis situations.

CHILD CARE SERVICES • Child care services are provided in some industries and corporations. Such services allow parents to be near their child or children. They can see their children at breaks and lunch periods (Figure 15-12). Such child care reassures workers of the type of care for their children. This reassurance removes worry from workers who can concentrate more on the job. Child care services in the workplace are seldom free, but fees are usually minimal.

For parents of young children, appropriate day care is a major factor in interrelating work and family. The following are important questions to consider when assessing a child care center.

1. Can the place be reached easily?
2. Are there plenty of good and varied toys and equipment for fun and learning?
3. Is the place safe, attractive, and comfortable?
4. Are there nutritious, tasty meals and snacks?
5. Do children and staff members communicate happily and easily?
6. Is each child respected as an individual?
7. To what extent is the caregiver(s) dependable, responsible?
8. Does each child have the opportunity for a wide variety of activities?
9. How are children's illnesses, vacations, and emergencies handled?
10. Can you afford the fees at this care service?

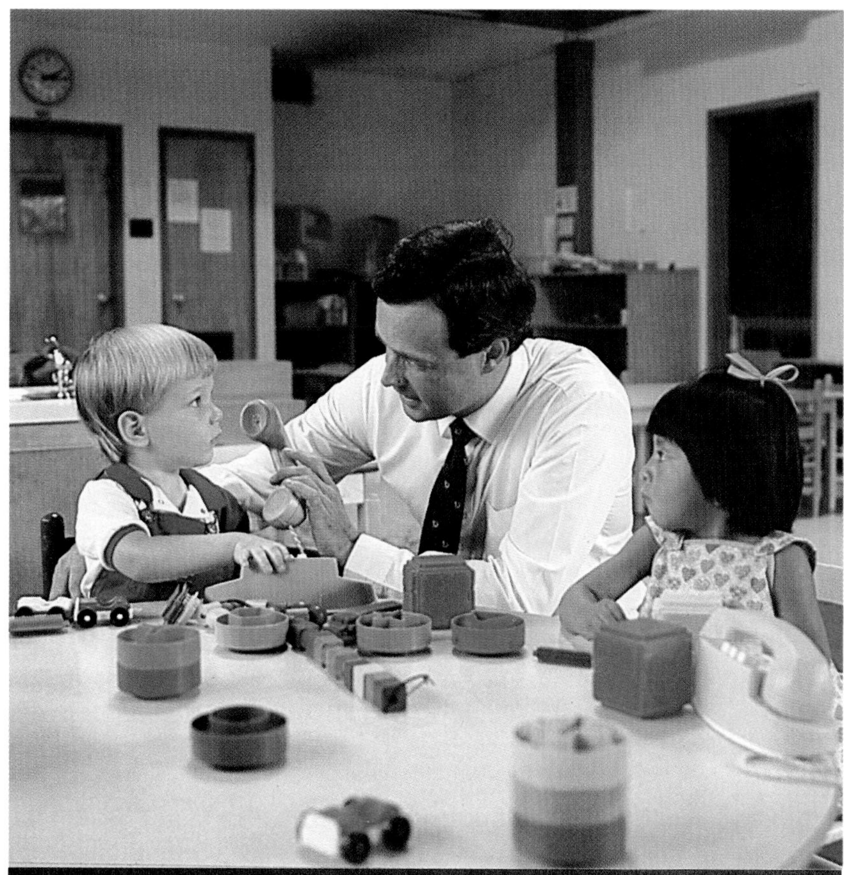

Figure 15-12
The quality of day-care services available to working parents is a major factor in the interaction of work and family.

PARENTAL LEAVES • Parental leaves allow parents to leave the work place for planned activities—children's doctor and dental appointments, school activities, etc. Some employers allow workers the option of fewer days of sick leave to allow days of parental leave. Parental leave can also include maternity and paternity leaves. Paternity leave can be several days or several weeks. During this time, the father assists with the care of the new baby. Maternity leave is more common, and sometimes lasts as long as six months.

LIMITED TRANSFERS • Limited transfers have become a policy for many corporations. Employers are beginning to give more consideration to requiring transfers that affect family members. More employers realize that relocations cost the corporations large sums of money and may bring about low morale of employees. Limited transfer policies involve careful consideration before workers are relocated.

Special assistance to workers and their families is offered in some large corporations.

Counseling for various family and personal concerns or for alcohol or drug abuse are increasingly offered to workers. Such services have direct benefits to workers and indirect benefits to employers. Employees with fewer problems that interfere with work are more productive workers.

Not all businesses are ready and willing to provide supportive benefits for workers and their families. However, as various unions and worker groups request and/or demand such services, greater consideration will be given to these benefits and supports. In times of difficult economic conditions, provision of such benefits may be made in lieu of pay increases or to supplement low increases.

In several studies of desired employee benefits, it was found that flexible hours ranked number one, family leave as number two, and day care for children as number three. Single-parent families with young children unanimously chose day care as the number one benefit desired.

Balancing the work world and family world is of growing importance to today's families as well as today's business and industry. Success in one world is often dependent on success in the other. Efforts to improve management, meet individual needs, and develop support systems can be of benefit to families and the economy.

WRAPPING IT UP

Our work and family lives are closely intertwined. What happens to us during the day on our jobs has both direct and indirect effects on our relationships with our family members. Likewise, family relationships influence our ability to be productive workers on the job.

In regard to the effect of work on family life, work provides the money for a family's *economic existence*. Food, clothing, and shelter are the basic needs that paid employment helps us to meet. Personal satisfaction at work and the *status* we gain can have positive effects on family relationships. Likewise, problems and frustrations at work can spill over into the home to create stress in family relationships. Many jobs also require *relocation* of an employee to a different city or state. Such moves can be stressful for family members, particularly in dual-worker families where the jobs of both workers are affected. Work schedules influence family relationships by setting constraints on how family members manage their time. Mealtimes, bedtimes, vacations, leisure activities, and participation in religious, social, and community activities are affected by the demands of one's work schedule.

In regard to the effects of family life on the work world, families provide competent workers to the work force. The skills necessary for work are related to the family's ability to teach interpersonal skills of communication and cooperation to its members. Families help to mold a person's attitudes toward work and his or her values on responsibility, promptness, and productivity. Families also help to restore workers' mental and physical well-being during the time that they spend at home. Rest, nutrition, relaxation, and emotional nurturance are all crucial for the continued productivity of the worker. Worker productivity can be harmed, however, by relationship problems and conflicts in the family. Drug and alcohol abuse, divorce, separation, and major illness in the family can have particularly severe negative effects on a person's performance on the job.

The way in which family and work life is balanced varies from one family to the next. The balance depends on the family's values and goals related to work. To help achieve a satisfactory balance between work and family life, families should consider developing a system of time management to handle scheduling needs and conflicts. Families must also consider the need for high quality communication in order to maintain satisfying relationships. Priorities may have to be set, and standards for low priority activities may have to be lowered, in order to achieve a satisfactory work-family balance. Other means include delegating new responsibilities to family members, and developing support systems of friends, neighbors, and community groups.

Employers, too, can assist families in achieving a satisfactory balance between work and family life. Allowing employees to choose flexible workweek schedules, *job sharing*, and compressed workweeks can ease the scheduling conflicts families may have in attempting to balance work and home commitments. Such supportive benefits as child care in the workplace, leaves of absence for parents, and limiting the number of times employees are transferred to another location are additional ways in which employers can help families to create a satisfying home life at the same time that they have a fulfilling work life.

Exploring Dimensions of Chapter Fifteen

For Review

1• Describe three aspects of the work world that affect the family world. Are these aspects positive, negative, or both?

2• Explain how the family sphere affects the work sphere.

3• Describe three local established systems of support for families. Describe three support systems that could be developed within an individual family.

4• List three management techniques that could assist in balancing work life and family life.
5• What is meant by "degree of family absorption in work"? Give an example.

For Consideration

1• In small groups discuss several television or movie families and determine if they are primarily income-oriented, primarily career-oriented, or integrated. Determine the degree of family absorption in work for each of the families.
2• Consider school work as your work world and establish a plan for a support system to assist you.
3• Determine at least two values related to work. Consider how you react to these values. What goals have they helped you form? How have they affected your behavior?
4• Create an example of the effects of work concerns and frustrations on the family. Create another example showing family concerns and frustration affecting work.
5• Select an occupation at random and establish a work schedule that you would consider most beneficial for both work and family. What factors would make this schedule positive? What negative aspects are involved in this schedule? What values and goals are reflected in your selection?

For Application

1• Using the chart of Interaction of Work and Family (Figure 15-2a-2b), describe a particular family giving examples of impact on the work sphere and family sphere.
2• Survey businesses in the community to determine support systems established to help families. Discover what action brought about these systems of assistance. Discover why such systems of support have not been established.
3• Develop a booklet or checklist of management techniques or hints to assist families in managing the interaction of their work/family life.
4• Create an example of the effects of work concerns and frustrations on the family. Create another example showing family concerns and frustration affecting work.

5. Determine how other cultures deal with interactions of work and family. Do they have more or less structured roles? Are certain family members designated to care for children? Are extended family members involved? How do the values and goals of a culture affect their dealing with work and family interactions?

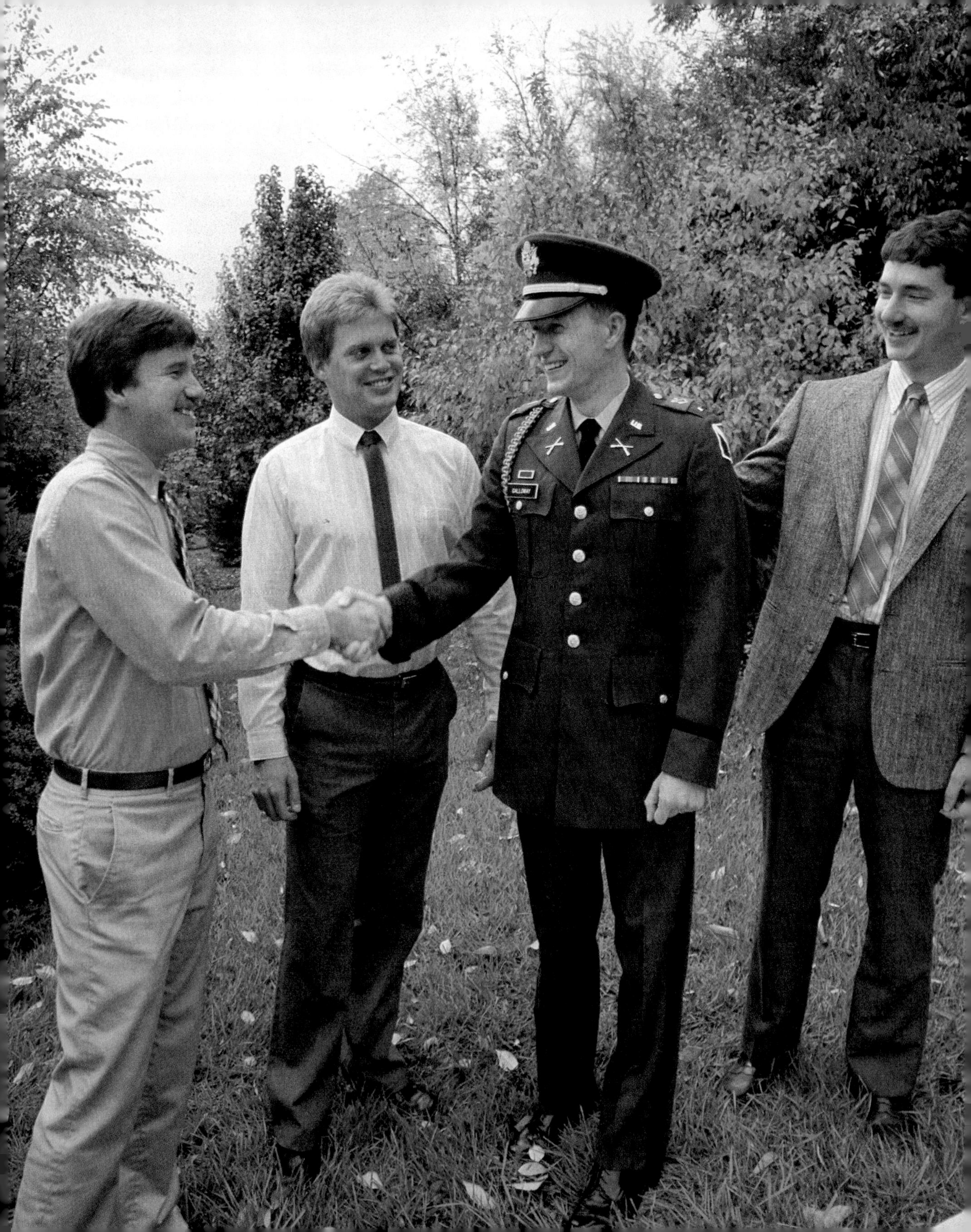

sixteen

MAKING OCCUPATIONAL AND CAREER DECISIONS

This chapter provides information that will help you to:

- Gather information about yourself.
- Gather information about occupations and careers.
- Consider family factors related to occupational and career decisions.
- Evaluate your experiences related to occupations and careers.
- Successfully get a job and keep it.

Gaining and keeping a job is part of the reality of life. A job may be the first step to a highly skilled occupation and a life-long career. A job may provide both temporary income and experience to reach a higher occupational goal. A job can allow the opportunity to explore an occupation or career before making a major commitment.

Regardless of the reason for seeking a job, occupational and career decisions need to be made. Information related to personal and family life must be gained, factors must be considered, and techniques must be applied in order to gain and keep a job that meets individual needs.

Figure 16-1

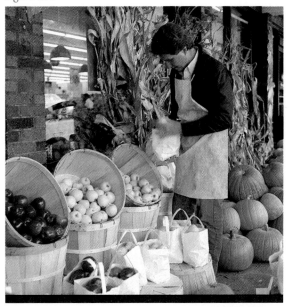

Actual work experience while still attending school may help in determining a future career.

GATHERING INFORMATION

One of the first steps in making decisions is gathering information. Whether making decisions about a temporary job or a life-long occupation, information is necessary. One way of gathering information about a career is to get a job while still in school that is related to your career interests, or area of study (Figure 16-1). Many unsuccessful or unsatisfactory careers are outcomes of too little knowledge about the particular occupation or career. A quick glimpse of a single aspect of a particular job may make the job appear exciting and interesting. Further investigation may show that the job has many aspects unsuitable to some individuals. Consider Susan's experience.

CASE IN POINT

Susan met an accountant who worked on a project for her father's business. Maria, the accountant, was well-dressed and professional. Susan was impressed. Susan began to think of accounting as a possible career. She considered herself well-organized and a logical thinker. She also had good grades in math. Susan signed up for a basic accounting class which included on-the-job training three times a week. Though Susan found the work and the class within her skill level, she began to realize that much of the job involved working alone. Only a small percentage of time was spent meeting and working with other people. Susan is beginning to see accounting from a different viewpoint. She may decide to change her area of study, or she may look for accounting jobs that involve a higher degree of contact with people.

What information is needed to help make occupational or career decisions? Information is needed about *you* and about the *occupation* or *career* in order to find the best match of job and individual. Much like a puzzle, the person and job must be put together carefully and accurately in order to get the desired fit.

Information about Yourself

You are an important source of information about yourself. Self-investigation is necessary in order to match personal traits with job traits. Individuals need to be aware of and consider their own special, unique qualities. Without this personal consideration, individuals can easily find themselves in a job that doesn't suit them. Consider Wilson and Melodie.

CASE IN POINT

Wilson: "My mother always wanted me to be a teacher. Her parents were both teachers, and she teaches too. Well, I thought that's what I would like, but I was wrong. We had to do volunteer helping in the classroom during my first year of college, and I realized I just didn't enjoy being around kids. They made me nervous, and I found them irritating. I didn't like going over the same material class after class. I've switched majors and plan to go into business. I'm just not cut out for teaching."

Melodie: "I've been a salesperson for almost a year now, but it doesn't suit me. I like creating things and being original. I didn't realize I would grow so bored with sales work."

Getting to know yourself before choosing an occupation or career might save you from unhappy experiences like those of Wilson and Melodie. Five kinds of information can help you know yourself better.

- your interests
- your values
- your skills and abilities
- your job preferences
- your personality

INTERESTS • The things you enjoy doing and being involved with are your interests. Your hobbies and social activities reflect your interests (Figure 16-2).

Figure 16-2

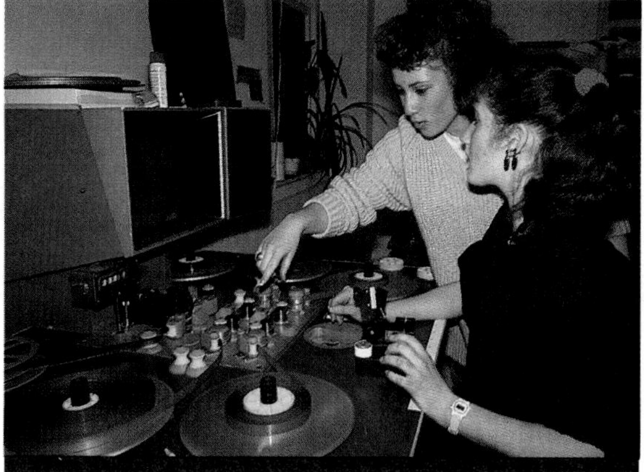

Extracurricular activities and outside skills and abilities help develop career interests.
Arlene Collins/Monkmeyer Press

VALUES • Those things considered to be of importance or worth are values. They are the things you hold dear.

SKILLS AND ABILITIES • The things you can do well are your skills and abilities. You may have achieved or performed in some areas that reflect your skills and abilities. You may never have had the opportunity to develop other skills and abilities.

WORK PREFERENCES • The feelings or ideas you have about certain kinds of job activities or conditions in which you work are your work preferences. For example, could you work in a job that was dirty such as garbage collecting? Could you work in a job that was dangerous such as window washing (Figure 16-3)? Level

Figure 16-3

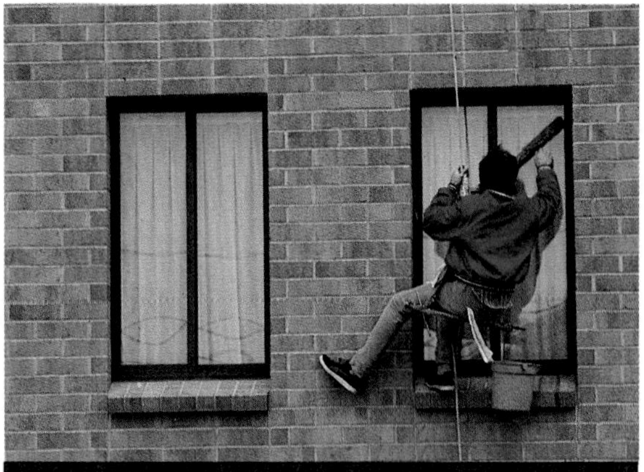

Could you do this job or would it be too dangerous?

of routine, degree of challenge, and degree of contact with others are some of the factors in job preferences.

YOUR PERSONALITY • Several aspects of your personality are important to consider in making job decisions. Do you prefer to be a leader or a follower? Would you rather work alone or in a group of people? Are you an introvert (quiet, reserved person) or an extrovert (outgoing, talkative person)? Are you patient with yourself and with others, or do you become easily frustrated and discouraged if things don't go your way? The kind of person you are will be a good match for some kinds of jobs and a poor match for other jobs. What kind of personality would best match the following types of jobs:

- police officer
- lawyer
- accountant
- school teacher
- doctor
- auto mechanic
- computer programmer

When you combine these five categories of information about yourself, you are better able to decide on the kind of work you will excel in and enjoy most. But how do you find out about these aspects of yourself? What sources are available to help you learn about you?

SOURCES OF INFORMATION • Who is a better expert on you than you? Your expertise can be clouded, however, by taking your personal traits for granted and overlooking your outstanding qualities. As you assess yourself, be sure to consider your long-term abilities and skills, such as the ability to play the piano or your skills in talking before a group. Such skills and abilities could be used well in the work world.

Start with a **self-inventory**. Write a description of your interests, values, skills, abilities, and job preferences. Recall things you've done that you liked or disliked. Think of things that have always drawn your attention or aroused your interest. Were some tasks you've performed boring or disagreeable to you? Do you like working alone or in groups? Do you prefer noisy work places to quiet, nonchaotic work places? Consider choices you've made that might reveal your values. Did you choose a quiet picnic site instead of a noisy crowded beach area? Did you prefer helping aging community members rather than working with young children?

Other sources for gaining information about yourself are people who know you well. Parents, siblings, and good friends can give you insights about yourself. Teachers and employers who know you well can help to complete your view of yourself. Valuable information can be gained through contact with an employer. Your self-concept may be altered significantly when you hear several people who know you well indicate that you have an outstanding skill or ability in a particular area.

Other beneficial sources for learning about yourself include grades and school records. Grades, teachers' comments, and general progress can point out important facts about your areas of ability and interest. Subjects in which you have a history of high grades will indicate a possible area to consider in occupational/career decision making.

Results of tests and check sheets can also provide information for occupational decision making. You've taken many tests through your school years that reflect your achievement, aptitudes, and ability. You may also have taken interest tests. Ask your guidance counselor to show you test results and explain their meaning. The guidance counselor may also have additional tests and inventories to assist you in assessing yourself.

Realize that you must use a *total* of information gained from yourself, others who know you well, grades, school records, and test scores. One grade, one person's information, or the outcome of one test are not strong enough evidence. All pieces of the puzzle must fit in order to give you the whole picture.

Remember that in your investigation of yourself you'll likely discover some things that are unpleasant to hear. Someone may tell you that you're not comfortable to talk with, yet you want to be a counselor. You may have a very low grade in chemistry, yet you want to study marine biology. Don't let one item or point discourage you. Investigate further while being realistic. The following show predictions that were proven wrong:

- Thomas Edison, inventor of the light bulb, was told by his teachers that he was too stupid to learn anything.
- A newspaper editor fired Walt Disney because he had "no good ideas."
- Louisa May Alcott, author of *Little Women*, was told she could never write anything that had popular appeal.
- Beethoven's music teacher once said of him, "As a composer he is hopeless."[1]

The following self-assessment scales are helpful in determining your work values, abilities, work preferences, and interests:

IDENTIFYING YOUR WORK PREFERENCES

A. How would you rank the following types of work:
Working with people
Working with things
Working with information (ideas, facts, numbers)

B. Which work situation would you prefer in each pair?
Working alone
Working with others

Doing the same thing each day
Doing something different each day

Giving others directions
Taking directions from others

C. Which working condition or task do you dislike so much that you would probably

[1]Adapted from Milton E. Larson, "Humbling Cases for Career Counselors," *Phi Delta Kappan*, February, 1973.

not take a job that included such conditions?

Loud noise or vibrations
Work that involved record keeping
Work in a large city
Work in the country
Frequent travel
Sitting for long periods of time
Standing for long periods of time
Not making many decisions
Making many decisions
Working under many deadlines
Getting messy and dirty
Inside work
Outdoor work
Having to work overtime
Wearing a uniform
Dressing casually
Dressing formally
Arranging your own time schedule
Dangerous work
Heavy physical work

RATING YOUR WORK VALUES

Are the following statements true, false, sometimes true, or sometimes false?

My work must be enjoyable and fun (value—enjoyment).

I must have a job in which I can help others (value—service to others).

I must have a steady, stable job (value—stability).

My work must allow me to be creative (value—creativity).

My job must be a position of power in which I direct others and make decisions (value—power).

I must have a job where people know about me and my work (value—fame).

I want a job with evenings and weekends free (value—personal time).

RATING YOUR ABILITIES

Indicate which level (High, Medium, or Low) you feel best describes your ability.

Coordination—able to use feet, hands, and fingers with skill.

Endurance—able to withstand physical and mental hardship or stress.

Reasoning—able to understand and solve problems.

Persistence—able to stick with a situation or problem.

Perception—able to see differences and similarities in things around you.

Numerical—able to understand and work with numbers quickly and accurately.

Verbal—able to understand and use words and ideas in writing and speaking.

Information about Occupations and Careers

Greater awareness of occupations and careers is necessary to make wise decisions about future occupations. Exploration to assist with the decision-making process should include job descriptions, requirements for the job, job future, and fringe benefits.

JOB DESCRIPTION • A job description is an explanation of the duties and the working conditions of a particular job. For example, a librarian's duties include selecting and organizing collections of books and other publications, assisting readers, and researching various technical problems. Duties vary for research librarians, school librarians, and technical librarians. Working conditions are mostly indoors and in relatively quiet surroundings. Skills needed include intellectual curiosity and interest in helping others.

A flight attendant's duties include making the airline passenger's flight safe, comfortable, and enjoyable. The attendant greets passengers, checks supplies and emergency gear, assists with preparing and serving meals, and aids people who become ill. Skills needed include poise, tact, and good rapport with people.

A group of jobs that share general characteristics or traits are called **career clusters**. These clusters are important aspects related to job descriptions. Several jobs within a career cluster may require similar skills and knowledge. Thus, though you may not be sure of a specific occupation or career, you can still study skills and gain knowledge about the cluster area. At a later point, a specific area in the cluster may become of greatest interest. The *Dictionary of Occupational Titles* categorizes careers and occupations into nine major areas.[2]

- Professional, technical, and managerial
- Clerical and sales occupations
- Service occupations
- Agricultural, fishery, forestry, and related occupations
- Processing occupations
- Machine trades occupations
- Benchwork occupations
- Structural work occupations
- Miscellaneous occupations

[2]U.S. Department of Labor, Employment and Training Administration, *Dictionary of Occupational Titles*, 4th ed., 1982 supplement, Washington: U.S. Government Printing Office, 1977.

Often an individual begins with an interest in one job but moves to another job within the career cluster.

CASE IN POINT

Alex had several jobs as manager of reception desks in small hotels. Later he moved to his present job as arts and crafts director at a large state lodge. Both of these jobs are within the service occupations career cluster. Tasks and skills learned in one job can be related to the other.

JOB REQUIREMENTS • All those things a person needs in order to get a job are **job requirements**. These include a specific amount of training or education, special abilities and/or work experience, or special licensing. Specific abilities and skills may be needed for a job. For example, you must be able to read blueprints to be an architect; you must be highly skilled in languages to be an interpreter. Special licensing or certification is necessary for jobs such as psychologist, truck driver, beautician, and dental hygienist.

Knowledge of job requirements is extremely important when considering or planning for the future. Time and financial commitment to gain necessary training and/or licensing are major considerations for most people. For example, a librarian needs a bachelor's degree and often a master's degree. A flight attendant needs two years of college plus training by the airlines or an airline school.

JOB FUTURE • The employment outlook for an occupation and the chances for advancement within the occupation are referred to as the **job future**. An employment outlook tells how much particular careers will still be needed when education and training are complete. Some careers and occupations have a more positive outlook than others. For example, computer programmers continue to be in demand (Figure 16-4), while the demand for railroad workers has decreased.

Figure 16-4

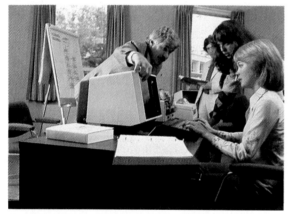

Some career areas have limited opportunities while others have potential for future career growth. Prepare yourself for a career that has a positive future.
NEC Corporation

Chances for advancement are the opportunities for moving up in a job. Chances for advancement are not good in all jobs. Librarians have fairly good opportunities to advance in highly technical library fields. However, flight attendants have more limited chances to advance other than to flight supervisors.

Advancement in a job can be placed on an imaginary ladder called a **career ladder**. The lowest rung on the ladder represents those jobs which require little or no skill or education. These are called entry-level jobs. More experience, more ability, and more education are usually necessary to move up the ladder. The further up the ladder, the greater the challenges provided by the job and the greater the pay. As you consider a job, you must look at the career cluster and the possible movement up the career ladder.

FRINGE BENEFITS • The added positive features or advantages (other than salary) included in a job are called fringe benefits. Basic fringe benefits include insurance plans, paid vacation time, and sick leave. Fringes could also include travel, expense accounts, company car, and workers' facilities such as gym rooms or dining rooms. Librarians receive basic fringe benefits; flight attendants receive basic fringe benefits plus travel and expense accounts and reduced air fare for families.

SOURCES OF INFORMATION • There are many good sources of information about occupations and careers. Your information about particular occupations or career clusters will be more complete if you use as many different sources as possible. The following actions on your part can provide a firm knowledge of occupations or careers in which you have interest.

Talk with people in the career or occupation • Even if you do not personally know these people, you can politely request a conversation. Most people like to talk about their work. *Talk with people who hire workers* in the occupations or careers in which you have interest. These people have a lot of valuable information about who is hired and why.

Confer with your school guidance counselor or occupational specialist for information about occupations and careers • These people have personal knowledge about the many occupations and careers as well as references to help you. They can assist you in locating computerized career guidance information. Such computerized information is up-to-date and usually specific to your state or locality. Additional information provided by computerized systems includes wages and salaries, physical requirements, work settings, education, and employment possibilities in the present and future.

Observe workers on the job • This can be done casually for some jobs such as waitress, police officer, or nurse. A more formal way of observing is by **shadowing** a particular worker. Some schools arrange for students to spend a day or a week with workers. During this time the student can see firsthand the duties performed, working conditions, and daily activities of the workers in a chosen field.

Write to professional agencies for information • Addresses of professional agencies should be available in your school library or from the guidance counselor. For example, if you are interested in the following occupations or careers you could write to the following agencies:

Law: Information Service
The American Bar Association
1155 East 60th Street
Chicago, Illinois 60637

Cosmetology: National Beauty
Career Center
3839 White Plains Rd.
Bronx, New York 10467

Printing: Printing Industries of
America, Inc.
1730 North Lynn Street
New York, New York 10020

Read information about occupations and careers • Books and magazines are good sources of information about occupations and careers. Your school librarian can assist you in selecting helpful sources. Two printed sources are likely to be available:

- *Dictionary of Occupational Titles*
- *Occupational Outlook Handbook*

The *Dictionary of Occupational Titles*, sometimes referred to as the DOT, is printed by the United States Department of Labor. Using coded numbers, it describes about 35,000 jobs. It explains the type of work performed, worker requirements, training required, physical demands, and working conditions.

The *Occupational Outlook Handbook* also describes jobs. It explains job requirements, places of employment, and employment outlook including present and future earnings.

These two sources and others provided by guidance personnel can assist you in gaining objective, unbiased information.

Know where to look for job openings • It is one thing to know what kind of job or occupation you would like to have. It is quite another task to know what jobs are currently available at the time you begin looking for employment. Finding a good job is easier if you know where to look!

Perhaps the most common source for finding out about jobs is the local newspaper's want-ads. However, not all job opportunities are advertised in the newspaper. Sometimes you will hear about a job opportunity by word-of-mouth. Friends, relatives, parents' friends, school counselors, teachers, neighbors, and church clergy comprise a valuable network of contacts for getting job leads. Sometimes such contacts can put in a good word for you and help to arrange a job interview if they should happen to know the employer or someone who works at the place of employment.

It pays to be creative in searching for a job. For example, you might consider putting an advertisement in the newspaper yourself, stating briefly the kind of job you are seeking and your qualifications. (In fact, that is how Jorgensen, one of the authors of this book, landed his first job as a teenager.) You might also open up the Yellow Pages of the telephone directory to locate potential employers for whom you would like to work. Your local Chamber of Commerce, your high school office, a college placement office, or government offices (city, state, and federal) might also have bulletin boards or listings of available jobs for you to scan (Figure 16-5). Finally, countless youth have found their first employment with the assistance of a parent or relative who owns a business. While having an employer who is also your mother or father may create some role definition problems, such an arrangement is often an excellent means for initiating a teenager's work experience.

Figure 16-5

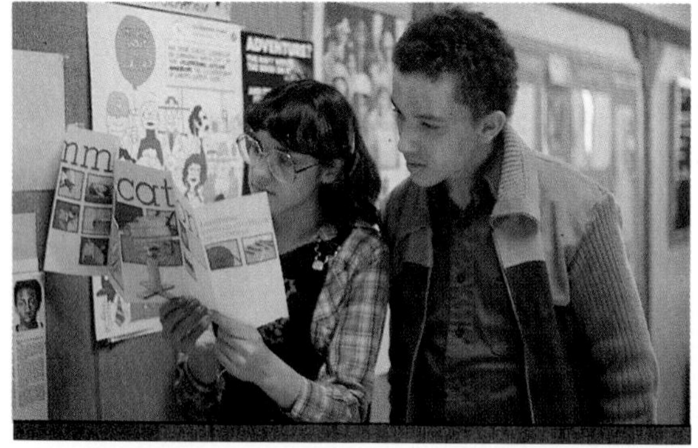

Many sources of job information are illustrated here. It is important to know where to look!

Additional avenues for job searching will open up after high school, when full-time careers or occupations are being sought. These include newspapers from other communities, trade and business publications (newsletters, magazines, journals), employment agencies, college or technical school placement services, and co-workers. With the exception of private employment agencies, which charge a fee for using their services to locate a job, these sources and the others listed above cost virtually nothing to the job seeker.

Whether you are searching for your first job as a high school student or a full-time career position after high school, the most important point to remember is to check out as many of these avenues as possible. Rarely will a job come searching for you! You must take the initiative by asking people, looking in newspapers, calling potential employers, and tracking down job listings in placement services and government agencies. Successful job seekers are those who expend the time and energy to locate job openings of interest to them. Assertiveness and abundant energy are personal characteristics that will pay off in the job search.

CONSIDERING FAMILY FACTORS

After you have gained information about occupations and careers, consider how these careers and occupations relate to family life. Handbooks and informative materials give many details about specific and cluster jobs.

However, little information is offered with respect to how certain jobs may or may not affect family life.

Clearly, in times of high unemployment, less thought is given to job selection. In such situations, a job may be accepted even though it affects family life negatively. In good economic times and for young people at early occupational and career stages, people can afford to be more selective. Efforts can be made to choose work areas that fit most closely to a preferred family lifestyle.

What Aspects Relayed in the Job Description Could Impact on the Family?

When reviewing duties, salary, or working conditions, consider the effect on individual family members and the family as a whole. The salary level may not be sufficient to support family members.

When assessing the fit of salary level to lifestyle, be aware of career ladders and how they relate to salary. Few young people can earn enough to support themselves and their family members. Yet, as movement up the career ladder brings more income, the likelihood of supporting additional members increases.

Working conditions may have direct and indirect effects on family members. Safety factors such as greater likelihood of injury or death are major considerations for worker and family. Employment that is life-threatening—race-car driving, doing construction work on skyscrapers, transporting poisonous chemicals, and work that is highly stressful—must be considered in terms of effect on the family.

Duties of a particular job can affect family members if the work must be performed in times or places that infringe on family time. For example, ministers, real estate agents, and insurance salespeople must use evening hours for work. Flight attendants must be away from home for significant time periods. Depending on a person's desired lifestyle and stage of family life cycle, these could be positive or negative features.

Spotlight on issues

Careers in the Family Services Field

Much of this book is devoted to the study of families—how they function, grow, and influence the development of people. After reading this book you will have learned about the tremendous amount of stress and strain that is placed on families in our contemporary society. You will have read about such stresses as inadequate income and poverty, unemployment, family violence and child abuse, drug and alcohol abuse, divorce, remarriage and step-parenting, and other types of family crises. Families do experience serious problems, and they often need help solving them.

Because of the vital role that families play in promoting our individual well-being, it is in the best interest of our society to help keep our family units as strong as they possibly can be. Government agencies at all levels (local, state, regional, and national), religious organizations, private foundations, hospitals, and other health-care services are just some of the groups that provide services to help families survive stressful periods and to resolve crises.

Were you aware of the growing number of career opportunities in the field of family services? Consider the following list of places that provide services to families. Some of these provide help in solving the problems and stresses that families are facing, while others serve families under any circumstances.

- Human service agencies (child protective services, abused women's shelters, rape crisis and counseling centers, and police departments)
- Marriage and family counseling services
- Government agencies that protect the rights of consumers by investigating consumer fraud
- Community service agencies (Red Cross, YMCA/YWCA, Cooperative Extension Service, and Parents Without Partners)
- Senior citizens centers
- Churches and other religious organizations (Lutheran Social Services, Catholic Family Services)
- Adoption agencies and maternity homes
- Hospitals and medical clinics
- Mental health centers
- Substance abuse treatment centers (treating drug addiction and alcoholism)
- Housing agencies and developers
- Day care centers, preschools, schools, and youth services
- Rehabilitation centers

This is only a partial list of agencies that serve families. Employment opportunities in them may be attractive to you. What are the qualifications and personal characteristics necessary to work in the field of family services? The following list should give you an idea of what is expected:

- College degree, either a bachelor's or master's, in a field related to family services (home economics, social work, sociology, psychology, human services, law, rehabilitation, or community health)
- Genuine desire to help people solve their problems
- Effective communication, problem-solving, and conflict resolution skills
- Pleasant, outgoing personality
- Willingness to accept the fact that family services occupations often are not the highest paying jobs
- Strong character with a firm commitment to values of integrity, honesty, and respect for the rights of other human beings
- Inner "toughness" that allows you to deal with emotional problems of others without becoming overly involved with your own emotions.

Occupations in the family services field are essential to the welfare of society. Yet, not everyone has the personality or skills necessary to be an effective employee in this field. If you are interested in working in these areas, you should consider discussing the possibilities with your high school vocational counselor, your home economics teacher, or possibly a representative from your local college or university. They can help you decide what your prospects might be for future employment in this important field.

What Aspects Related to Job Requirements Could Impact on the Family?

Job requirements that include special abilities, knowledge of equipment, work experience, and licensing can impact on family members. The financial and time commitments to meet these job requirements can infringe on a person's chosen family lifestyle. Yet, many such job requirements are needed early in a career and are achieved prior to a person's marriage or children. Also, working together to meet the job requirements of family members can have a positive impact.

Consider the following job requirements and how they might affect families.

- Nat has been taking classes in auto mechanics. He needs to have his own hand tools before applying for a job.
- Lorna is very interested in becoming a licensed practical nurse but it requires two years of training.
- Venetia must pass the state cosmetology exam in order to start work as a hairdresser.
- In order to be the department head, Nancy must complete a master's degree.
- Karl must increase his typing speed to qualify for a secretarial job. He'll have to rent a typewriter to practice.

Meeting job requirements is not only necessary at the entry stage of occupations.

Throughout your career, requirements will need to be met in order to advance or excel in your work. In your own school, many staff members are probably working and studying to advance their careers by meeting additional requirements. Many occupations and careers require a continuous updating of knowledge. Achieving these requirements for advancement often requires the involvement and assistance of family members. Check newspapers for announcements of training courses, workshops, or in-service sessions completed by workers in various jobs.

What Aspects of Job Future Could Impact on the Family?

As you think about family lifestyle desired now and in the future, job future becomes highly important. If the employment outlook is dim in a specific job or job cluster, there is less likelihood a person can provide for family members. This is complicated by the changing job market in which some jobs are growing in demand, while other jobs are becoming increasingly obsolete. Possibilities for advancement may require actions that are in opposition to desired family lifestyle. For example, advancement in some corporations requires change of residence from one city to another. There may be required visits to the site that take the worker away from home for extensive periods. On the other hand, advancement and longevity in some jobs may be positive for family life. For example, airline pilots with experience and advancement have more choice of assignments and can select schedules to accommodate family needs and goals.

What Aspects about Yourself Need Consideration?

The information gathered about yourself (abilities, interests, work preferences, and values) also needs consideration when making decisions about careers and occupations. These aspects about yourself are a fairly stable part of you. You may need to mold your career/occupation decisions around these personal factors. Consider how Manuel and Shelia used the information about themselves to eliminate certain occupations and to consider others.

CASE IN POINT

Shelia used the *Dictionary of Occupational Titles* to gain information about a career as a librarian. She understands the job description, job requirements, and job future. The job future and job requirements were acceptable to Shelia, but she had no personal interest in the duties of a librarian. Even after reading more thoroughly, she gained no interest. Shelia will consider another career since her interests do not lie in the area of library work.

Manuel researched the occupation of flight attendant. He realized this career was opening up for males, and he enjoyed traveling. However, Manuel enjoys being outdoors; he feels confined in small spaces. Clearly Manuel's work preferences will not allow him to consider the occupation of flight attendant.

Some aspects about yourself can and will change. Your preference for certain types of work and your interests may change. Your abilities will probably grow, and your values may alter. However, your personal traits are basically a part of you and need to be considered as they are now. The selection of occupation or career needs to be molded to you.

GETTING AND KEEPING A JOB

Now that we have identified the types of information that are useful in making decisions about careers and occupations, how can we apply our knowledge to successfully land and keep a job? A number of guidelines can help you search for employment. These apply to you as a teenager searching for your first paid job, as well as to older individuals who are seeking employment on a long-term basis. You must be able to accurately evaluate your prior work-related experience. You must be able to communicate your experience to a potential employer who is considering the possibility of hiring you. The process of interviewing for a job is perhaps the most important step in getting a job. Your personal characteristics, interpersonal skills, and work habits all combine to help you keep your job and possibly advance in your work field.

Evaluate Your Experiences

Experiences are an important part of obtaining a job. Prospective employers look closely at the work experience of a job candidate.

Too often people underrate or overlook their experiences. This mistake is common when people mentally assess their experiences or relay experiences to employers. People who have never been employed or who have been unemployed for a long time tend to consider themselves without work experiences.

Experiences do not have to be *paid* work experiences. Employers are usually interested in maturity, managerial ability, and willingness to handle responsibility. These qualities can be demonstrated by means of various activities and experiences, not just by paid employment.

HOME EXPERIENCES • Many responsibilities and activities in the home provide experiences that could be beneficial to many jobs. Would care of a family's or neighbor's pet be an experience valuable for working at an animal shelter? Could care of young siblings be a beneficial experience in day care center work? Might managing a household budget (including rent, food, and clothing money) be an important experience for some occupations? Consider how differently Erin and Annette responded to a prospective employer's questions about work experiences.

Employer: What work experiences have you had?

Erin: None. I've never worked before.

Employer: What work experiences have you had?

Annette: I've not yet had a paying job, but I've had quite a few unpaid responsibilities. I managed our home while my parents were out of town for three weeks. I supervised my younger sister and brother and kept the financial business in order.

Employer: What exactly did you do?

Annette: I made sure my sister and brother got to school and to extracurricular activities. I purchased and prepared all of our food, kept things clean, did laundry, supervised their homework, and kept the bills paid. Of course, I was in school at the time and had to manage my classwork too.

Annette's answer relayed that she had held a position of responsibility even though she had not been formally employed. Home and family experiences can count if related to prospective employers. Work in family-operated businesses, farming activities, and daily household tasks can be important factors when employers consider your work experience.

SOCIAL ACTIVITIES AND VOLUNTEER EXPERIENCE • Activities in which you have participated provide a good chance to try out various types of work. Such activities also provide experiences that reflect your responsibility and skills. Serving as a visual aids assistant in high school, being chairperson of a school fund-raising activity, being a volunteer in a nursing home, or participating in a sport are activities that can be related to a prospective employer. These activities can reflect maturity, perseverance, ability to manage and organize, and responsibility (Figure 16-6).

Figure 16-6

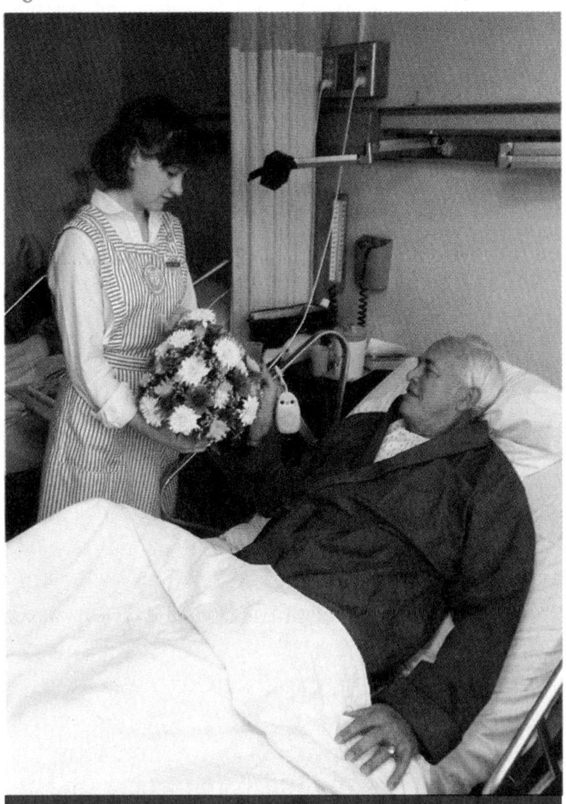

Volunteer work provides valuable work experience, allows you to "try on" a particular career, and can reveal various abilities that you posses.

Paul Conklin/Monkmeyer Press

Develop a Résumé

Once you have identified and evaluated your experiences, whether paid or unpaid, you must be able to clearly communicate them to a potential employer. One way to do this is to verbally tell the employer all about you and your qualifications for the job. However, in most job situations, an employer will not even talk to you until he or she has seen a written statement about your experiences and qualifications for the job you are seeking.

The best way to do this is to have a clearly written **résumé**. *Résumé* is a French word meaning ***brief history***. It is a quick and efficient way to tell an employer about your qualifications for the job. A complete and accurate résumé is an important tool for getting a job.

Your résumé usually represents the first impression an employer has of you. A neat, well-organized, and easy-to-read résumé indicates that you are conscientious and well-organized. A sloppy, unorganized résumé that has misspelled words or errors in grammar reflects poorly on you as a potential employee. If you are sloppy and careless in assembling your résumé, then an employer may assume that you will be a sloppy, careless employee as well. Résumés should be typewritten on good quality paper. If you have access to a computer, a letter-quality printer should be used.

While good résumés may vary in format and style of presentation, the following should be included:

- Your full name
- Your mailing address
- Your telephone number
- Your educational experience (high school attended, year of graduation, colleges and universities attended, degrees earned)
- A chronological list of paid and unpaid work experiences, including the dates of those experiences
- Special skills that you have acquired such as typing, writing, artistic or industrial arts skills (wood working, automobile engine repair, metal working)
- A list of your hobbies and special interests
- Special honors and awards that you have received (such as National Honor Society, Academic Honor Roll, 4-H Officer, Student Council Representative, or Tennis Team Captain)
- The names, addresses, and telephone numbers of two or three references (people who can be contacted to provide information to the employer about your skills and abilities, your personality, and your qualifications for the job)

Figure 16-7 is a résumé for Annette Foster. Note that she has included on her résumé her work-related experiences at home and in social and volunteer activities, even though she was not paid for these experiences. She has also included other information that will help an employer decide if Annette is a good employment prospect. Because Annette's résumé is complete and well-organized, she has increased her chances of receiving a job interview. Remember that this is an example of only one type of résumé format. Other formats are perfectly acceptable, depending on the job field of interest.

Interviewing for a Job

Getting the job you want usually depends on more than just submitting your written résumé to the employer. If you have a well-written résumé and your qualifications seem to fit what the employer is looking for, you may be asked to appear in person for a job interview. The job interview is a most important step in getting a job, and should be taken very seriously.

CASE IN POINT

Julie was about to graduate from high school in June. She planned to attend college in September. She wanted to get a full-time job for the summer in order to save money for books and living expenses. Although her best friends already had jobs lined up, Julie was relatively shy and a little bit afraid of all that had to be done to get a job. She was nervous about asking any employer for an interview and the possibility of being rejected. She was even more nervous about being in an interview situation. She was afraid that she would say the wrong things or that she would not know the answers to questions that would be asked of her. As summer drew near, Julie was afraid that she would not have the courage to search for and land a job.

When Julie told her friend, Ann, how reluctant she was to look for a job, Ann encouraged Julie to take a risk. Ann conveyed how she had been rejected by

RESUME'

for

Annette Marie Foster

ADDRESS: 4721 Cherry Hill Road
Spring Hill, IL 61907

TELEPHONE: (312) 555-5555

EDUCATIONAL EXPERIENCE:

Cherry Hill High School, 1986-1989
Graduation Date: May 24, 1989

National Leadership Workshop
National Honor Society
July 14 - July 28, 1988
Washington, D.C.

WORK EXPERIENCE:

Sole responsibility for siblings, self, and home while parents out of town.
Responsibilities: Supervised two younger siblings, purchased and prepared food, cared for home, coordinated home/school activities for a three-week period, June 18 - July 10, 1987.

Chairperson of Cherry Hill High School Muscular Dystrophy Drive.
Responsibilities: Leadership for planning and implementing student fund-raising bazaar and dance. Coordination of committee of 15 members; 750 students participated (unpaid position), January 20 - February 18, 1988.

Volunteer Service at Cartwright Senior Citizen Center.
Responsibilities: Volunteered two hours each week at center for aging. Activities consisted of reading and writing letters for residents; feeding incapacitated residents; distributing refreshments; assisting with group activities; and filing patient medical records, March 10 - March 20, 1988.

Retail Sales, Martin Book Store.
Responsibilities: Direct sales to store customers; taking stock of store inventory; helping to reconcile end-of-day cash register receipts, typing of orders, May 25, 1989 - August 20, 1989.

Figure 16-7
Developing a résumé is an important step in getting a job.

Figure 16-7 (continued)

SPECIAL SKILLS:	Typing (55 words per minute) Able to read Spanish for comprehension. Experience in working with computers and computer programming.
HOBBIES AND INTERESTS:	Water skiing Reading mystery novels Horseback riding Swimming
SPECIAL HONORS:	Elected Junior Class Vice-President Cherry Hill High School October, 1987
	Elected to the National Honor Society November, 1987
	Track Team Co-Captain February, 1989 - May, 1989
PERSONAL REFERENCES:	Sandra Martin, Owner Martin Book Store 2211 Oak Street Cherry Hill, IL 61927
	William McCartney, Head Track Coach Cherry Hill High School 507 North Market Street Cherry Hill, IL 61902
	Juanita Granado, Volunteer Coordinator Cartwright Senior Citizen Center 813 Broadway Avenue Cherry Hill, IL 61922

one employer in her job search, but that many others were kind and helpful. Ann applied for several jobs. The job she took at the local book store was one of three job offers that she had received. She convinced Julie that by thinking positively and relaxing, Julie, too, could successfully land a job.

Ann helped Julie by rehearsing job interview situations with her, similar to those that Ann had experienced. She let Julie know what her strong and weak points were in the interview. They then worked on correcting them in subsequent rehearsals. Ann concentrated on helping Julie to relax and to be herself.

Julie soon realized that the questions were not that difficult to answer. She gained confidence and developed an attitude that she, too, like her friends, could do many different types of jobs and could do them well. She decided to take the risk and sent her résumé to several different employers. Her new-found confidence paid off when she was offered a job as a summer camp counselor for a local church. Julie was happy that she took the risk.

The job interview has several purposes for the employer. First, the interview gives the employer a chance to confirm the first impressions of you presented in your written résumé. If your résumé claims that you have certain knowledge or skills, the employer may follow up in person to see just how much you know or how skilled you are. This is why it is important never to "pad" your résumé with false information or things you have not really done.

Second, the interview allows the employer to explain the nature of the job to you. Your questions about pay, benefits, working conditions, and hours can be answered. If the employer is really interested in you as a possible employee, he or she will want to make a good impression on you, too.

Finally, the employer gets to meet you personally. It is likely that your physical appearance, personality, and such social skills as communication and problem solving will be observed. An employer will be eager to find out how you relate to other people and how you respond to questions about yourself and the work that you will be doing if hired. Do you have a pleasant disposition? Do you seem like the kind of person with whom the employer and others in the workplace could get along? Can you "think on your feet"? How do you seem to respond under the pressure of a job interview situation?

Consider the following example of Ryan and Mitchell. They have listed identical job skills and experience on their résumés. Each has applied for a sales clerk job with the local hardware store. Mr. DiMarco, the hardware store manager, has set up an interview with each of them. Who would you hire? How do you think Mr. DiMarco responded to each of them during their interviews?

Mr. DiMarco: Ryan, your résumé says that you helped your uncle in his roofing business last summer. Did you like that experience?

Ryan (*looking down at the floor, avoiding eye contact with Mr. DiMarco*): It was o.k. I got kinda' tired of it though.

Mr. DiMarco: Well, Ryan, what makes you want this job in my store?

Ryan (*still looking at the floor and getting nervous*): I don't know. I guess I could use the extra money. Besides, my dad says I should try to get a job.

Mr. DiMarco: Ryan, tell me what you would do if one of my customers came into the store to return a defective power saw purchased here.

Ryan (*laughing nervously, trying to make a joke*): I guess I'd ask the guy when he dropped it and broke it!

Mr. DiMarco: Mitchell, your résumé says that you helped your uncle in his roofing business last summer. Did you like that experience?

Mitchell (*smiling and answering with confidence*): Yes, sir, I liked most of the things I learned to do. At times the hard work made me tired, but overall, it was a good experience for me. I'm glad I did it!

Mr. DiMarco: Well, Mitchell, what makes you want this job at my store?

Mitchell (*looking directly into Mr. DiMarco's eyes*): I guess I'm like everyone else—I can really use some extra spending money. But I also want to get some experience in the hardware business. I like to work with tools and I like to be around people. What better place is there to accomplish all these things?

Mr. DiMarco: Mitchell, tell me what you would do if one of my customers came into the store to return a defective power saw that was purchased here.

Mitchell (*with confidence*): I'd first ask the customer to explain the exact nature of the problem. If it seemed like the saw was really defective, I'd talk to you about what I should do. I imagine that you would try to help the customer by replacing or fixing the saw, wouldn't you, Mr. DiMarco?

Mr. DiMarco: Yes, Mitchell, I always try to satisfy the customer who has a legitimate complaint. Satisfied customers come back.

What specific things did Ryan say or do to create a negative impression during the interview? What could he have done differently? In what ways did Mitchell impress Mr. DiMarco?

The job interview also has important purposes for the job applicant. The interview gives the applicant a chance to find out more about the job and its conditions. You may learn during the course of the interview that you really don't want the job. You may not want to do the kind of work that is expected. You might not like the hours or may feel that the pay is not high enough. In addition, the job interview allows you to meet the people with whom you will work. You too must therefore decide if the job involves work with people with whom you can get along. Finally, the job interview gives you a chance to verbally elaborate on the qualifications listed on your résumé. Whereas the résumé provides only a brief outline of experiences and qualifications, the interview allows you to explain these things in greater detail.

Successful job interviewing depends on a few "rules of thumb." Try to arrange a date and time for the interview that fits into your schedule. Try not to repeatedly cancel interview appointments because you have scheduling conflicts. Be on time to the interview. If possible, be a little early! If you find that you are going to be late, call the employer to explain the situation. This is an important courtesy. Reschedule the appointment, if necessary. This is better than showing up late without any prior warning or explanation.

Also, it is essential to present yourself in a well-groomed manner. Wild hairstyles, excessive make-up, or outlandish clothing generally do not make a good impression for most jobs. Try to present yourself in a way that shows you are responsible and conscientious. Remember that first impressions created by your physical appearance can set a positive tone for the balance of the interview.

Prepare yourself for the interview. Find out something about the business or company that is considering you for a job. Prepare in advance the questions you have about the job. Write them down and take them with you to the interview. Anticipate some of the questions that might be asked of you, and mentally prepare possible responses. If possible, ask a friend or a parent to rehearse an interview situation with you.

Finally, follow-up the interview by sending a thank-you note to the employer. Thank the employer for the interest shown in you and for taking the time to interview you. You must realize, too, that some interviews go well while others do not. Try to learn from your mistakes and do better in the next interview. Don't be devastated if you are rejected for a job. *Everyone* is rejected at one time or another. This challenges our self-esteem and confidence. Bounce back, learn from your mistakes, and go after the next opportunity.

It may first appear that stating your experiences verbally or on a résumé is boastful. However, the only way an employer can get this valuable knowledge is from you. By knowing the fund-raising chairship activities of Annette Foster in Figure 16-7, an employer realizes that she has organizational skills, is responsible, and has the ability to work with others. The volunteer experience tells an employer that Annette has patience with people, commitment to a job even though it is unpaid, ability to work with others, and trustworthiness (handling of patients and medical records). Such information can be influential in getting a job. Do not be afraid to emphasize your strong points!

Keeping a Job

Once you have successfully landed a job, your employer will be interested in seeing that you satisfactorily perform the duties that the job involves. Recall from Chapter 14 that unsatisfactory job performance is one cause of unemployment. Your ability to keep a job, usually referred to as **job security**, depends in large part on your job performance. While jobs vary in terms of their duties and employers' expectations, there are a few standard guidelines that apply to just about any job situation. In looking at the following list, note that the behaviors on the left-hand side are helpful in keeping a job while those on the right-hand side are harmful to job security.[3]

[3]*Life Skills and Opportunities Curriculum*, Volume 22 P/PV, 1987.

HELPFUL BEHAVIORS	HARMFUL BEHAVIORS
A. Physical Appearance	
1• Neat clothing and careful self-grooming	1• Sloppy clothing or self-grooming
2• Trendy, but non-extreme, hair-styles and make-up	2• Extreme hair-styles or make-up
3• Contemporary, but non-extreme, clothing styles	3• Faddish or extreme clothing
B. Language	
1• Speaking clearly	1• Using a lot of slang words and phrases
2• Using proper English	2• Using incorrect English
3• Asking for clarification when instructions are not understood	3• Using profanity
C. Work Habits on the Job	
1• Being on time to work	1• Being late to work and taking longer breaks than allowed
2• Staying busy	2• Being very slow
3• Listening carefully and following directions	3• Fooling around a lot so that work does not get done on time or in the correct way

HELPFUL BEHAVIORS	HARMFUL BEHAVIORS
4• Being organized	4• Gossipping
5• Completing tasks on time and in the correct manner	5• Being dishonest
6• Being dependable	6• Inappropriate behavior toward co-workers, such as making sexual advances
7• Being honest and sincere in relationships with supervisors and co-workers	7• Being insincere or deceptive with co-workers and supervisors
	8• Failing to call in if you are going to be late or absent
	9• Being unable to accept reasonable criticism
	10• Overemphasis on money earned from the job

D. Attitudes

1• Being willing to work above and beyond the call of duty	1• Only willing to do what is necessary to get by on the job
2• Being cooperative and friendly in dealing with co-workers and supervisors	2• Being argumentative and negative in relationships with co-workers and supervisors
3• Wanting to learn more and being eager to advance	3• Having an attitude that conveys you are bored
	4• Being defensive

Employers seek to hire people who can contribute productively to the operation of the business or company. An employee who demonstrates too many of the "harmful" behaviors is not likely to be seen as productive and may be dismissed from the job. Remember that even *one* of these behaviors may be "too many" for some employers (Figure 16-8a and b).

Employees who concentrate their efforts in more productive ways, as outlined above in the list of "helpful" attitudes and behaviors, may find that they are rewarded with much more than just keeping their current job. Employers reward good job performance with raises in pay, promotions to higher level positions, and extra benefits. Your personal success in the world of work is strongly influenced by the type of worker you are. Opportunities for advancement in occupational fields are open to those who exhibit productive work habits and positive attitudes toward their work.

WRAPPING IT UP

There are many roads to getting a job and several reasons for doing so. Teenagers might want a job for temporary income as well as to gain experience for subsequent career pursuits. Adults must make important occupational and career decisions in order to meet

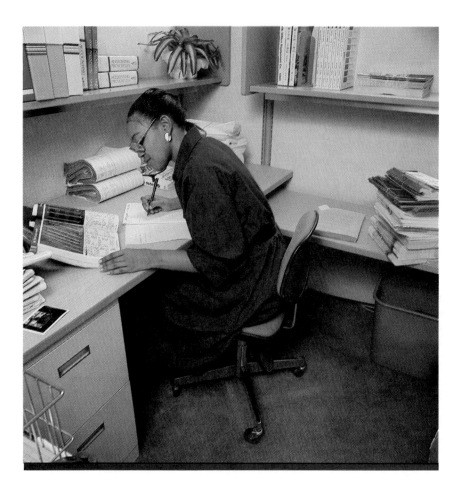

Figure 16-8a
Employees who concentrate their efforts in productive ways are often rewarded with increases in pay, extra benefits, and promotions.

their work goals and, in most instances, to provide economic support for their families.

In making occupational decisions, it is important to gather information to determine the best match between you and possible occupations. Self-evaluation of personal values, interests, skills, and work preferences should be accomplished prior to gathering information about particular careers. A realistic and honest self-assessment will help to narrow the range of possible occupations for you. Particular occupations can then be investigated by looking at job descriptions and considering their requirements, future opportunities for employment and advancement, and fringe benefits. Also to be considered are the ways in which jobs influence family life. This includes working conditions, required duties, and salary levels. Many sources of information are available for learning about particular jobs and their current availability in your community. Gathering such information involves a concerted effort and commitment of time and energy.

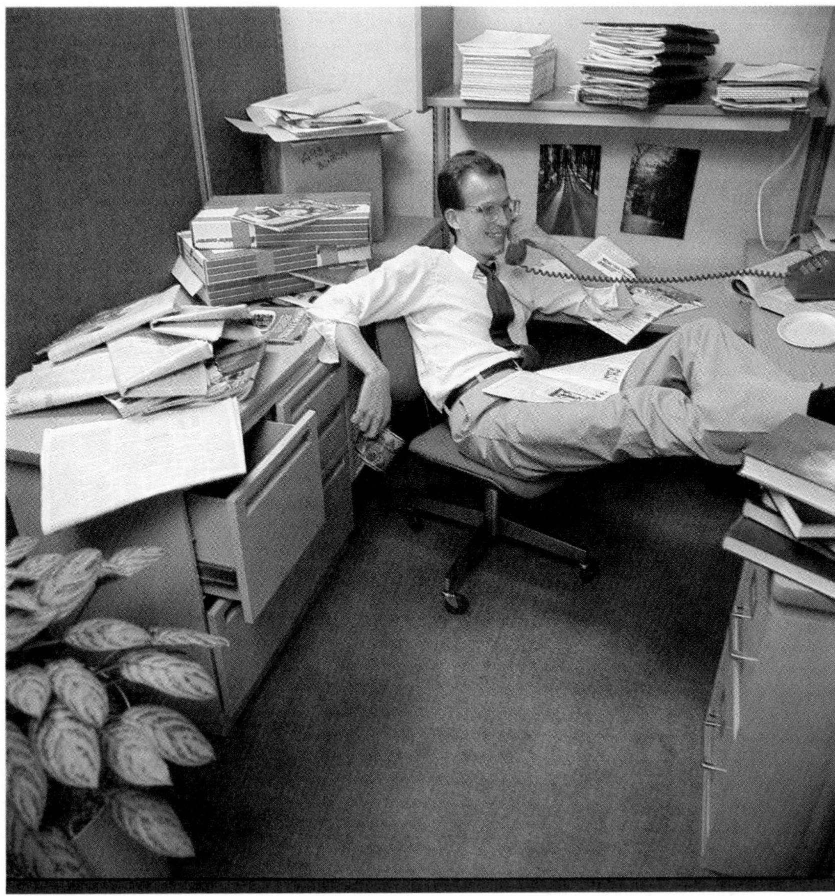

Figure 16-8b Employers want workers who are productive. A lazy employee may end up without a job!

There are many exciting careers and occupations that fit your needs and blend harmoniously with your family lifestyle. Having information about yourself, about occupations and careers, and realizing experiences you have had can help you attain the best job.

Getting the job you want requires careful planning and the accomplishment of certain tasks. You must first be able to recognize and honestly evaluate your work-related experiences. These experiences may be paid or unpaid. Your experiences must then be communicated to a potential employer who might consider hiring you for a particular job. One way of doing this is to develop a written ***résumé*** that clearly communicates your experiences and qualifications. If your résumé conveys to an employer that you are qualified to do a certain job, then you may be asked to appear for a personal interview. The interview will allow you to verbally elaborate on the qualifications summarized in your résumé. The interview also gives the employer a chance to evaluate your appearance, personality, and job-related skills. The interview is usually the pivotal point at which an employer decides if you should be offered the job and at which you decide if you want the job.

Keeping the job you have depends on many factors. Your work habits, performance of the required tasks, physical appearance, attitudes, and language all contribute to an employer's decision about whether or not to retain you as an employee. Productive employees who work well with other people are rewarded with raises in pay, extra benefits, and promotions to high-level positions.

Exploring Dimensions of Chapter Sixteen

For Review

1• What information about yourself could be helpful in making occupational and career decisions?
2• What information about occupations and careers could be helpful in making decisions?
3• What is a career ladder? Give an example.
4• "In order to enter firefighting training you must pass an extensive physical examination." This is an example of what type of information?
5• What is a résumé? How is it used?
6• What are the major purposes of a job interview?
7• What factors are helpful in keeping a job? What factors are harmful to job security?

For Consideration

1• Give an example of how fringe benefits can be a positive aspect of a job. Give another example of a negative aspect of a job.
2• You are in the midst of a two-year training program. You learn that the specific occupation you are training for has reduced job vacancies and is likely to continue reducing job vacancies. What do you do to not waste the year's study?
3• Consider a particular job. List home experiences, social experiences, and volunteer experiences that could provide knowledge about the job as well as experiences to indicate in a job interview.
4• Give several examples of how job requirements in a particular occupation could affect family life. Include both positive and negative effects.

5. A friend looks at a résumé you have written and says, "Wow, you really do brag about yourself! Why did you say all these things?" How would you respond?
6. You find out that you are going to be late for a job interview. What would you do?
7. Make a list of places in your community that you could go to identify job openings. What other sources of information are available to you?

For Application

1. Using the *Dictionary of Occupational Titles*, look up three occupations in which you have at least some degree of interest. List two positive features and two negative features of each.
2. Interview a person or people in an occupation in which you have interest. Ask them about the job description, job requirements, job future, and fringe benefits. Ask how this job interferes with or enhances family life. Ask what kind of home and family experiences might prepare people for this job.
3. Write a résumé for yourself. Even though it may be brief at the present time, outline your personal experiences, qualifications, skills, and characteristics that would reflect favorably upon you should you submit your résumé to an employer.
4. Visit an agency in your community that provides family services. Set up an appointment to interview the agency director and/or one of the employees. What do they see as the benefits of their employment? What is stressful for them? How did they become involved in this line of work?

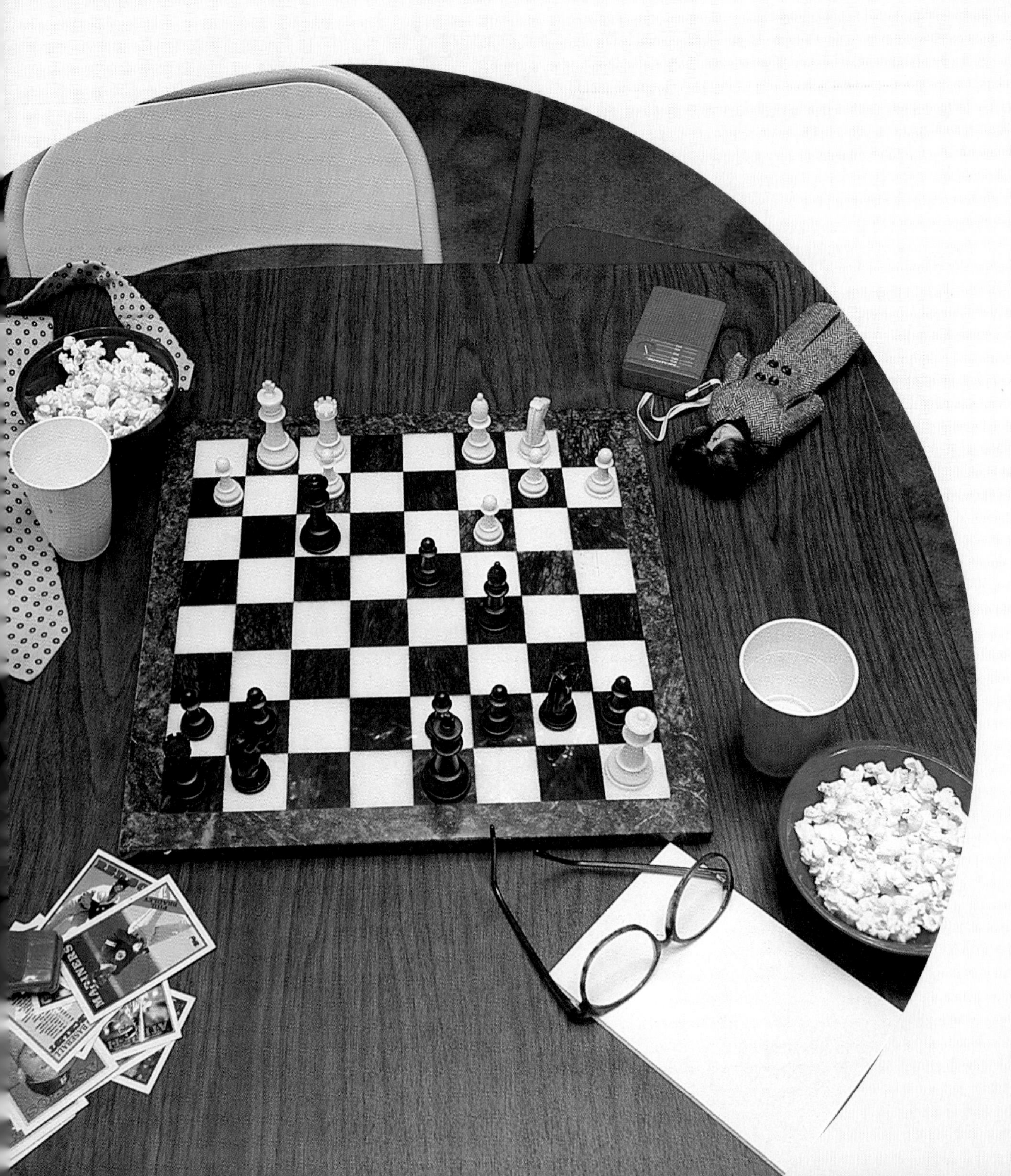
MARINERS

part six

Enhancing Family Functioning

As you have learned, realizing goals and meeting expectations in family relationships are made difficult by many things. Interpersonal skills must be learned. We are not born as experts in communication, decision making, and conflict management. Furthermore, work roles, parenting roles, and roles as marriage partners can conflict with each other, causing great stress on relationships within the family. Also, people change over time, regardless of whether they are in the childhood, adolescent, or adulthood stage of the human life.

Even though the United States is among the wealthiest and most affluent societies in the world, simple economic survival continues to be an issue for millions of low-income and poverty-stricken families. The growing number of homeless individuals during the 1980s is testimony to the financial stress that many undergo in providing an adequate income for food, clothing, and shelter. However, unemployment, inflation, and insurmountable debt are potential threats to any family unit regardless of income level.

In Chapter 17, we will look at the financial resources of families and discuss ways to manage them effectively. Effective financial management involves knowing your rights as a consumer in our current economic system. The family unit is the primary unit for the consumption of goods and services in our society. It is therefore important to understand the family's rights and obligations as a consumer.

Financial problems are just one of the many stressful conditions that families encounter. In Chapter 18, we will explore ways of strengthening family relationships across a wide range of stressful events. Effective stress management goes hand-in-hand with maintaining strong and fulfilling family relationships that endure over time.

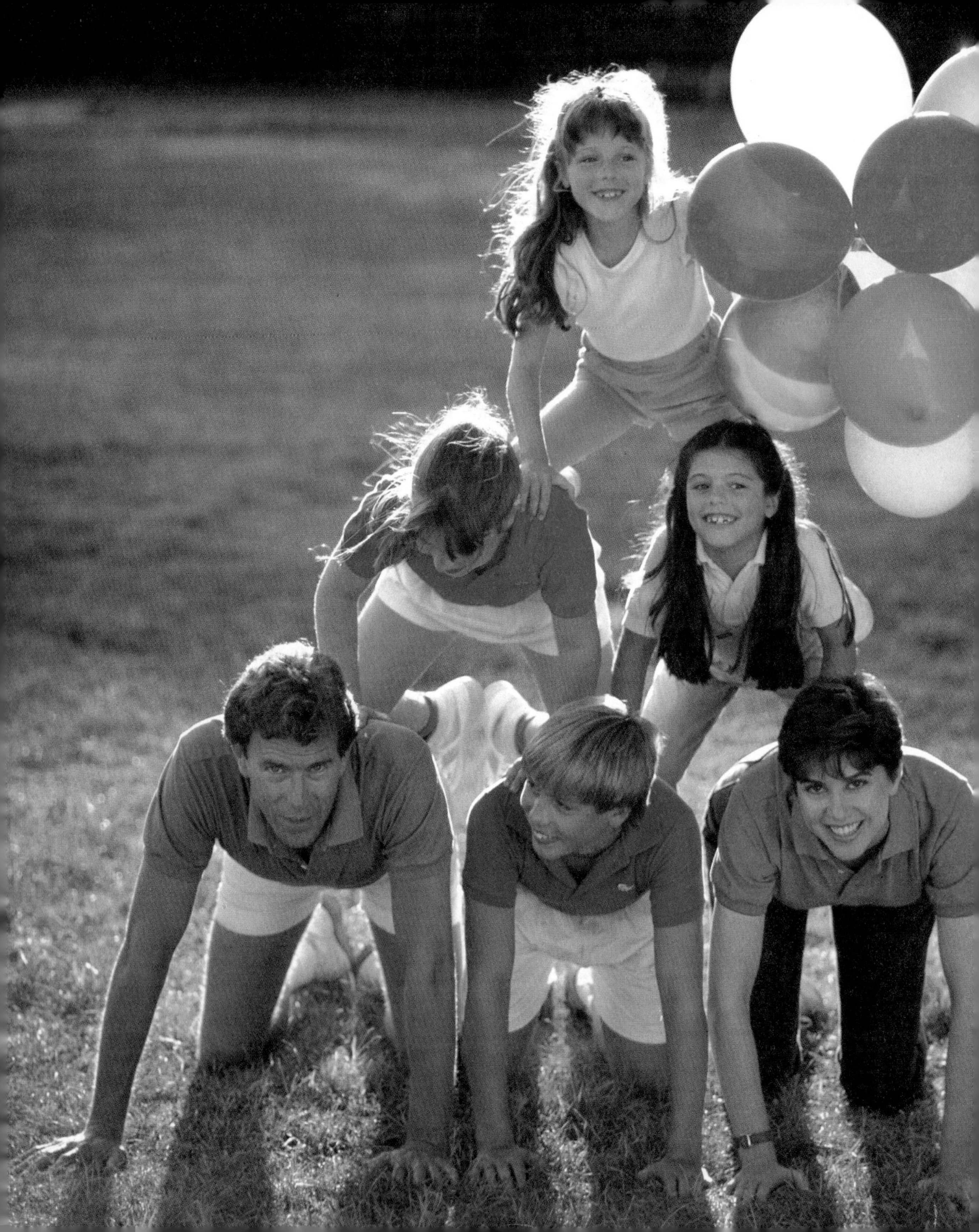

seventeen

MANAGING FAMILY FINANCIAL RESOURCES

This chapter provides information that will help you to:

- Understand the concepts of level and standard of living.
- Recognize the changing financial needs of families over the life cycle.
- Realize the importance of financial planning by families.
- Recognize the problems frequent credit users face.
- Know the rights of families as consumers.
- Empathize with low-income families and those with handicapped members.

Resources are the means by which families meet their goals and satisfy the demands that are placed on them by individual family members and by society. Resources include anything that the family can use to help itself function more effectively (see Chapter 10 for a review of the functions that families fulfill).

In previous chapters we discussed many resources that are important for establishing and maintaining effective interpersonal relationships, both within and outside the family. These resources fall into two classes: **human resources** and **material resources**. Human resources such as time, energy, and the interpersonal skills of communication, conflict management, and decision making are all helpful to individuals and families as they strive to reach their goals. A person's health and general level of intelligence (cognitive development) are also important human resources.

Material resources include the goods that family members consume such as food, clothing, and appliances (televisions, washing machines, ovens, etc.). Money is also a material resource that must be managed in families if members are to realize their goals and expectations. The amount of money that a family has at its disposal determines, in large part, the family's ability to acquire other material resources. This includes the type and quality of affordable housing that can meet the family's need for shelter.

Most families acquire their incomes from members who work outside the home. This salary or wage is contributed to the family bank account. However, family income also can be acquired in other ways. For example, some families inherit money from relatives who have died. Others invest money in stocks, bonds, or other commodities and earn dividends that these investments yield. Families with low incomes may rely on government agencies to provide income subsidies in order to maintain a minimum standard of living.

No matter what the source of income and regardless of the amount, today's families must engage in sound practices of financial management if they are to meet their economic goals. In this chapter we discuss the more important principles for effective financial resource management.

LEVELS AND STANDARDS OF LIVING

To a large degree, family financial resources determine the family's level of living. **Level of living** refers to the actual number and types of goods and services that a family currently has. The **standard of living** is the quality of life that a family *desires* in terms of material resources. Consider the following indicators of level and standard of living:

- The quality of one's neighborhood (crime rate, safety, number of run-down houses, quality of public schools)
- The number or type of cars that the family owns
- The amount and type of leisure-time activities that a family is able to enjoy (going to a restaurant for dinner, going on vacations, traveling)
- The ability of the family to maintain the health of its members (regular medical care, hospitalization, health insurance)
- The adequacy of clothing and nutritious food supply for family members

Undoubtedly, you could think of other indicators. An important point, though, concerns the gap that might exist between one's standard of living and the actual level of living experienced. Individuals and families vary widely in terms of their standards of living.

Some aspire to have much more than they currently have in terms of material goods. Others may have lower expectations that are more in line with what they currently have. Generally speaking, the more the standard of living falls short of the actual level of living, the greater the degree of disappointment with the family's financial situation.

We acquire our standard of living from a variety of sources. Perhaps the most important source is from the family in which we grew up. Many people aspire to live at a level that is equal to or greater than that enjoyed in the parental family. Our standard of living is also influenced by our observations of friends', relatives', and neighbors' levels of living and perhaps even by the levels of living portrayed in the media—movies, magazines, television, etc. How closely we come to actually reaching our standard of living depends on the income we earn and how that money is managed.

Figure 17-1a

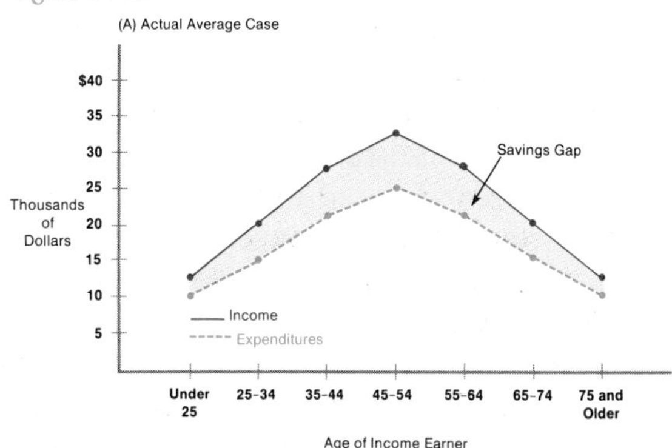

Figure 17-1b

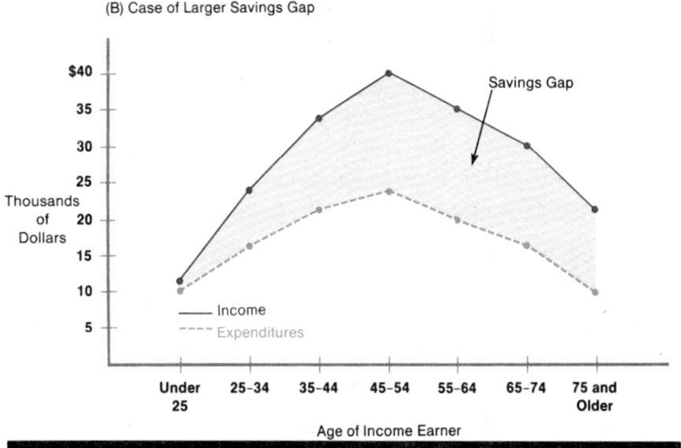

FINANCIAL RESOURCES OVER THE LIFE CYCLE

As families move through the stages of the family life cycle they realize changes in two important areas: the level of financial resources available and the level of expenditures demanded by the developing family. This fact is illustrated in Figure 17-1. The top portion of this figure shows the *average* trend in income and expenditures in the American family. Both begin quite low and peak about the time that families have teenagers and are entering the launching stage of the life cycle. Note that, on the average, income increases slightly more than expenditures during the middle stages. This difference represents a

Figure 17-1c

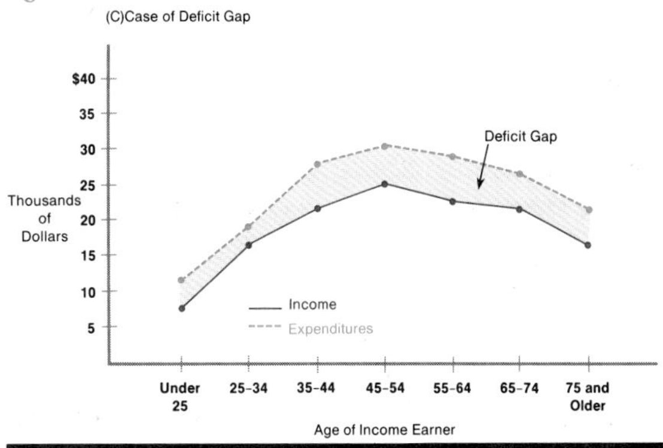

savings gap which allows the family to accumulate some financial reserves. During later life cycle stages the income and expenditure curves both drop and converge. Income drops with retirement and expenditures drop when children are launched from the family.

It must be understood that the top part of Figure 17-1a represents a statistical average. Families vary in their ability to save money and accumulate resources. Some have larger savings gaps than others (Figure 17-1b, middle panel). Some families are barely able to make ends meet. They find themselves spending all of the money that is earned. Still others find that they spend more than they earn, thereby encountering financial difficulties as they realize a **deficit gap** in their situation (Figure 17-1c, bottom panel). Income and expenditures can form any of a number of combinations to produce a family's financial condition.

Figure 17-2

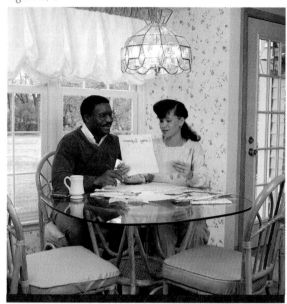

Financial planning begins with setting specific goals. If it is your goal to save for a down payment on a home, your plan would be different than if your goal were to purchase a second car.

THE IMPORTANCE OF PLANNING

A key aspect of financial management is the ability to plan. **Planning** involves a deliberate effort to make decisions in the present that will affect the future in a positive manner (Figure 17-2). You have probably learned that when you have a major exam in school, you do better if you have planned your study time adequately. You also may have learned that family vacations run more smoothly when they have been planned carefully, *before* the day of departure!

Effective planning involves a number of steps. These include the following, which apply to financial planning as well as to other types of planning.

Setting a Clearly Defined Goal

To plan effectively, you must have a reasonably clear picture of what you hope to achieve or accomplish with the plan. The goal you set must be realistic. If you plan to go on a diet to lose weight, it is best to set a goal for a specific number of pounds to lose in a specific time frame. For example, you might set a goal of losing ten pounds in the next six weeks. However, it would be unrealistic to set a goal of losing ten pounds in the next five days! Also, it is too ambiguous to say that you are going on a diet to lose "several pounds sometime this summer."

Financial planning requires specific goal setting. If you work after school, you may decide to save some of your paycheck in a savings account. You may set a goal of saving $500 by the time school lets out in the spring. In setting this goal, you calculate that it will take a minimum deposit of $25 per week to accomplish this goal. Your goal is clearly defined and realistic and you have taken an important step toward effective financial planning (review Chapter 3 for further discussion of goal setting).

Assessing Your Resources

Planning requires that you understand the potential and the limitations of the resources you have available to reach your goal.

CASE IN POINT

Jerry's friends planned a summer trip to Europe that would cost $1,500. Jerry looked at all of the resources he had available to determine if he would be able to afford to go with them. He looked at his savings account. He then determined how much additional money he would be able to earn from his part-time job and he asked his parents if they would be able to contribute any additional money.

However, Jerry was saving money to help pay for a new car and the insurance it required. In weighing the alternatives, he decided that the new car was a higher priority and that his major resource, his savings account, would be better spent to reach that goal. Because the other resources he had available were not enough to be able to afford the trip to Europe, Jerry decided not to plan for it.

Being in Control of Time

Time orientation is important in the actual effort to carry out the plan. This means that you have accurately gauged the amount of time that it might take to carry out the plan, and that you have the necessary time available to you. As you assess your total available resources, time should be included as one of them.

CASE IN POINT

Jana agreed to help collect money for the heart foundation by walking door-to-door in her neighborhood. She thought she would have plenty of time in the next week to complete the task. However, she did not stop to think of the amount of time that the task would take. Nor did she consider the major geography test at school, practice for the track team on three afternoons, and a prior commitment to care for the neighbor's children on Saturday. As the week was drawing to a close, Jana panicked when she realized that she had too much to do with too little time in which to do it. She was unable to carry out her plan to collect money for the heart foundation.

Effective planning requires **foresight**. This is the ability to anticipate future events accurately. The most successful businesses are those that are able to look ahead and to anticipate what consumers will want to buy or what services they will want to have in the future. They design and manufacture products based on their view of the future, rather than on what consumers appear to want at present. Financial planning in families also requires foresight.

CASE IN POINT

Terese and Edward were thinking about having their first child. They discussed the future and the financial needs they would have after the birth of their child. They agreed that they would need to have at least $3,000 in a savings account for possible emergencies that might arise. They also reviewed their life insurance coverage, knowing that their child would need to be supported in the event that one or both of them should die. They also realized that their one-bedroom house was too small to accommodate a growing family. They decided to postpone parenthood until these aspects of their plan were handled. They had the foresight to recognize that the future will bring financial challenges when children are added to the family.

Effective time management, whether it involves the ability to assess time resources or foresight, is an important component of effective planning.

Motivation and the Ability to Carry Out the Plan

A plan is only as good as the person's motivation and ability to carry out the necessary actions to meet the plan's objective. Some people are great at formulating plans that sound good on paper. However, they fall short of actually following through in implementing the plan. While they may have the necessary resources to follow through, they may lack the initiative to do so.

CASE IN POINT

Pete and Rosa made a plan to save money to build a new house that they had always dreamed about. They needed to save $200 a month for two years in order to have enough money for the down payment. However, they were unable to change their buying habits in order to save the money. They charged a number of expensive items on credit cards and continued to spend more than they really had for their groceries. Pete accompanied his friends from work on a fishing trip, which cost $500, while Rosa purchased an airline ticket to visit her parents in another city. They dug themselves so far into debt that they had to take the money they wanted to save for the new house to pay their bills. Their house remained a dream because they did not exercise adequate self-discipline to make it become a reality.

There are several other important features of effective planning. These include having as much pertinent information as possible as you make your plan, being flexible in altering your plan if resources are insufficient or if finding new resources is necessary, and working effectively with other people with whom the plan is being made. This last feature is particularly important for effective financial planning in families. Cooperation, communication, and strong problem-solving skills are essential ingredients of a successful planning effort.

ACHIEVING FAMILY FINANCIAL SECURITY

Family financial security is achieved when the family has adequate resources to meet members' basic needs for food, shelter, clothing, safety, and health. The income that is earned from work is a major part of establishing financial security.

However, income alone is not enough. Financial security also depends on how income and other resources are managed. Financial security is achieved when financial and other resources are managed in a way that allows the family to reach its desired standard of living. For example, one family might live at a comfortable standard of living on a $30,000 per year income, while another family may be debt-ridden and go into bankruptcy on a $60,000 annual income.

In this section we will explore several keys to successful financial management in families. These include budgeting, investment, wise credit use, and insurance. Each involves the ability to *plan* for the future.

Establishing a Budget

Budgeting is a way to plan the expenditure of money in a wise manner. A budget helps to assure that income earned adequately covers the expenses that the family faces. A budget not only helps a family to meet their financial goals on a month-to-month basis, but it also assists in the achievement of long-range financial goals.

A budget has two objectives: (1) to create discipline in the family's spending and (2) to reduce the amount of money wasted through needless spending. The first objective involves developing a plan of spending so that the family does not run out of money before all of the expenses have been covered. The plan must accurately reflect the actual monthly income and expenditures of the family.

Any budget must be periodically revised to take into account rising prices of goods and services (known in economic terms as **inflation**), and to reflect significant changes in family income and expenses that might take place. To develop a useful budget, you must be aware of your spending patterns and be willing to keep track of them from month to month.

The second objective of a budget means that the family must reach agreement about expenditures: necessary expenses, expenses that are important but not essential, or unnecessary expenses. Many family budgets are rendered useless when impulse purchases are made for unnecessary expensive items.

CASE IN POINT

Martin went to the local shopping center to buy a special tool to fix his television. Electronics was his hobby so he decided to fix his own television because it would be easier on his budget. However, while at the store he noticed that the most recent model of a video camera was on sale for only $1,200. His eyes grew wide when he saw it, yet he knew that his budget could not handle it. Just the same, Martin could not resist the temptation to buy the camera. He wrote a check for $200 and placed the balance on his store charge account. Martin succumbed to the impulse to buy even though he will regret it later when he finds that his budget is $200 short for groceries and rent, and when he has to make his first credit payment.

To handle the urge to buy on impulse, a family budget may set aside a certain amount of money, sometimes referred to as **mad money**, to allow for occasional impulse purchases. In this way, the necessary items in the budget are not affected and family members do not feel guilty about buying an item that was not part of the budget.

In order to develop the necessary awareness of expenses and income, a form like the one in Figure 17-3 might be used. After several months of record keeping, this form can be converted into a permanent monthly guide that can be revised as the need arises. While it is important to keep regular records of dollar amounts, it is not necessary to account for every penny and dime spent.

In considering budget priorities, it is helpful to know where the typical family in the United States today spends its monthly income. This is illustrated in Figure 17-4. Monthly expenditures for taxes, food, and housing (rent, mortgage) account for one half of the family's entire budget.

Because of the large percentage of the typical budget consumed by these three items, all of which involve *necessary* expenditures, a family must engage in *setting priorities* for the remaining budget categories. For example, many people desire to have many things—a car, a house, furniture, vacations, and several visits per week to their favorite restaurant—only they can't afford them but want them now. They begin to spend money they don't have, often by borrowing or through the use of a twentieth century invention—the credit card. Before they know it, they are drowning in a sea of debt.

Effective budgeting means establishing priorities among such desired goods. These goods may then be purchased one at a time without overspending in any of the monthly budget categories. Of course, the top priority should be those items which meet basic physical needs for food, clothing, health care, and housing. Another top priority should be on *saving* a certain amount regularly (weekly or monthly). A savings account provides a safeguard when unexpected emergencies such as unemployment, sudden illness of a family member, or a major household repair arise.

Effective budgeting involves many abilities: planning, communication, conflict management, and decision making. It also involves a cooperative mood and a willingness to compromise. A budget is a tool used by the family to achieve financial stability.

Investment

Once a family's necessary expenses have been covered, including an adequate cushion in a savings account, the practice of investment might be considered. **Investment** is simply a way of using money to make more money.

In considering possible investments, a number of factors should be considered:

1• *Risk*—the chances of losing your money from the investment
2• *Return*—the approximate percentage of dollars to be earned for every dollar invested
3• *Liquidity*—the ease with which your money invested can be converted back into cash, if you should need it
4• *Effort*—the amount of personal time, expertise, and energy required to manage your investment
5• *Maturity*—the amount of time it takes to realize the rate of return that is expected from the investment
6• *Power*—the protection that your investment provides against rising prices (inflation)
7• *Taxes*—the extent to which your investment is taxable by your local, state, or federal governments

Figure 17-3

Example of Monthly Budget Form

Item	Jan.	Feb.	Dec.	Total
Total money income				
Major fixed expenses: Taxes: Federal				
State				
Property				
Auto				
Rent or mortgage payment				
Insurance: Medical (including prepaid care)				
Life				
Property				
Auto				
Debt payments: Auto				
Other				
Savings for: Emergency fund				
Flexible expenses: Food and beverages				
Utilities and maintenance (household supplies and services				
Furnishings and equipment				
Clothing				
Personal care				
Auto upkeep, gas, oil				
Fares, tolls, other				
Medical care (not prepaid or reimbursed)				
Recreation and education				
Gifts and contributions				
Total Spending				

SOURCE: U.S. Department of Agriculture, "A Guide to Budgeting for the Young Couple." *Home and Garden Bulletin*, Number 98, July, 1977, p. 7.

Figure 17-4

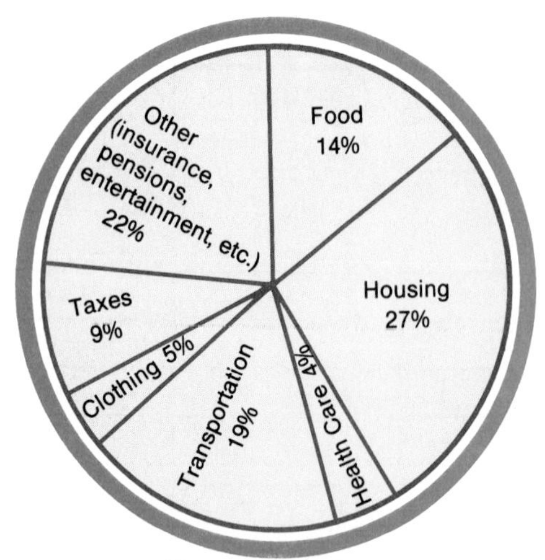

SOURCE: ***Statistical Abstract of the United States***, 1988. Washington, D.C.: U.S. Department of Commerce, 1987, p. 420.

Figure 17-5

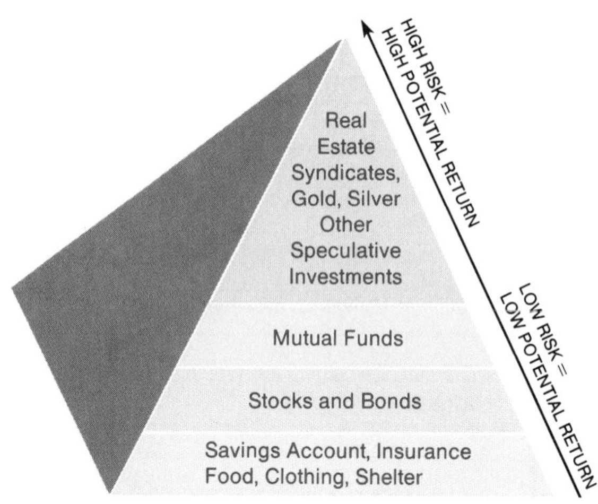

There are many types of investment options open to anyone. They are identified in the investment pyramid depicted in Figure 17-5. As this figure shows, the degree of ***risk*** in an investment varies in a direct manner with the potential return that an investment can provide. That is, the riskier the investment in terms of your chances of losing money, the greater the potential return should the investment turn out to be a good one.

For example, purchasing shares in the stock market or state and municipal bonds will generally yield greater return per dollar invested than will a standard savings account. However, the investor is also more likely to lose money on the stock and bond markets than is the case for a savings account. Mutual funds, which involve a pooling of funds by several people in an investment company, are managed by the company on behalf of the investors. If poorly managed, the investors can lose a great deal. If managed well, however, a good return on the dollars invested can be realized. Precious stones and metals (gold, silver, diamonds), along with speculative real estate investments, comprise some of the riskiest investments. They pose the highest risk, yet also carry the greatest potential return.

Figure 17-5 also indicates that the base of the pyramid should be achieved first, before the family makes riskier investments. Before investing one dime of your earnings, it is essential that you are able to afford the money that must be tied up in the investment. You must first assure that the family is taken care of in terms of adequate income for food, clothing, housing, and health care. Cash on hand in a savings account is essential to meet unexpected financial problems such as accidents or illness. You must also have adequate insurance to protect the family should a major calamity such as a fire, natural disaster (floods, storms, etc.), serious illness, or unexpected death of an income provider occur.

Once the base of the pyramid is covered, you may consider investing extra income, known as **discretionary income**, in the lower risk investments. Then, you may increase the number of riskier investments as your budget allows. Remember, the riskier the investment, the more you stand to gain *or* lose. Also, riskier investments cause your money to be tied up longer before they yield a profit (that is, they are less liquid).

The Use of Credit

"Drive now, pay later."

"Small down payment, no monthly payments for two months."

"All major credit cards accepted."

"Low monthly payments."

These are common phrases in our society today. Much of what we buy is through the use of credit. Credit allows a person to purchase something without having the cash on hand. It is a form of borrowing money from a bank, other financial institution (savings and loan, credit union), or the store from which the item is purchased. In fact, the vast majority of all large purchases—cars, boats, vacations, furniture, household appliances, and houses—are made without cash; that is, they are purchased on credit.

Using credit allows the purchaser to enjoy goods and services before enough money has been saved to buy them. The credit user then pays back a certain amount of the borrowed money (known as the **principal** of the loan) each month, for a predetermined amount of time until the loan is completely paid.

However, it is important to know that using credit is not free. The borrower must also pay a service charge known as **interest**, which covers the cost of using the lender's money for that period of time. Thus, the consumer ends up paying more for the item purchased than it actually cost in the first place. For example, if you were to charge a $500 stereo system on credit and took one year to pay the charge, you could end up paying between $550 and $575 for the stereo (depending upon the interest rate and how much of the loan principal you actually paid per month).

The actual interest you pay varies from one type of credit or loan to the next. Interest rates usually vary between 10 and 25 percent for most types of credit purchases. However, an interest rate difference of even 1 percent can mean a substantial amount of money on large purchases, such as a house or car (see Figure 17-6). In Figure 17-6, as is the case with most home mortgages, a 30-year period is allowed to the home buyer to repay the loan. As you can see, a small change in interest rate means an extra cost of thousands of dollars in the final purchase price. Monthly payments go up, as does the total amount of interest that the buyer will eventually pay over the 30-year period.

Before you buy anything on credit, it is important that you know the exact interest rate. It is also important to know the terms of the credit agreement. That is, how often are you expected to make payments? monthly? weekly? How much are the minimum payments that you are expected to make? Are all payments to be equal size? How long do you have to pay back the loan? Are you allowed to pay the entire balance of the loan early without having to pay an extra penalty? How much interest will you have paid once the entire loan has been paid? These facts should be stated in writing in an agreement that you sign with the lender.

Figure 17-6

Example of Monthly Payments and Actual Total Interest Charges for a $60,000 Home Mortgage at Different Annual Interest Rates

Interest Rate	Monthly Payment (principal and interest)	Total Finance Charge for 30-year Loan Period
8%	$440.26	$ 98,493.60
10	526.55	129,558.00
12	617.17	162,181.20
14	710.93	195,934.80
16	806.86	230,469.60
18	904.26	265,533.60

SOURCE: Robert O. Hermann, *Consumer Choice in the American Economy* (Cincinnati: South-Western Publishing Co., 1988), p. 357.

CREDIT CARDS • More than half of all retail sales in the United States are handled by the use of credit cards (Figure 17-7). Gasoline companies allow customers to make purchases with credit cards. VISA, MasterCard, American Express, and other credit card companies provide the consumer with the ability to purchase a wide variety of products by charging them with credit cards. The amount of interest charged for credit card purchases varies, but it is usually between 18 and 21 percent of the unpaid balance of the charge. These interest rates are higher than most loans a person might obtain from a bank, savings and loan, or credit union.

Figure 17-7

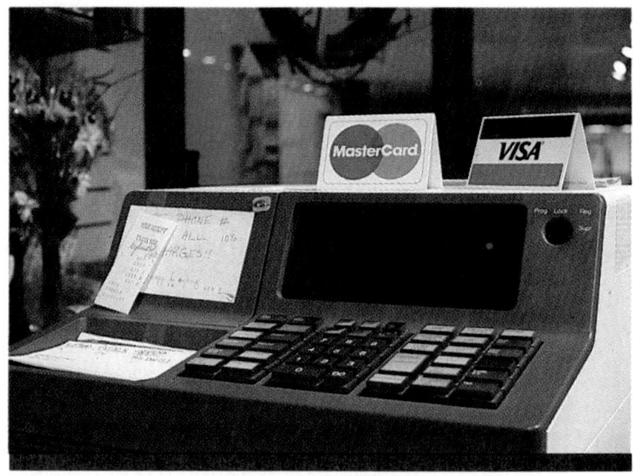

Using credit cards to purchase goods is very common in our society.

USING CREDIT WISELY • In order to continue receiving credit, a person must have an acceptable **credit rating**. A good credit rating is established by reliably making payments on loans and credit cards. A poor credit rating is established when you are consistently late in making loan or credit card payments, or if you should fail to pay them altogether (this is known as **defaulting on the loan**). When you have a poor credit rating, it becomes more difficult, and at times impossible, to borrow money or to get your credit card renewed for future use. Thus, if you desire to use credit,

Spotlight on issues

Credit Laws

The federal government has enacted many laws to protect the rights and specify the responsibilities of both credit users and lenders. These laws are enforced by federal and state agencies authorized to prevent consumer fraud as well as consumer abuse of the credit system.

The Truth-in-Lending Act and Fair Credit Billing laws are designed to prevent the lender from deceiving the borrower or user of credit. For example, before entering into a credit agreement, the consumer must be informed in writing of all conditions of the credit agreement, including the actual interest rate. The consumer has the right to question the accuracy of any billing statement issued by the lender. Also, the lender must inform the consumer of the proper channels for filing an inquiry about the accuracy of a bill. The consumer is not responsible for payment of the amount in question until the matter is resolved. However, the consumer is obligated to follow the proper procedures in finding out about and resolving the disputed charges.

The Equal Credit Opportunity Act states that discrimination on the basis of race, sex, age, religion, national origin, or marital status against anyone seeking credit is prohibited. At one time, being a divorced woman was a "black mark" on a credit history. Lenders did not consider such women good "credit risks," and denied them credit. Often such women had not established a credit history because their ex-husbands had taken out loans and used credit in the husbands' names only. Also, being Hispanic, black, or of another ethnic minority was also used as an excuse to deny credit to certain people. Such practices today are illegal. Equal weight must be given to all credit applications regardless of the applicant's sex, marital status, or race. Women of all marital statuses have the right to establish a separate credit rating in their own names.

There are other laws which protect the rights and specify the responsibilities of credit users and lenders. Some of these relate to your *credit rating*, which is used by lenders in deciding whether or not to approve your loan application or your request for a credit card. Your credit rating is on file in one or more local and national credit bureaus. Your credit rating goes down when you have defaulted on prior loans (been unable to pay), if you don't make your scheduled payments on time, or if you have otherwise abused your prior credit privileges.

You have the right to know what is contained in your credit file in the credit bureau. You also have the right to challenge inaccuracies and have incorrect information removed from your file. Access to your credit file is limited to yourself and those who have a legitimate need to evaluate your credit rating: insurance companies, banks, potential employers, or those to whom you currently owe money (creditors). This is an important right to privacy that all people have. Stiff penalties will be applied to anyone who seeks information from a person's credit file under false pretenses.

it is important that you do so in a responsible manner.

Anyone using credit should be aware of laws that exist to protect the rights of you—the consumer and credit user (see *Spotlight on issues*). Thus, not only is the credit user expected to act in a responsible manner when taking out loans or using credit cards, the lender must also act in a way that is fair to the borrower.

Credit use has advantages for the consumer. You are able to buy certain things that might otherwise take years to acquire—at least as long as it would take to save enough money to buy them. Think how long it would take to save the $75,000 needed to buy the house you want for your family or the $18,000 needed to purchase the car you would like to have. By taking out a loan for such things, the consumer can enjoy them now while paying back the lender over a period of time.

However, despite its advantages, credit use can also be a dangerous tool. You can get in serious financial trouble by borrowing too much money or by borrowing money too frequently. The higher the interest rate you pay, the more serious the problem. Credit cards, for example, can be *too* convenient for some people. They can easily be viewed as just "plastic money" that at the time of the purchase is not real. Before long, the frequent credit card user finds that the monthly payments required from the use of four, five, or six different credit cards are simply too high for the budget to handle. When the monthly bills arrive, the person is shocked to realize that there is not enough money left over to pay for food and other necessary items.

The result of too much credit use is negative. Payments may be made late or you may have to default on one or more of your loans altogether. Your credit rating will suffer and you will find it more difficult to obtain credit in the future. In extreme cases, a person or family may have to declare **bankruptcy**. In such cases, a judge determines the extent to which one is able to pay back any debts. A person may lose possession of his or her car, house, and other assets that may be required to help pay off the debt. Bankruptcy is a major black mark on a person's credit rating.

Some credit users literally drown in a sea of debt. How can you avoid the danger of too much credit use? The first hint is to use credit only when absolutely necessary. When you can purchase an item with cash or money you have saved, you pay less than if you borrowed the money because there is no interest payment. Also, try not to use credit to purchase items that are a regular part of your budget. This includes food, utilities, clothing, and entertainment. Finally, every time you borrow money, include the monthly payment as part of your monthly budget. Keep track of your credit purchases, especially if they are made with a credit card. Several purchases that seem small at first may add up quickly. Before you realize it, you have many payments to make each month and not enough income to cover them and all of your other necessary expenses.

Wise credit use requires the skill of planning. You must have foresight as well as the ability to accurately evaluate your available resources. You must be motivated to limit your credit use in a way that allows you to reach your goals, but that also keeps you from going too deeply in debt.

FAMILIES AS CONSUMERS[1]

In earlier generations, families often produced many of the goods that they consumed. Such goods as clothing, food products, and even housing were often produced by families who benefited by their use.

Today, however, individuals and families produce little of what they consume. We are a society of consumers of goods and services that others produce. The food we eat as well as the clothing we wear is produced and processed by private businesses and industries. Our economy thrives on the spending of consumers who must rely on the marketplace to buy the goods and services that are needed or desired. Much of this consumer spending takes place in the family context.

Consumer Rights and Responsibilities

Although we all play the role of consumer on a continuing basis, few people understand the rights and responsibilities of consumers in our society. Many rights and responsibilities are enforced by laws designed to bring justice to the relationship between consumers and producers. The following are ***rights*** that consumers have in relation to producers and sellers of goods and services.

THE RIGHT TO ACCURATE INFORMATION • Consumers have the right to accurate information about a product or service. This means that the consumer should not be subject to misleading, deceptive, difficult-to-understand, or fraudulent information about a product. If an automobile salesperson tells you that the car you are buying has a certain type and quality of engine, then you have the right to expect that it does have such an engine.

Consumers are bombarded daily by advertising that makes fantastic claims about a product's quality: "Our product is the best." "No other product can match our quality." Such claims are not considered to be factual because they are difficult, if not impossible, to prove. They are commonly known as **advertising hype**. Thus, such claims are not considered to be factually deceptive or misleading since the consumer is assumed to

[1]Much of the information presented in this section is based on the excellent treatment of the subject given by Robert O. Hermann, *Consumer Choice in the American Economy* (Cincinnati: South-Western Publishing Co., 1988).

be leary of such exaggerations so typical of product advertising. Only when certain facts about the product's characteristics or what it can and cannot do are falsely presented is the consumer's right to accurate information violated. For example, some years ago a certain mouthwash product claimed to prevent colds when medical experts concluded it really did not. The federal government required the mouthwash manufacturer to remove that claim from the label of the product.

THE RIGHT TO SAFETY IN USING A PRODUCT • Some products may be potentially hazardous to the consumer's health or otherwise dangerous to the user (for example, there may be a risk of physical injury). If such hazards or dangers are likely, then the consumer has the right to be informed of the risks involved in the product's use.

One well-known example of this is the warning label that cigarette manufacturers place on cigarette packages and include in cigarette advertising. Because it has been determined that cigarette smoking causes certain diseases of the heart and lung, the government required that the consumer be informed that such potentially hazardous side effects exist. Another example involves the use of electrical appliances near water. Warning labels are attached to such devices to alert the consumer of potential hazards such as electrical shock.

If used in the correct and intended manner, no product should pose an unexpected threat to the consumer's well-being. If it does, the product comes under scrutiny by governmental agencies and such agencies may remove it from the market.

THE RIGHT TO BE FREE FROM A POLLUTED ENVIRONMENT • Air and water pollution are major environmental issues today. Waste products from automobiles, factories, and individual carelessness (littering, improper disposal of chemicals, metal and glass containers, etc.) threaten the integrity and safety of our living environment. Consumers have the right to be protected from these hazards. To be adequately protected, however, consumers must share this responsibility with business and industry. It is everyone's responsibility to protect our environment and to keep it clean and safe.

THE RIGHT TO A FREE CHOICE AMONG PRODUCTS • Our economic marketplace in the United States thrives on the idea of free and open competition among various products. Competition encourages increased quality of a product to be sold at more reasonable prices than might occur if product choice was limited. For example, if only one company manufactured automobile stereo systems, there would be little incentive to produce a high quality product at a reasonable price. However, with many types of car stereos on the market, the various manufacturers must compete to make a quality product at a price that the consumer will decide is worth it relative to the other stereos available.

THE RIGHT TO REDRESS • This means that any consumer has the right to fair treatment by the seller or manufacturer of a product should a problem arise that is the fault of the seller or the manufacturer. Many of us know someone who purchased a new or used car that turned out to be a "lemon." Something was always going wrong with it, often within days of the purchase. Others have purchased appliances or other products that failed to work as they should—or failed to work at all!

Assuming that they are not due to the consumer's misuse or mistreatment of the product, consumers have the right to have such problems remedied by the seller or manufacturer. Refunds, replacements, or repairs are means by which such problems can be fixed.

THE RIGHT TO INVOLVEMENT IN GOVERNMENT POLICIES AFFECTING CONSUMERS • Consumers have the right to participate in public agencies that protect the interests of consumers. Federal agencies include the Consumer Product Safety Commission, the Food and Drug Administration, and the Federal Trade Commission. Numerous state and local consumer protection agencies also exist such as the Better Business Bureau and offices of the local and state attorney general. Individual consumers have the right to become involved in setting program priorities and in changing agency policies in ways that better meet the needs of consumers.

As is true in many areas of life, the rights of an individual are accompanied by certain responsibilities. Consumers have responsibilities in each of the above-mentioned areas. For example, consumers have the responsibility to be informed about products they buy. Consumers should not take everything they hear about a product through advertising, or from the seller, on face value alone. This means that the consumer should make every reasonable effort to find out about the quality of a service or product *before* it is purchased. A publication such as *Consumer Reports* provides useful information and quality ratings of many products such as cars, stereos, major household appliances, and even life insurance policies. Before purchasing a product, you might also talk to other people to see how satisfied they are with the one they bought.

Consumers have the responsibility to use products in a safe manner and in a way intended by the manufacturer. This is particularly true for products that may be hazardous if used incorrectly. It is also the consumer's responsibility to protect the environment. Examples of this include the person who recycles glass and aluminum cans, the person who deposits litter and trash in proper containers, and the person who tries not to abuse such natural resources as lakes, rivers, and forests.

Finally, it is the consumer's responsibility to seek redress from a seller or manufacturer when a product or service is unsatisfactory. Unless a dissatisfied consumer brings a problem to the attention of the seller, there is nothing the seller can do to correct the problem and, perhaps, prevent it from happening again. Satisfied customers are an important source of additional business. Dissatisfied customers can hurt business. One common example of this principle occurs when eating a meal in a restaurant. If your meal or service is unsatisfactory in some way, the restaurant manager will want to know about it. Not only will it give the restaurant a second chance to please you, but it will also help to correct a problem that might cause dissatisfaction among future restaurant customers.

Resources for Consumers

We have already identified a few of the resources that individuals and families have available to become better consumers. For example, many communities have Better

Business Bureaus (BBB). The BBB provides information about businesses in the community and the products or services they sell. The BBB maintains a file on any complaints businesses may have received from consumers, as well as information regarding how the complaints might have been resolved. If you are considering a major purchase or if you are planning to deal with a business that is unfamiliar to you, it would be wise to contact your local BBB to see if they have any information about whether others have complained about the business and how any complaints might have been resolved. If your community does not have a BBB, then the local Chamber of Commerce may be a good alternative source of information.

Many consumer publications are available to help provide information about the quality and costs of various products. As mentioned earlier, an excellent publication is *Consumer Reports*. This magazine provides consumers with objective information about the relative costs, safety, durability, and performance of various products. Local, state, and federal government agencies also have many publications designed to aid the consumer in making wise purchasing decisions. Usually these are available at no cost.

If a consumer has a complaint that cannot be resolved with the seller or manufacturer and if the local Better Business Bureau is unable to resolve the problem, then the consumer may need to contact the consumer affairs division of the local or state government (sometimes these are referred to as consumer protection agencies). There are legal avenues that can be followed in order to resolve a consumer dispute. Dissatisfied consumers have the right to seek a resolution in a court of law, if necessary. Fortunately, most disputes never make it this far. Usually the manufacturer or seller is more than willing to keep a customer satisfied by resolving *bona fide* consumer complaints.

FAMILIES WITH SPECIAL NEEDS

Families differ in their available resources to meet goals and satisfy needs of family members. Some families have special needs which place an extra strain on their resources, or which reduce the number of resources at their disposal. In this section we will examine the resource needs of such families. We will also explore the ways in which financial, energy, and time resources are managed in special-need families in order to better cope with the challenges they face.

Low-Income Families

As affluent a society as the United States has become, many families must cope with economic resources far below what is necessary to maintain an acceptable level of living. A sizable number of American families live in poverty, while others live on the edge of the poverty line as officially defined by the United States government. For example, in 1982 there were 34.4 million people living below the poverty level, which amounted to 15 percent of the entire American population. Black families, particularly those that are headed by a single-parent mother, are much more likely to live in poverty than are white families. In 1980, single-parent families of both races were more likely to live in poverty (44 percent) than families headed by two parents (7 percent).

What does it mean to live with such low levels of economic resources? It usually involves any one or a combination of the following factors:

- Unemployment of one or both of the adult members of the household
- Inadequate supply of nutritious food for family members
- Substandard housing that often involves overcrowding of family members
- A growing threat of homelessness due to unemployment and the inability to pay rent or mortgage
- Reliance on governmental assistance in the form of welfare payments, food stamps, and cash subsidies in order to survive
- Lost family pride and sense of personal embarrassment in being unable to keep a respectable job, home, and level of living
- Inability to establish and use credit, or having to pay higher interest rates and go deeper into debt when borrowing
- Being unable to pay for adequate life or health insurance, thereby being more at risk of catastrophic illness and other crises

In brief, low-income families must live with far fewer financial resources in a society that is among the richest in the world. For some, this is a short-term experience that may not last more than a year or two. For others, however, the low-income status is more permanent. Many families continue to live in a poverty-stricken status from one generation to the next. They are unable to break the vicious grip that poverty can have on people who lack the resources necessary to escape it.

There are many myths about those who live at low-income levels. One of these myths is that people who live in poverty do so because they are lazy or lack the motivation to "get a good job." The fact is that most people who live in low-income situations encounter major barriers that prevent them from escaping the cycle of poverty that has been established. Racial discrimination and prejudice help to account for the fact that a greater proportion of black families than white families are low income. Divorce and desertion leave single-parent mothers in the difficult position of having to raise a family on only one income, which often is quite low relative to what a man may earn. Being unable to afford a college education or attending schools that inadequately prepare young people with the skills necessary to succeed in higher paying jobs also contribute to the perpetuation of poverty. Low-income people often lack the basic resources necessary to generate additional financial resources.

Given their difficult situation, what can low-income families do to better cope with meager economic resources? There are no simple answers to this question. However, the following steps can be taken to help alleviate the situation:

- Establish mutually supportive networks of friends and relatives to assist with child care, transportation, home repairs, and other needs when the parent(s) must work.
- Know what community resources are available to help families with low incomes. These might include special health care, food and clothing allocation, and educational programs. Low-income families are often entitled to free or extremely low-cost legal services.
- Find ways to stretch limited resources. For example, start and maintain a savings account, no matter how small at first, to help

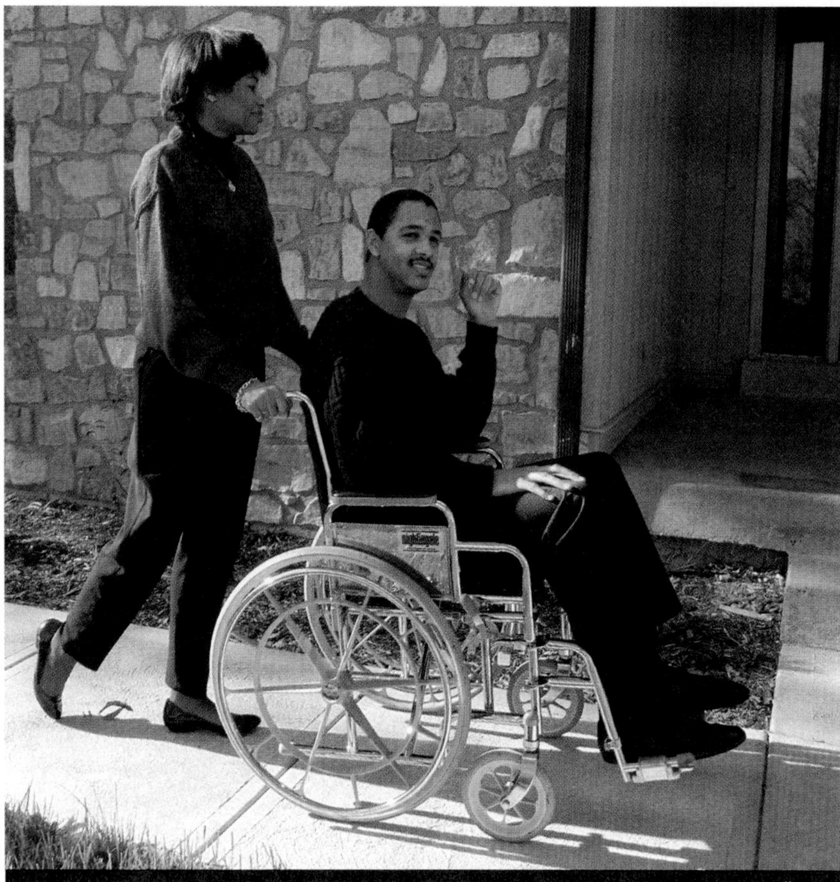

Figure 17-8
Families with handicapped members face challenges that other families do not. If a handicap limits a person's ability to earn an income, that person's family may experience financial stress.

later on. Also, some money might be saved by establishing a budget and carefully monitoring spending for items such as food.
- Attempt to undertake further education in order to complete the high school degree (for those who dropped out). Additional employment skills can be gained by enrolling in vocational education programs.

Families with fewer economic resources than others must rely on marshalling their *other* resources to assist them. These include utilizing their social networks along with applying their abilities to plan, communicate, and make decisions.

Families with Handicapped Members

Families with handicapped members face challenges that other families do not have (Figure 17-8). A **handicap** is any condition which limits a person's ability to function in such areas as work, school, and normal physical activity.

In the United States, nearly 25 million people have such disabling conditions. These include such physical handicaps as chronic illness; illnesses that have crippling effects (arthritis, polio, multiple sclerosis, and muscular dystrophy, for example); loss of a limb (arm or leg); deafness, blindness, or other defect in sensory organs; and birth defects. Mental illness and mental retardation are other handicaps that create stress on family resource management. Some individuals have learning disabilities which hinder the acquisition of literacy skills necessary to function in society (such as basic reading, writing, and mathematical skills).

Handicap conditions can put a burden on the financial resources of families. The amount depends upon the particular disability. For example, handicaps caused by illness or injury may involve extensive medical bills over an extended period of time. The costs of doctors and hospitals today can be overwhelming, particularly if the family's health insurance does not cover them adequately. Crippling conditions may require substantial costs if special equipment is needed such as leg braces, wheel chairs, and special beds and furniture.

If the disabled family member is one who would otherwise have a job to bring income into the family, the loss of that income is another blow to the family's financial stability. Even if they are employed, the income that a disabled person earns is, on the average, less than a healthy person would earn. Also, employers often discriminate against the disabled person, believing that he or she is incapable of performing tasks required in higher paying jobs. However, the fact is that many handicapped individuals are fully capable of doing many things that others do not realize.

The resources of families with handicapped members are stressed in other ways. Interpersonal relationships can be stressed due to the special attention that the handicapped member requires. The disability may take time and energy resources that would otherwise be placed elsewhere, as the following case illustrates.

CASE IN POINT

Carl's brother, Andy, was recently diagnosed as having muscular dystrophy, a crippling disease that requires some hospitalization and which eventually will cause Andy to be confined to a wheel chair. All the attention Andy has received from his parents, friends, and relatives has caused Carl to feel neglected. He is resentful of all the time and energy that his parents are lavishing on Andy. At times Carl strikes out in anger toward other family members, including Andy.

In the case of Carl and Andy, perhaps their parents did not realize how Carl was feeling. In such cases, parents may also be stressed to the point of finding it difficult to maintain satisfaction in their own marital relationship. Disabling conditions are likely to affect *all* relationships in the family, not just those involving the handicapped member. Adjustments have to be made, but this is difficult when those taking care of the disabled person find their time and energy resources being drained by the constant attention he or she may require.

Some families cope quite effectively with handicapping conditions, while others have more difficulty. Those who are more effective often have a supportive network of friends, relatives, and possibly even employers who offer help. The availability of community services to help the family cope with the disabled member is also a benefit. For example, many communities have support groups for families with members who have certain types of diseases or conditions such as blindness or deafness. Families who avail themselves of these services often find that they are better able to adjust to the disabling condition. Finally, the basic interpersonal skills of communication, conflict management, problem solving, and planning that we have discussed at many points in this book are important. If families can apply these skills and be flexible and adaptive in dealing with the disabling condition, then they are likely to cope better than families who lack these skills.

WRAPPING IT UP

Both *human resources* and *material resources* assist families in meeting their goals. Human resources include time, energy, and interpersonal skills. Material resources include food, clothing, housing, and the money that it takes to acquire these resources. The level of a family's resources determines their *level of living* and the degree to which they are able to meet their desired level or *standard of living*.

Financial resources are necessary in today's consumption-oriented society. As families develop through the stages of the family life cycle, both financial demands and financial resources vary. If demands grow faster than resources, then the family may find itself in debt. If, on the other hand, family financial resources accumulate faster than demands, then saving and additional resource accumulation are possible.

Because of the uncertain financial status that most families face today, the concept of financial planning assumes great importance. *Planning* involves the clear identification of a goal, an accurate assessment of current resources, and an ability to think in terms of future wants, needs, and income-earning potential. Planning also requires the motivation to implement the plan once it is established.

An important part of financial planning is the family budget. *Budgeting* helps to discipline family spending. It also helps to reduce the amount of money unwisely or needlessly spent. Budgeting forces the family to establish priorities for spending and provides a written guide for acting on those priorities.

Other important features of family financial planning include *investment*, saving, and wise use of credit. Many investment opportunities exist as a way to use money to make more money. However, investments tie up your money for a period of time. Some investments may require that you leave your money in them for several years. Therefore, before investing your money, you must be certain that you have an adequate savings account, life and health insurance, and adequate income to cover the basic physical needs of the family for food, clothing, and shelter.

Many families find they are unable to control their use of credit. This keeps them in debt. While convenient, credit use can be expensive in terms of the *interest* payments that must be paid along with the *principal* of the original loan. Although being able to make monthly payments in order to have a desired product now is attractive to many, we get into credit trouble when we take too many loans and wind up with many monthly payments that our income does not cover.

Families, as consumers, have a number of rights and responsibilities relative to the manufacturer and seller of goods and services. These include being given accurate information about products purchased; safely using products that are safe to use; maintaining a pollution-free environment; making free choices among a number of available products; seeking redress when a product or service is unsatisfactory; and participating in government policy formation as it affects consumer rights and responsibilities. Many resources are available to assist the consumer in realizing these rights and responsibilities both before and after problems arise with manufacturers and sellers of goods and services.

Some families have special resource needs. Low-income families find it difficult to provide for the essential physical needs of family members, often due to unemployment or working in low-paying jobs. Particularly prone to low-income status are minority group families and those headed by single-parent mothers. Such families, if they are to survive, must rely on community and government resources, creative means of stretching resources, and additional education and vocational training if they are to break the vicious cycle of poverty in which they find themselves.

Families with handicapped members also have special needs. Not only do handicapped members create economic hardship, but the handicapping condition can stress interpersonal resources and relationships. To function more effectively, such families can access the system of community resources available to support the particular disabling condition that they are dealing with. Supportive friends and relatives, as well as employers who make adjustments to accommodate the disabling condition, can also help. The more flexible such families are, and the better able they are to apply basic interpersonal skills, the better able they will be to cope with the handicapping condition.

Exploring Dimensions of Chapter Seventeen

For Review

1. Define the concept of standard of living. Explain how it is related to level of living and the economic resources of a family.

2. Identify and explain the major components of planning. What can families do to assist themselves in financial planning?
3. What is credit? Explain the difference between wise credit use and unwise credit use.
4. Identify the basic rights and responsibilities of consumers.
5. In what ways are low-income families affected by their financial condition? How are families with handicapped members affected by their special situation?

For Consideration

1. Make a chart which lists all of the normal expenditures that a married couple without children are likely to have every month. Then make a chart listing all of the expenditures that a family with three teenage children are likely to have. Estimate the monthly amount needed for each expense item listed.
2. Your friend, Beth, tells you that she is going to borrow a large sum of money from the bank to purchase a new car. What advice would you give to Beth before she borrows the money? What information should she have before she accepts the loan from the bank?
3. Look at the advertising in a number of different magazines. Identify those claims in ads that are statements of fact and those which are advertising hype. Explain why you identified some as "facts" and others as "hype."
4. Your friend tells you that all poor people are lazy and wouldn't be poor if they didn't want to be. How would you respond?

For Application

1. Visit your local Better Business Bureau. Interview the staff who work there. Obtain information about how to file a complaint, and what happens once a complaint is filed.
2. Invite a professional investment counselor or expert in family financial planning to your class. Have them present information about how different investments work, along with their relative risks and benefits.
3. As a class project, identify all agencies in your community which help to support families with handicapped members. Invite one or more representatives of these agencies to your class to discuss their activities and the types of families they help.

4. Obtain a number of credit card application forms for different types of credit cards (cards like VISA, MasterCard, and American Express; department store cards; gasoline cards; etc.). Make a list of the rules and regulations governing the use of these cards. Compare the interest rates. How are the various cards similar? different?

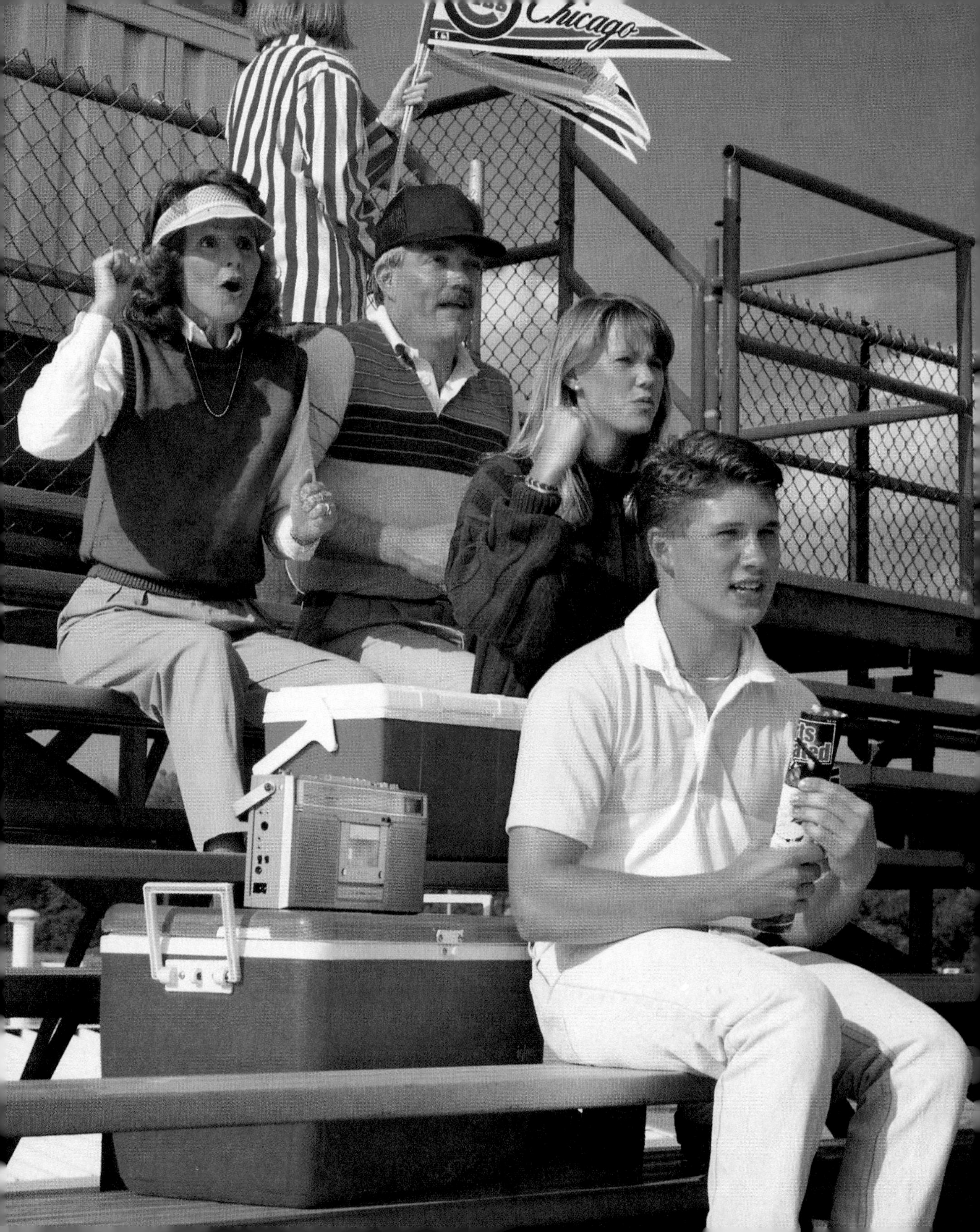
Chicago

eighteen

STRENGTHENING FAMILIES

This chapter provides information that will help you to:

- Understand reactive vs. proactive behavior related to family strength.
- Realize unique aspects of communication in families.
- Be aware of ways to manage stress and control stressors.
- Apply family enrichment techniques.

Many of the problems that occur in today's families are dealt with only after the frustrations have developed to crisis proportions. Too often family concerns are not discussed until divorce lawyers have been consulted or police have been called in. Too often family members begin to communicate only after a child runs away, parents separate, or a family member chooses escape through drugs or alcohol. These are **reactive behaviors**. Reactive ways of dealing with family problems are actions or responses to a problem after the problem surfaces.

Proactive ways of dealing with problems are preventive actions. **Proactive behaviors** enhance positive family relationships and strengthen families. These proactive behaviors will be discussed in this chapter.

COMMUNICATION

It would be impossible to talk about proactive ways to strengthen families without talking about communication. Strong understanding, mutual concern, and intimacy are the building blocks that strengthen the family structure. Without communication, family members can't gain understanding, express mutual concern, or reflect and share intimate feelings.

Information on communicating effectively was presented in Chapter 5. Emphasis was given to building positive interaction by using specific communication skills. These skills can be applied to family communication. In addition, there are unique aspects of communication in families that are helpful in applying these skills and thereby gaining more positive family interaction.

General Communication Skills

- Make intentions clear.
- Understand context.
- Send I-messages.
- Listen.
- Give feedback.

Unique Aspects of Family Communication

- Family communication stretches across the life cycle.
- Family members take each other for granted.
- There are multiple purposes in family communication.
- Family communication involves intergenerational interaction.
- Family communication involves risk taking.

By using general communication skills and being aware of unique aspects of family communication, you can gain a high quality of family communication.

Communication across the Life Cycle

You exist in a family throughout all stages of your life. Even after you leave your family home and establish a home of your own, communication with family members is important. Communication patterns established at early stages must often be altered as family members mature. Behaviors at certain periods of the life cycle—striving for independence, forming strong peer relationships, acceptance of mid-life achievement—may require alterations in the style or pattern of communication. Though the basic communication skills apply throughout the life cycle, the ways in which we apply these skills may need to vary over time.

A good example of the necessary alteration occurs in adolescence and young adulthood. Parent-child communication changes to become a situation of mutual sharing and mature understanding. Less communication is based on the parent as teacher and director, and the child as learner and follower. More communication is based on adult interactions with equal participation by child and parent. Frequently, this communication fluctuates. A parent may return to the former pattern if it seems necessary. The young adult may return to the child role when it seems safer or more secure. This process of moving back and forth in communication patterns can cause confusion and frustration, yet it is a necessary part of making the transition from one stage to another.

CASE IN POINT

Lou has related well with his father during the last ten months. Most of the arguments that occurred between them when Lou was younger seem to have passed. Lou's job, his sports activities, and his future plans have provided communication that has been based on adult sharing.

Last week, Lou had a party in his parents' home and a lamp and some china figurines were broken. Lou's father was very angry and criticized Lou's behavior, calling it childish and irresponsible. Lou also became angry, resenting his father's attitude. Lou felt like a scolded child, rather than an adult who had behaved foolishly.

Both Lou and his father feel uncomfortable in this movement back and forth in their communication patterns. The transition from adult-child communication to adult-adult communication takes time and patience.

Unlike communication with nonfamily members where the life cycle stages are less pronounced, communication in families operates in a slow but continuous process of change. In transitions from one life stage to another, there are communication difficulties. Processes for communication with family members must be reworked and re-established.

Family Members Take Each Other for Granted

There is a tendency for family members to take each other for granted. By seeing each other day after day and year after year, family members accept each other's presence. This acceptance is positive until it reaches a point where members do not see each other's personal needs. Many of the communication skills are based on meeting mutual personal needs. Overlooking needs of family members—taking family members for granted—often leads to overlooking the communication skills. Often a communication skill is used in a situation with a nonfamily member while the skill is overlooked when dealing with a family member in a similar situation (Figure 18-1).

For example, a magazine you have just purchased is on the coffee table. A friend begins leafing through the magazine, wrinkles the pages, and treats it roughly. You are

Figure 18-1

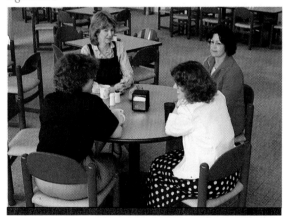

Conversations with nonfamily members often differ from conversations among family members.

irritated because the magazine was expensive and you haven't looked at it yet. Consider how you communicate your feelings to your friend. Then consider how you would communicate to a sibling or parent who had done the same thing to your magazine. Chances are great that you would use more concern and care in communicating with your friend. You might apply an I-message statement such as, "I haven't seen that magazine, yet. I would hate to have it ruined." You would probably consider a way to state your feelings without harming the relationship. You would probably try to meet your friend's needs. In contrast, you probably give less thought to applying communication skills when reacting to a family member. You might say, "Hey, stop wrecking my magazine!" or "Keep your hands off my stuff if you're going to ruin it."

Too often, little or no thought is given to personal needs of family members. The importance of maintaining a strong relationship may be overlooked. Family members and the family relationships are frequently taken for granted.

Communication with family members contains some of the most important communication that you will experience. Efforts need to be made to consider each family member an important person and each communication an opportunity to strengthen a relationship.

Multiple Purposes in Communication

The communication that occurs in the family has several different purposes or functions. You communicate with family members to build a positive relationship; that is, to gain understanding, express your care and concern, and to show your intimate feelings.

> Thanks, Dad. I really needed your support in talking with Mr. Putnam.
>
> Pete, we care about you. I know we've said it before but we really are concerned and want to help.
>
> I understand how you feel.

You also communicate for teaching-learning purposes. Such interactions take place continuously in families. Teaching facts, values, and skills is an important aspect of family communication.

> Stir the gelatin thoroughly when you add the hot water so it can dissolve.
>
> Put the accelerator to the floor before you start the car on cold mornings.
>
> I feel it is my responsibility to vote even in an off-year election when it may seem that my vote won't matter.

Family communication occurs for general managerial and maintenance purposes. Much of the interaction that occurs in the home is this type of communication.

> I'll need the car tomorrow.
>
> We've run out of eggs.
>
> The upstairs bathroom is filthy. Who can clean it before our friends arrive?

The multiple purposes of family communication are factors in some family conflict situations. Consider these statements of frustrated family members:

> My teacher and I communicate better than my mother and I.
>
> The boy who delivers our paper is more kind and considerate than my own son.

> People are nice to me in the park. They stop to talk and ask why my family isn't more concerned about an old man like me.

The communications cited above are examples of a *single*-purpose communication. Multiple purpose communication in families presents greater opportunities for frustration and requires more patience and understanding than single-purpose communication.

Efforts may need to be made to distinguish the purpose of communication. For example, a mother says to her teenage son, "Are you wearing your jacket today?" She may be asking because she plans to stop at the dry cleaners and would take his jacket if he is not planning to wear it. The son may assume that she is being overly protective and is indicating that he is not yet able to know when to wear a jacket. He may answer rudely and thereby generate an argument. By clarifying her statement ("I'm stopping at the dry cleaners. Do you want me to take your jacket?") a conflict might be prevented.

Intergenerational Interaction

Parent-child, grandparent-child, or parent-grandparent-child relationships involve situations wherein one person may have dominance and power. Older people often feel that their experience is a force that should take leadership in the topic or issue discussed. ("I know; I've been there." "I've gone through this; I know what I'm talking about.") Younger people often feel they are more aware of current situations and that this awareness can counteract experience. ("That idea is old; nobody thinks like that anymore." "You have to live in today's world, not in ancient times.") Each party wants to tell the other how things really are and how the situation or issue should be handled. In such situations, it is easy to forget to use I-messages; telling becomes more important than listening.

Family communication that allows both generations to put forth their ideas and concerns is more likely to be successful. The most positive communication patterns are those that minimize dominance and power and allow open sharing of ideas. The communication skills, if applied, can be highly beneficial to intergenerational communication.

Personal, Intimate, and Emotional Concerns

Because families involve people who love and care for each other, communication will reflect personal, intimate, and emotional concerns. Sometimes you may find that a counselor or friend may be able to discuss a topic more openly and objectively. This is probably because the person sees you as a person rather than as a child, grandchild, or sibling. The nonfamily person may help you to view your concern more clearly. A parent, sibling, or grandparent may be too involved to have an objective conversation. Yet, it is important to be aware of the emotional-personal feelings that relatives have. Their emotions and intimate feelings exist and can have a strong impact on you.

It is often helpful to have both kinds of communication—subjective and objective—when dealing with certain topics. This is especially true when important decisions are being made. Some family members can communicate their objective and unbiased thinking as well as their subjective and emotional feelings.

Nancy Phillips: "Dad, my guidance counselor said that the University of California would definitely be the best of the three colleges that accepted me."

Ed Phillips: "California! Nancy, that's clear across the country! I had no idea you were seriously thinking about going to school in California."

Nancy: "It only makes sense if that's where I would get the best training."

Ed: "Look, Nancy, I can understand that. Your counselor may very well be right. But you're the only daughter I have! I would hate having you so far away. I know I'll miss you. I would like you to go to school somewhere closer."

In this conversation, the father relayed both his objective and subjective thoughts. If family members are unable to do this and can only communicate their emotional, biased viewpoints, then additional sources of information can be sought to assist decision making.

Personal, intimate, and emotional concerns and issues do exist in families. Being able to accept other family members' feelings and to express such feelings to others is a part of mature family communication.

Risk Taking

When you share personal ideas and feelings, you take a risk that people may relay the shared information with others. There is a risk that your personal thoughts, fears, or feelings may be laughed at or ridiculed. This risk is present in nonfamily communication but may be stronger in families.

Families have a high level of intimacy, which provides many opportunities for sharing personal thoughts. Family members are often teased in fun or anger. This teasing process may result in revealing ideas and thoughts that were once shared only in private. Family members may recall and reveal private communication shared years earlier and then assume that the information is no longer important.

Remember when you were afraid of the dark and you would scream and cry.

She wet the bed until she was in school. She had a terrible problem.

Dad went through that depression a few years ago. He just sat around worrying about losing his job.

All of these family situations could cause embarrassment, humiliation, and anger. Revealing private thoughts and actions may prevent further communication. If the risk of humiliation and embarrassment becomes too great, sharing will not continue.

Families must establish guidelines for respecting the privacy of family members. Family members need to feel that their shared personal thoughts, ideas, and feelings will not become public knowledge without permission.

Families today have limited time for communicating. Interactions must stress quality (clear, meaningful exchanges) rather than quantity (frequent, lengthy interactions). Basic communication skills along with awareness of unique aspects of communication in families encourages positive, quality family communication.

FAMILY STRESS MANAGEMENT

This chapter describes proactive or preventive approaches for family concerns (one of which is positive family communication). How, then, can managing stress be discussed? Why not focus on preventing stress? Isn't managing family stress a reactive behavior?

This confusion is based on a misunderstanding of stress. Usually people think of stress as harmful (see Figure 18-2). They try to avoid or prevent stress. It's true that too much stress damages the body. However, there are positive aspects of stress. You might not achieve a good score or win an athletic event without some stress. We need stress. When stress stops, we know we are no longer mentally or physically responsive to the demands of life.

Stress is the body's response to any demand made on it. These responses include helpful emotions such as love and happiness. They also include fear, anger, and general physical changes. The following physical reactions are typical stress reactions:

- Increased heart rate
- Increased breathing rate
- Dilation of pupils
- Increased perspiration
- Slower digestion
- Increased hormone production

The stress-producing situation or **stressor** may be pleasant or unpleasant, frightening, anger-producing, or full of sadness. Consider these examples of stressors:

- Someone following you home after dark
- You narrowly miss being hit by a truck as you jaywalk across the street
- Your cat is killed by a car
- You learn that you got an A instead of a C on a test
- You enter a room where friends have gathered to surprise you on your birthday

Figure 18-2

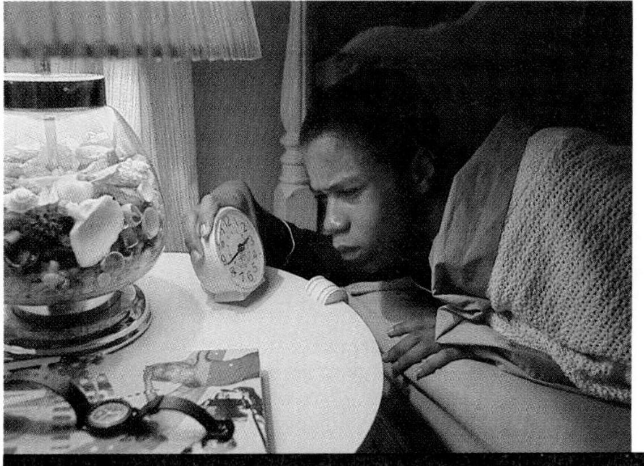

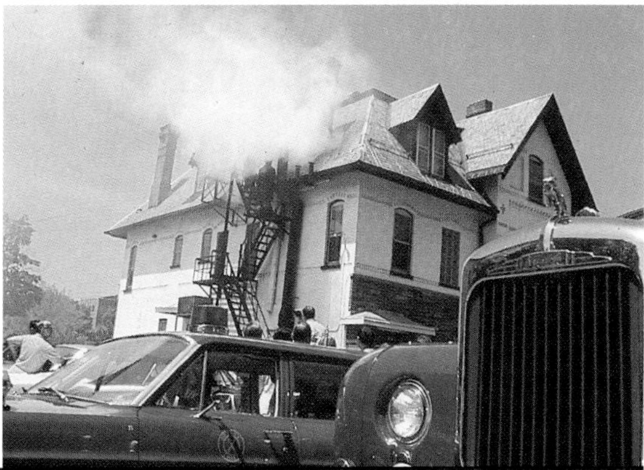

An event doesn't have to be life-threatening before it creates stress. Simple life changes, such as getting out of bed earlier than normal, can create stress.

Aetna Life and Casualty Company

The process of stress is illustrated in Figure 18-3. The stressor, the way the individual perceives stress, the stress itself, and the result of the stress are all important parts of the stress process.

Since stress can bring about positive results, freedom from stress is not a realistic goal. Stress cannot and probably should not be prevented. The levels or degrees of stress can be managed in order to prevent destructive stress. When possible, stressors can be controlled. The management of stress levels and control of stressors are proactive ways to deal with stress.

The outcome of stress is frequently positive. For example, the stressor of severe weather may cause physical reactions that increase alertness and allow an automobile driver to respond more alertly to driving hazards. Many people find the stressor of a major test, performance, or other important situation to initiate positive action. The stress created by the event can cause action (increased study, improved practice) that yields positive results. In such situations, the stress process is the same but the final outcome is positive.

Both positive and negative life events cause stress. Stressful events require readjustments. In a study of hundreds of people, it was found that certain life events require greater amounts of readjustment than others. The results of this study are shown below. The most stressful events—death of spouse and divorce—are listed first.

READJUSTMENT TO STRESS

Life Event

1• Death of spouse
2• Divorce
3• Marital separation
4• Jail term
5• Death of close family member
6• Personal injury or illness
7• Marriage
8• Fired at work
9• Marital reconciliation
10• Retirement
11• Change in health of family member
12• Pregnancy
13• Sex difficulties
14• Gain of new family member

Figure 18-3

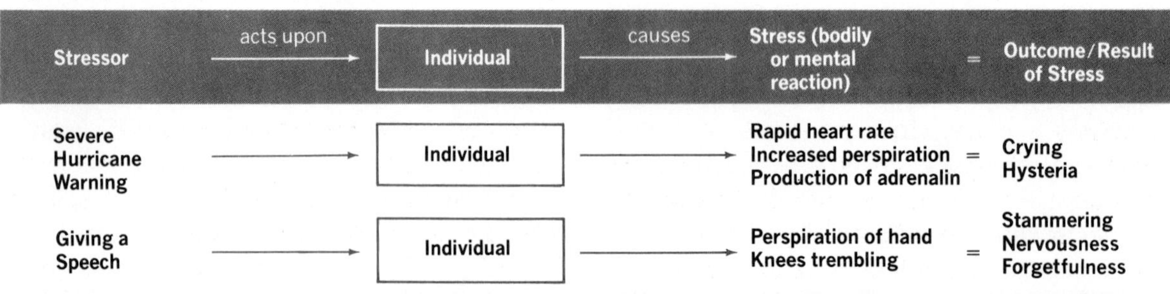

The stress process involves the stressor, the individual, the stress itself, and the outcome of the stress.

15• Business readjustment
16• Change in financial state
17• Death of close friend
18• Change to different line of work
19• Change in number of arguments with spouse
20• A high mortgage payment
21• Foreclosure of mortgage or loan
22• Change in responsibilities at work
23• Son or daughter leaving home
24• Trouble with in-laws
25• Outstanding personal achievement
26• Spouse begins or stops work
27• Begin or end school
28• Change in living conditions
29• Revision of personal habits
30• Trouble with boss
31• Change in work hours or conditions
32• Change in residence
33• Change in schools
34• Change in recreation
35• Change in church activities
36• Change in social activities
37• Change in sleeping habits
38• Change in number of family get-togethers
39• Change in eating habits
40• Vacation
41• Christmas/other holidays
42• Minor violations of the law

Stress and the Family

The close, personal relationships among family members and the close proximity in which members exist cause stress to spread from one member to the family as a whole. In general, if one member is affected by stress, other members are also affected. Managing stress, then, becomes a major task in preventing family problems.

Families are involved in the process of stress in several ways. Family action may be a stressor. That is, the behaviors and actions of the family as a whole cause stress. The stress may be in individual members or in the family as a whole. The resultant behavior(s) may also be reflected from one member to another or from the family to society and the world as a whole.

Families also function as recipients of stress from outside the family. The outside stressor acts on the family as a whole or on individual family members who then act on the family. Either way, stress within the family occurs and results in particular behavior (Figure 18-4).

FAMILY REACTIONS TO STRESS AND STRESSORS • Families differ in their reactions to stress. Some families are challenged by stress. Other families live in fear of their own stress reactions. The differences in behavior from family to family are based on perception, tolerance, and skill.

PERCEPTION • How events or stressors are interpreted will affect resultant stress. If stress is to occur, the family members must perceive the situation as stressful in the first place. For example, one family may consider unemployment or unpaid bills a cause of stress. Other families may consider these situations typical and not stress-producing.

A family's feelings about a particular stressor depend on its belief system. If family members consider family life unrewarding and dull, each new stressor will be viewed in that context. Each new occurrence will be seen as adding new stress to an already troubled situation. Yet, if family life is seen as challenging, meaningful, and rewarding, stressors will be viewed less severely.

Figure 18-4

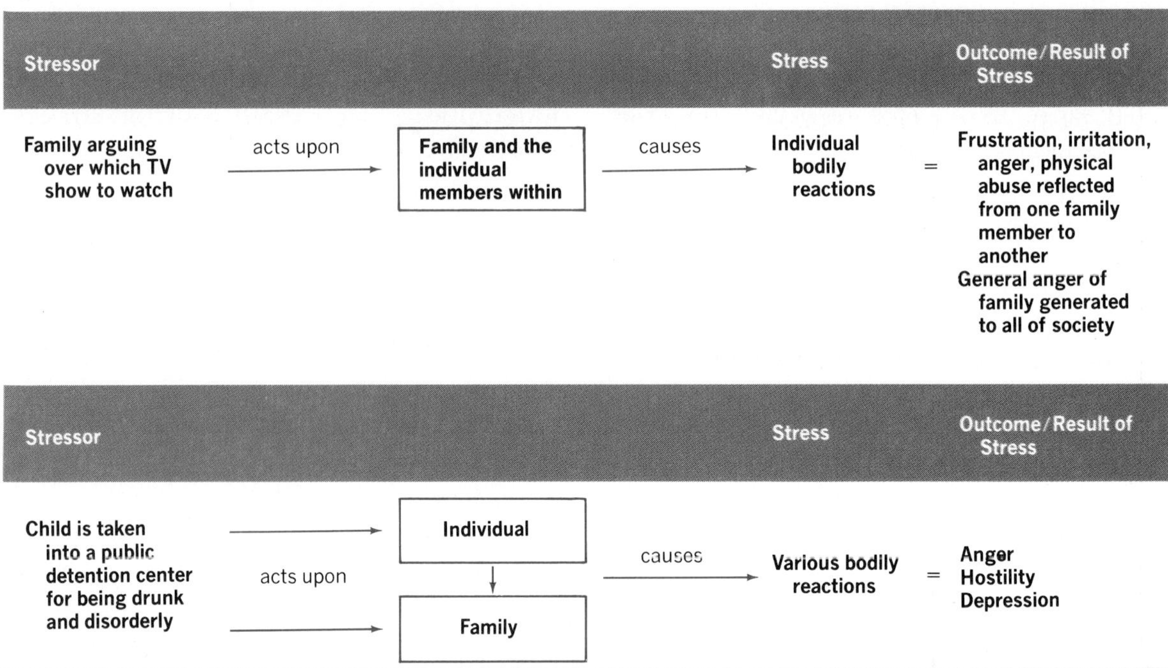

Like individuals, families receive the outcomes of the stress process. The stressor may act on an individual or on the family as a whole.

TOLERANCE • Stress tolerance is the capacity to withstand the stressor. It is also the amount of stress the family can withstand before their abilities are seriously impaired. Some families can withstand multiple stressors and not show much stress. Another family becomes extremely stressful over one seemingly minor stressor. One family may become overwrought and hyperactive to the point of severe physical illness with only minor stress. Tolerance levels for stress in another family may be high with large amounts of stress operating without serious problems.

SKILLS • Some families have many skills and resources to overcome the stress process, while other families have few skills, resources, and assistance. The ways in which a family views its own skills are also important. If a family feels confident and expects to solve its problems, the stress will be less severe than if they feel defeated and at the mercy of the stressor.

FAMILY STRESS FACTORS • There are several factors or principles that relate to stress and/or stressors:

- The more important the event (stressor), the greater the stress that is felt (for example, death, severe crippling, or a major illness).

- Events that occur suddenly or unexpectedly cause a greater feeling of stress (for example, a cyclone or unexpected death).
- The longer an event takes place, the greater will be the stress (for example, unemployment or alcoholism).
- The more simultaneous the stressful events, the greater will be the stress (for example, a house fire, a car accident, and the death of a relative occurring at the same time).
- The likelihood of stress is greater during a period of change (for example, relocating, new job, or new school).

Family Stress Management Techniques

Managing stress consists of both controlling stressors and dealing with stress. Both of these actions include attitude changes in the family members (inner changes) and changes of situations outside the family (outer changes). Consider Figure 18-5 where these outer and inner changes are plotted with the stressor and the stress.

Families that are good managers of stress have several characteristics in common. These families:

- Have self-awareness. They know their strengths, skills, and weaknesses. They plan for the future. They never bite off more than they can chew.
- Use a variety of techniques. They utilize many stress-reducing techniques as the situation dictates.

Figure 18-5

Changing attitudes and situations may help families to manage stress.

	Inner Changes (Attitudes)	*Outer Changes (Situational Changes)*
STRESSOR	**(A)** Changes in your view or perception of the situation (develop family self-awareness) (awareness of network of assistance)	**(B)** Changes in the situation that alter the prospective stressor. (improved management in the home) (environmental changes)
STRESS	**(C)** Changes in feelings and responses to the stress. (reframe the stressor) (realization that physical and mental reactions are closely related)	**(D)** Changes in situation to help cope with stress. (environmental changes) (exercise, physical movement) (use problem solving)

- Have many interests. They are able to draw on several sources for personal satisfaction—hobbies, recreation, family.
- Are active and productive. They make things happen and practice stress management during the bad and good times.
- Use support. They develop friendships with others for help and comfort during periods of stress.

TECHNIQUES FOR INNER CHANGE • Attitude plays an important role in what is perceived as stressful to a family. Though many stressors are beyond a family's control (inflation, crime, world politics), how a family perceives these situations can be controlled to some degree. Box A in Figure 18-5 represents the way the family views particular situations. Some families may consider any situation other than a standard routine to be stressful. Modifying a family's or individual's view of situations can lessen the number of possible stressors.

Likewise, a family's feelings and responses to the actual stress (bodily or mental changes) are related to attitude. This is represented in Box C. Some family members refuse to recognize physical or mental changes, such as nervousness and irritability, as a reaction to stress. There may be a hesitancy to respect the close nature of physical and mental reactions to stressful situations. Modifying a family's or individual's view of the stress taking place (in the family or individual) may limit the degree of stress reaction.

REFRAMING • When you reframe, you put things in a different order. You place situations in different boundaries. For example, a family member can reframe a blownout tire by thinking, "I'm glad this didn't happen on the freeway." Increased numbers of social activities of family members (as possible stressors) can be reframed to consider "All of our family is interested and concerned with the community and school."

This is not merely a "looking at the world through rose-colored glasses" approach. It is an attempt to see what is a possible stressor and put it in its proper perspective. Rather than presenting only problems from family members, stressful events can also be reframed as opportunities for enrichment or growth.

Stress Situation: Mother's Broken Leg:

It will cause our family to have medical bills. Mother will be in pain. We'll all have to wait on her.

Reframed Situation:

Though it will be difficult for all, Mother's condition will provide us with time to spend together. We can have some good discussions and enjoy each other's company.

DISASTER ROLE PLAYING • Worrying about disasters that might occur can create stress about something that does not really exist. Disaster role playing—acting out what might happen and how to deal with it—can alter the perception of the situation. Preparation for a disaster or difficult situation may lessen the impact if the disaster occurs. It can eliminate the stressor of worry about the impending disaster.

CASE IN POINT

Andrew and Ilsa live with their mother. Their father died seven months ago. The children worry about what will happen to them if their mother should die or be seriously injured and unable to work. By openly discussing this possible disaster, both the children and their mother gain security about how the children will manage and who will care for them. Knowledge of how the situation will be handled may prevent the situation from being perceived as a stressor.

Stress is usually more severe when it takes you by surprise. Disaster role playing is a way of planning ahead for problems. It is a way to remove the surprise element from stress.

BEING A GOOD WORRIER • If you are in a family of worriers, turn the worry to helpful situations. Instead of worrying and building stress about rain for the family reunion, consider, "What can we do to prepare for the chance of rain?" Turn worry into problem solving. "If this ever occurs again, how will we handle it better?" or "How shall we prevent this type of problem?"

DEVELOPING FAMILY SELF-AWARENESS • Families that are aware of their resources—both their strengths and weaknesses—are more likely to realistically view stressors and accompanying stress. When members know that they have the ability to take over each other's roles or if they have awareness of nonfamily people who can be of assistance to them, they will have less stress. They are less likely to waste their time and energy perceiving situations as stressors.

THE MINI-LETTER • Use whatever is handy to write a short letter about the things causing you stress. Explain how you are reacting to the stress. Tell how you feel and how you are upset. Re-read the letter and pass it on to another family member. This technique puts the stressor and stress into perspective. You begin to see it may not be as stressful as first perceived. It also allows other family members to realize your particular stress (Figure 18-6).

Figure 18-6

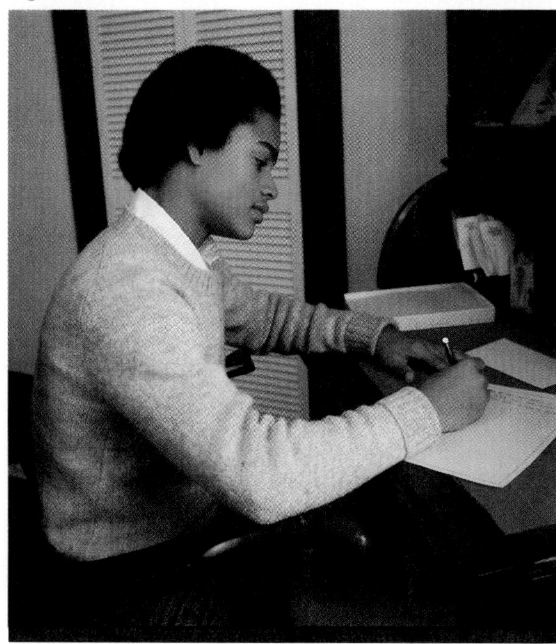

Writing about the things that cause you stress can help put the stress and stressor in perspective.

EMPHASIZE THE NONSTRESSFUL • When things are stressful, it is easy to forget or overlook the great number of situations functioning well. By thinking about and sharing with a family member those things that are not stressful, you may alter your response to stress. The stressful aspects of life appear less stressful. When things are stressful, an interesting mental exercise would be to think how happy you would be if you lost all that you have and then gained it back again.

TECHNIQUES FOR OUTER CHANGES • It seems like life would be easy if we could alter all the possible stressors. Wouldn't it be nice to eliminate homework, lower prices on clothes so you could have all you want, stop your boss from nagging, and have your friends and neighbors be more cooperative? How pleasant it would be if we could minimize stress levels and have only enough stress to keep us alert and energized but not stressed to detrimental levels. We know, however, that potential stressors will always be with us. Likewise, stress will always be felt. Yet, we can make efforts in the home and family to prevent prospective stressors (Figure 18-5, Box B). We can minimize the levels of stress with various techniques (Figure 18-5, Box D).

MANAGEMENT IN THE HOME • A highly chaotic environment can cause many situations to be perceived as stressors. A calm, relaxing environment allows family members to consider situations as they are rather than immediately considering them as stress producers. Planning and managing family activities and tasks can lessen chaos. A calm, chaos-free environment allows family members to perceive fewer situations as stressful.

DIVERSE FAMILY ACTIVITIES • A family needs management, yet it does not need a steadfast routine that won't permit variety in activities. Families with many interests can draw on various sources for satisfaction. Recreation, diversion, or even something as simple as a changed routine at mealtime can refresh members. This diversion or renewal can help families view situations more realistically rather than consider them stressors. It can relieve stress for short time periods.

PHYSICAL EXERCISE • Individuals and family members can use physical exercise and movement to relieve or lessen stress. Walking, skating, jogging, jumping rope, or any kind of physical exercise can help lessen physical and mental stress. This is especially important for family members who have minimal physical exercise in their jobs. It can also be beneficial in situations where there is a high level of family anger and frustration.

Stress can be lowered if members decide to stop and resume the argument or discussion at a later time. "Hey, I'm really angry. I'm going to take a walk and then let's talk some more." "Look, I know I'm angry and frustrated. Let me just go let off some steam." Such statements might help to curb violent outcomes of stress.

SOOTHING, CALMING ENVIRONMENT • Stress can be lessened by various controlled surroundings. Photos of peaceful and pleasant situations—a stream, a wooded area, a sunset—may reduce physical and mental stress. Soft music, a quiet corner, or a place to meditate can help regulate stressful feelings. Families need to be aware that members must have these altered environments in order to confront their stress. Respect of privacy is important in families.

Stressors and stress in families cannot be eliminated. Certain proactive techniques, however, can assist families in dealing with stress.

FAMILY ENRICHMENT

Many families exist without having major problems: they seem to manage their day-to-day family concerns. Yet, many of these family members would like to have closer, more satisfying family relationships. They would like to expand and enrich the interaction in their family. To enrich means to make stronger or to improve. Family enrichment is considered a major way to prevent family concerns and problems before they occur. Enriching families is a proactive behavior.

Ways to Enrich

When family members decide that they want to strengthen and enrich their family and are willing to commit time to the family, they need to consider ways to make their family stronger. The following methods for family enrichment have been used successfully by many families. Family members will want to decide together which methods appeal to them and which will best fit their needs. Not all methods work with all families (Figure 18-7). Age and maturity level of family members are determining factors. When a method or methods are decided on, the family members must make a commitment to devote real effort to following through with the method.

SPECIAL "AT HOME" NIGHT • Establish a special night. It may be a game night, music night, or just a quiet reading night. This means that the television, radio, and stereo are off and the family, together in one room, devotes time to playing some games, working together on a project, or playing musical instruments and singing. A continuing story could be read aloud together. Books such as *The Swiss Family Robinson*, *Treasure Island*, *I Remember Mama*, or some of James Thurber's humorous stories can relay adventures, sadness, and humor of family life.

Figure 18-7

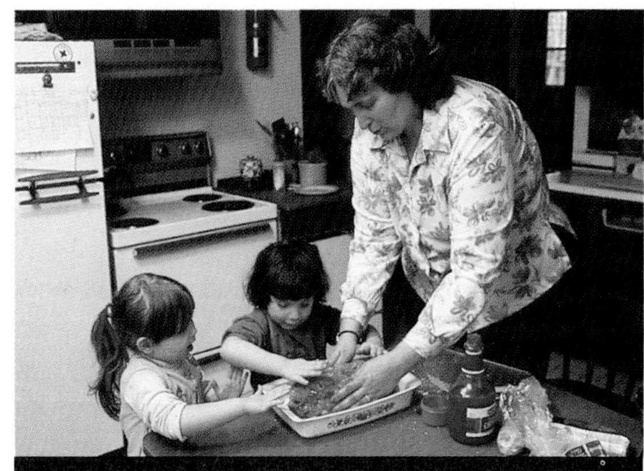

Although this family may find that preparing the evening meal together is a way to enrich family members, other families may prefer to find other ways to enrich.
USDA Photo

The choice of games, stories, or music depends on the age and talents of family members. Frequency of the special nights (weekly or biweekly) should also be established to fit each family. The important ingredient is that family members are together and sharing an activity.

CONTROLLED TELEVISION • Some families have found that even without a specified and planned activity, eliminating television for one night a week or for several hours each night has increased family interaction and sharing. Even avid television watchers could determine one evening that has little viewing pleasure.

Other families have discovered quality presentations on evening radio and have declared radio night once a week. They have found they can interact more by getting involved with and discussing the radio programs than they can with television programming.

NEW FAMILY TRADITIONS • Establish some new family traditions. These traditions need not be major or expensive, yet they can provide a continuing dependability and security in the family. Some families choose a special food night that becomes a lasting tradition—spaghetti night, Chinese food night, Mexican food night, etc. Family library night followed by a stop for ice cream or pizza, a special brunch following church or temple services, a trip to the zoo each spring, and a special treat after that annual leaf-raking in the yard are all traditions that can be established. They add feelings of continuity and togetherness. The actual event matters less than the thought behind it.

Major traditions can be highlighted and given greater emphasis. Holiday and seasonal activities and family celebrations such as birthdays and anniversaries can be capitalized on. Families can promote sharing and focus on the fun of being together.

FAMILY MEETINGS • One method to enrich families that has been successful for many people is holding family meetings. Family meetings or conferences are planned, established times in which the members meet together to discuss activities and share some time together. Some families establish rotating roles or responsibilities for the sessions: food organizer, activity or game arranger, moderator, and clean-up person. Discussion topics can include anything of importance to the family; for example, care of the family dog during vacation, how to decrease the grocery bill, or how to provide better security in the home. Such meetings can be as short as 15 to 20 minutes each month or several hours each week. The meetings must meet the needs of the individual family members both in time and in content. Families that have given these sessions a serious try have found them to be very helpful.

FAMILY SPORTS ACTIVITIES • Some families have chosen a sports activity in which all family members can take part. Sharing the experience of learning a sport new to all members can be very rewarding. Having one member teach or guide other family members in the sport the person has mastered can also be enjoyable. A family sport is healthy and provides means for shared activity and conversations. Biking, skiing, bowling, tennis, swimming, and hiking provide opportunity for family activities for members of nearly all ages.

PLANNED OUTINGS • A monthly planned outing is a method used by some families to insure family leisure time together. The outings need not be expensive. Most communities have many low-cost or no-cost sites such as parks, museums, historical sites, public gardens, zoos, and beaches. Each month a different family member can select the site, arrange details, and check times. It usually works best if a specific date (first Saturday of the month or second Sunday of the month) is established. Otherwise, the outings become too difficult to schedule. Many families find that establishing a monthly planned outing is enjoyable, educational, and encourages more family activities.

FAMILY GOAL SETTING • After family members feel comfortable about the efforts to improve family interaction, more specific approaches can be taken to strengthen the family unit. Family members can work together to decide on particular family goals. Goals can be in the physical, mental, or spiritual area with each member having individual goals as well as a central group goal. A goal may be a specific group achievement such as a major trip, a building project, or group task. Such goal setting fosters unity and shared family feelings.

These activities are only a few of the many things family members can do to strengthen their family unit. Such activities need not be limited to only your family members. Many of the activities can include another family or other persons who share your ideas and goals.

Roadblocks to Enrichment

Most people want stronger families. Most of us feel that our family relationships could be improved and could become more fulfilling. Yet, many families or individuals in the family fail to take action to strengthen or enrich the family unit. This seems strange when we think of how important families are to most people. As family members, we need to be reminded that a family is not just a convenience that we use. Rather, it is a highly important group of people to whom we must contribute our efforts, energies, and time.

There are three basic reasons why families don't spend more time taking positive steps to improve their family relationships. First, people sometimes feel an embarrassment about bringing up the topic. It might be awkward to say something like, "I wish we could do something about making our family closer" or "Let's think about how to strengthen our family." It may seem that someone might laugh or make fun of the idea. Actually, that's usually not what happens. Usually other family members have had similar feelings but have been hesitant to speak up. Sometimes there is a chuckle or smile. But after hearing that there is a desire for more family closeness and sharing, there is usually a nod of agreement from all family members. Parents who may have felt their children would think the idea silly are surprised at the positive reaction. Children who felt that their parents would not be interested are pleased to see their parents take an encouraging attitude (Figure 18-8).

Figure 18-8

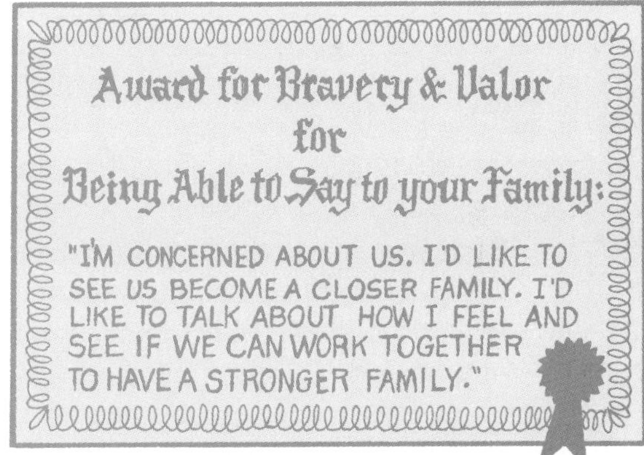

It takes courage and a certain amount of risk to tell your family that you'd like to work together to strengthen your family unit.

A second roadblock is that people sometimes feel uncomfortable with planned, organized activities in the family. It would seem natural to have such planning and structure in a classroom, community, or church group. Yet, these structured behaviors in the family setting don't feel quite right. True enough, it may take time to become comfortable with some of the skills and techniques which may seem "square" or "hokey." You may need to ask yourself if a stronger family is worth discomfort.

The third reason families may do nothing to strengthen the family unit is because of limited time. It is not uncommon to hear a family member say, "Sure, I would like to do something to help our family become closer, but just when do we find the time?"

It is true that families are busy. Active family schedules may leave little opportunity for working together to enrich the family. However, family time can be built into the schedule. A specific time can be established and other activities fitted around this time. This will be easier to do if the family members decide that a stronger family is something they really want and if they commit themselves to take action to strive for a stronger family. It will also be seen in the next section that some methods for family enrichment take only small amounts of time.

You may want to consider the following questions with respect to roadblocks to family enrichment. These are good thought provokers whether you are considering your future family or your current family.

Spotlight on issues

Family Mobility

Each year approximately 20 percent of American families move from one home to another. People migrate, sometimes in large groups, to locations where job possibilities exist. Families relocate because of job promotions or transfers. Family moves are also prompted by changing housing needs or desires to change homes or neighborhoods. These moves may be to a nearby area or to a different country.

Whatever the reason for the geographical relocation, there are some basic similarities in consequences. All moves cause some disorganization. Even when the move benefits most family members, there is stress on the family. New schools, a new home, new neighbors, and perhaps a whole new lifestyle can make people feel cut off and lonely.

Military families, though transferred often, experience several positive features in their mobility. Military personnel are usually provided with adequate housing facilities upon relocation, thus easing the strain of immediate house hunting. Military families can count on a close-knit network into which they are readily accepted by other military families. However, these advantages may be compromised by military duty that requires only the military members of the family to relocate while the rest of the family remains behind.

Families thrive on and are nurtured by a network of support in their community. That network is often broken by the move. Initially, this break can require family members to depend more on each other; in time, however, they will need to reach out to a wider community network. In new surroundings, this network can be tapped by reaching out to community groups and individuals. Family members who take part in welcome groups or new neighbor groups soon find themselves involved in the new community. Religious groups, hobby clubs, school activities, and informal athletic groups also provide good ways to become part of the new community.

Teens may have an especially hard time when families relocate. Because peers are of great importance to them, teens may find it very difficult to leave old friends and make new ones. Extracurricular school activities are one good way to get acquainted in a new setting. Providing or asking for homework assistance or working on class projects are also worthwhile when looking for new friends. Volunteer work and part-time jobs can help teens get to know their community and make new friends. The many discouraging aspects of relocating can be overcome by turning to other family members and by making an effort to reach out to the new community.

How worthwhile is a strong family to you? To what degree is improving family relationships a high priority item?

How much time are you willing to give to strengthening your family? Ten minutes a week? One evening a week? An hour each week?

How embarrassed would you be to tell your friends that you aren't able to go to a particular activity because you are doing something special with your family? Not embarrassed at all? Somewhat embarrassed? Wouldn't tell your friends?

How much would you give up to strengthen your family? One half-hour television show a week? One half-hour television show a night? One social activity a week? Fifteen minutes of telephone conversation a night?

How much effort would you put forth to convince another family member to work toward family enrichment? No effort? Some effort? A lot of effort?

Eliminating the roadblocks to family enrichment is probably the most difficult aspect of the enrichment process. Bringing the entire family to the point of wanting to strengthen relationships and being willing to devote effort and time is a major step. Sometimes one family member is less enthusiastic or lacks real interest in the effort. If this is the case, proceed without this person but continually encourage the person to join the family activities.

Remember that the goal of family enrichment is not for problem solving but rather for family strengthening by means of shared activities, interests, and ideas. Such sharing may prevent future concerns and problems. Enriching, strengthening, and giving family members greater opportunity to become close are proactive behaviors. Communicating positively, managing stress, and promoting family enrichment are proactive, preventive ways to strengthen families.

WRAPPING IT UP

Today's families are challenged in many ways. Often such challenges create stress, causing family members to react in unhealthy ways. Such ***reactive behaviors*** include drug and alcohol abuse, running away from home, marital separation, and divorce. However, families can take proactive steps to prevent problems from reaching such serious proportions. ***Proactive behaviors*** can strengthen family ties and enhance positive relationships within the family.

At the core of strengthening family relationships is the maintenance of healthy communication patterns over the life cycle. For example, the nature of parent-child communication is continually changing as both children and parents move through their respective developmental timetables. Family members must continually work to communicate in ways that show mutual respect, empathy, and caring.

Related to the difficulty in communication across the life cycle is the fact that family members tend to take each other for granted over the years of living together. We tend to forget the individual needs of family members. As a result, communication can take a less positive tone or, at times, might actually be hurtful in its consequences.

Enhancing family communication further involves recognizing the multiple purposes that such communication has for different members. Often communication must take place across generational lines, which creates significant differences in values, norms, and just where each generation "might be coming from." Because of the personal and intimate nature of family communication, emotional involvement can cloud the real issue and prevent effective communication from taking place.

Strong families are those that are able to handle stress effectively. Although stress may yield negative outcomes for a family, some stressor events may generate positive outcomes. Whether stress is positive or negative in its consequences depends, in part, on the degree of adjustment required by the particular stressor event. Some events (such as death in the family and divorce) are more stressful than others (such as changing residences or job responsibilities).

The degree to which families successfully cope with stress is a function of three things.

First, perception of the same stressor event may vary from one family to the next. For example, some families may find retirement of one or both workers to be highly stressful, while others may perceive the same thing as an expected and routine event. Second, some families are resilient in the face of stress. They are better able to tolerate severe or multiple stressor events. Third, families vary in their level of basic interpersonal skills, such as communication, problem solving, and conflict management. Those with stronger interpersonal skills are better equipped to cope with a stressful event.

There are a number of things families can do to better cope with the stress in their lives. These include reframing the problem, role playing, developing family self-awareness, and engaging in diverse activities and in physical exercise. Some families simply work to have a positive outlook on life; they avoid needless worrying. They emphasize the nonstressful aspects of their lives.

Many other activities can enrich family living. These include special "at-home nights," establishing new family traditions, controlled television viewing, family meetings, and frequent family recreational activities. Setting special family goals and working on a common project can bring a sense of unity to family life. To accomplish family enrichment, common roadblocks to positive action must be removed. These include overcoming the sense of embarrassment that might be felt when family enrichment is first suggested, overcoming the uncomfortable feeling that might be associated with increased structure in family life, and finding the time in a busy schedule to engage in family strengthening activities.

Most families find the investment of time and energy in family enrichment activities to yield substantial returns in the form of a more cohesive and fulfilling family environment. This principle applies to families of all types and structures—nuclear, blended, single-parent, single earner, dual earner, foster families, and step-families. As important as families are for the growth and development of individual members, there is much to be gained by fostering the most supportive atmosphere for achieving personal fulfillment of *all* family members—young and old alike!

Exploring Dimensions of Chapter Eighteen

For Review

1• Explain the meaning of proactive and reactive family behaviors. Give examples.

2• Describe at least four unique aspects of families with respect to communicating.
3• What is the difference between stress and a stressor?
4• List at least three ways to manage stress.
5• What is family enrichment? Explain at least two techniques to gain enrichment.

For Consideration

1• Write an advertisement for a proactive way to strengthen families. Tell why it is important to prevent as opposed to curing family problems and concerns.
2• Give a real-life example or create an example of how intimate, caring, personal relationships in families can interfere with objective communicating. Why does this happen? Can you eliminate this problem? Would you want to eliminate the problem if you could?
3• A magazine cover boasts that this issue will tell you how to "eliminate your stress." Do you believe this claim? Why or why not?
4• Help Steve with his concern. He would like his family to have more fun together. Though they have no big problems, the members of Steve's family do not interact much or do much together. Tell Steve about family enrichment and how to apply it.

For Application

1• Interview people who work with families (counselors, ministers, social workers, doctors) and ask why they feel families do not use proactive ways to gain strength. Ask them for suggestions for ways to get more people interested in proactive family behaviors.
2• After reviewing unique aspects of family communication, determine which aspect causes the most difficulty in your own family. Discuss this aspect with your family members, and establish guidelines to overcome this difficulty.
3• Create a list of stressors outside the family that impact on the family. Create a second list of stressors that are generated in the family. Decide which cannot be altered by you and your family and which can be limited or totally eliminated. Share these findings with your family.

4• Adapt one or several of the enrichment techniques to meet the needs of your family. Explain how you would like to see this technique applied. Tell how it might fit with your family's schedule and personality. Share this with your family.

glossary

active listening Listening which exhibits a high degree of verbal and nonverbal response; putting the speaker's message into the listener's own words and sending the message back to the speaker.

advertising hype Extravagant or exaggerated promotional gimmicks and claims.

aesthetic value A feeling or belief about beauty, about the way things look, feel, taste, sound, and smell.

aging family stage That stage of family life that takes place during the final years prior to death.

alimony The payment of money by the primary wage earner, ex-husband or ex-wife, during and after divorce.

altruism The regard for or devotion to interests of others; concern for human good and the betterment of society.

anger A strong feeling of displeasure or frustration; one of the core human emotions that begins to be exhibited by preschool-age children.

antisocial behavior Behavior marked by a lack of social skill and a negative, combative orientation toward others.

attachment Feelings of security, warmth, belonging, and trust fostered in infancy.

autonomy An aspect of the social development of children marked by a desire for independence from parents and other attachment figures.

bankruptcy A legally declared state of financial ruin that requires an individual to sell his or her assets for the purpose of repaying bad debts.

beginning family stage That stage in family life that begins with marriage and ends with the birth of the first child.

career cluster A group of occupations that share the same general characteristics.

career ladder Various careers arranged in ascending order, from entry-level positions to positions offering greater challenges and economic reward. For example: data-entry clerk; programmer trainee; programmer; systems designer; senior systems designer; database manager; vice-president, operations.

child bearing family stage That stage in family life that begins with the birth of the first child and ends with the birth of the last child. This stage often overlaps with the parenting family stage.

child support Financial assistance given by a parent to aid children until they reach age 18. After a divorce or legal separation, the primary wage earner—ex-husband or ex-wife—is usually responsible for such assistance.

chromosomes Microscopic strands that contain genetic material. In human biology, 23 matched pairs of chromosomes (46 total) are found in the nucleus of every cell, except sperm and egg cells, which contain only 23 unmatched chromosomes.

classification The ability of preoperational children to arrange objects in some logical fashion; for example, according to color.

cognitive ability A measure of an individual's overall intelligence, creativity, and problem-solving skill.

cognitive development *See* mental development.

communication Listening to and sharing information and feelings.

community property laws Laws dealing with how property is to be divided in case of divorce, which declare that property acquired during the marriage is to be shared equally by both marriage partners.

competent worker A worker whose job skills, level of education, and experience make him or her a valuable performer.

concrete operations A stage of cognitive development defined by Jean Piaget. Between the ages of 7 and 11, children acquire certain language, mathematical, and problem-solving skills that allow them to reason, use logic, retain information, and think more abstractly.

context The set of circumstances and conditions that surround an event or a particular communication.

continuum A line that is marked to represent degrees or levels of certain characteristics or issues. Values, for example, can be placed on a continuum to reflect one's feelings.

core emotions Fundamental human emotions: joy, sadness, anger, and fear.

credit rating The sum of information regarding a consumer's credit history used as the basis for granting or denying requests to borrow money now and pay for purchases later.

cultural learning The sum of the effect that society, culture, and environment has on an individual.

culture The social heritage of a group of people. It includes all the characteristic features, attitudes, values, traditions, customs, and rules of behavior of a particular group.

decentering The ability to focus on more than one aspect of a problem; a cognitive skill of concrete operational children.

defaulting on a loan The failure to repay borrowed money or to meet some financial obligation.

defective genes A gene associated with a certain disease. A number of health problems—cancer, blood disorders, alcoholism, etc.—can have genetic origins.

deoxyribonucleic acid (DNA) The chemical basis of heredity; the molecule that carries genetic information and controls the function of cells.

discretionary income Income left over after all bills are paid.

displaced homemaker Persons who have stayed out of the workforce to care for family members but who now find themselves less needed in the home, in need of employment, and without employable skills.

divorce The legal process that ends a marriage.

dyslexia A physical learning disability which causes an individual to reverse the order of words and letters, making normal reading impossible.

economic means of existence The specific work undertaken by family members that generates income and allows the family's economic function to take place.

economic need One of several types of motivations for working; the major reason people work. *See also* personal reasons; social reasons.

effective parenting The process of meeting the needs of another human being that demonstrates respect, care, and attention.

egg *See* ova.

egocentrism An aspect of an infant's cognitive ability that makes it impossible for him or her to distinguish objects or other persons from himself or herself.

electronic cottage A term used to describe the work-at-home lifestyle. Because the use of electronic equipment, such as computers, makes possible many types of at-home employment, some social scientists use *electronic cottage* to describe the work-at-home lifestyle.

embryo The developing human individual, from the time the fertilized egg is implanted in the mother's uterus until it is about eight weeks old.

emotional development The process of learning to control and express emotions.

emotional intimacy A measure of growth in a relationship marked by a willingness to trust and reveal feelings.

empathy The capacity to see issues as others see them; consideration of an issue from viewpoints of others; the ability to mentally participate in another person's feelings.

empty nest stage The family stage in which all children have been launched.

environment The set of social, cultural, and physical circumstances and conditions by which an individual is surrounded and influenced.

external evaluation The tendency to rate oneself and others on the basis of outward, nonessential rewards and possessions, such as good grades, expensive cars, or designer clothes, rather than on inner merit.

extrinsic value A belief or feeling that has worth because it is a means to gain other values or desired results.

family A group of people living together who are related by blood, marriage, and/or adoption (used by the U.S. Census Bureau). A group of people who reside together periodically and are related by blood, marriage, adoption, and/or common purpose (this definition is more comprehensive).

family boundaries Characteristics that separate the family from other people outside the family.

family rules Stated or unstated guidelines for behavior of persons belonging to a specific family.

fear A strong feeling of fright, panic, or terror that may be real or imaginary; one of the core human emotions that begins in infancy and develops over time.

fertilization The process in which sperm penetrates an egg cell, thereby initiating the development of a new individual.

fetal alcohol syndrome Presence of medical symptoms, such as facial deformity or mental retardation, in infants whose mothers consume large quantities of alcohol during pregnancy.

fetus Beginning about six to eight weeks after conception, a developing human is referred to as a *fetus*.

fixed income Income—money coming into the household—does not increase, even though the cost of housing, medical care, food, and clothing may rise.

foresight The ability to look forward. An important component of planning.

formal operations A stage of mental development in adolescents marked by higher levels of abstract thought and problem-solving skill.

fully functioning individual A term used by psychologist Carl Rogers to describe people who strive to develop themselves to their fullest potential.

gene A cluster of DNA (deoxyribonucleic acid) molecules; the primary factor of heredity that contains the code for specific human traits.

goal An end toward which effort is directed.

grief The pain, discomfort, and feelings that most people have after the death of someone they love.

group specific value A belief or feeling that differs among societies, groups, and subgroups. Values and attitudes about the importance of time, public behavior, eating habits, and the discipline of children can be specific to a given group.

growth hormone One of several hormones secreted by the pituitary gland at puberty that initiates and regulates physical growth.

guilt A strong feeling of self-disgrace or shame associated with the knowledge of having done something wrong; one of the core human emotions that begins in the preschool stage of development.

handicap A disadvantage, especially a physical disadvantage, that makes certain kinds of achievement unusually difficult.

healthy social development Behavior in children that exhibits maximum levels of prosocial skills and minimum levels of antisocial skills.

homogamy The similarity of individuals' backgrounds.

human life span The series of six stages that mark a person's physical development: prenatal, infancy, childhood, adolescent, adulthood, and aging.

human resources Capacities, such as time, energy, brain power, communication skill, and decision-making ability, that enable human beings to establish and maintain interpersonal relationships.

Human T Lymphocyte Virus III (HTLV III) A virus that causes Acquired Immune Deficiency Syndrome (AIDS).

I-messages A simple statement of fact about how one feels or thinks; for example, "I get worried when I see you so angry." I-messages allow individuals to disagree without threatening each other.

impaired fertility A condition present in 10 percent of American marriages where the couple finds it difficult to conceive a child for a variety of reasons.

infancy stage One of the six stages of human physical development that begins with birth and ends at two years.

inflation A measure of the increase in the prices of food, housing, clothing, transportation, etc.

integrated roles Shared work roles for males and females that allow family members to do what is necessary, regardless of traditional sex roles.

intellectual intimacy A measure of growth in a relationship that is characterized by the sharing of ideas and knowledge.

interest on loan The amount paid by a borrower to a lender for money used to finance purchases.

intimate distance An aspect of nonverbal communication; a distance of 18 inches or less that is usually reserved for communication between very close friends.

intimate relationship A relationship characterized by a high degree of closeness, sharing, and caring.

intrinsic value A belief or feeling that has worth in its own right.

investment An outlay of money for the purpose of earning a profit.

job frustrations Any of a number of stresses associated with work, including poor working conditions, dissatisfaction with a boss or coworker, insufficient reward, etc.

job future The employment outlook for an occupation and the chances for advancement within the occupation.

job requirements All those things a person needs in order to get a job; includes training, education, special abilities, work experience, and special licensing.

job security A measure of a worker's freedom from firings and layoffs.

job sharing Two people dividing the tasks and responsibilities of one full-time job.

Johari's Window A figurative tool that helps one look into four specific parts or arenas of self-concept or personality in relation to how much we reveal to others.

language acquisition The process of learning, understanding, and using verbal communication.

large muscle coordination The ability to move and manipulate large muscles, muscles that permit an individual to crawl, walk, jump, and play.

launching The process by which a family sends its children into the world to earn their own living and establish their own families.

launching family stage The family stage in which children go forth in the world to establish independence from their parents, gain an education, earn their own living, and form families of their own.

level of living Number and types of goods and services (necessities and luxuries) that a family currently enjoys.

long-term goal An object that is to be achieved over a long period of time.

mad money Income that is reserved for an extravagant or unnecessary purpose.

marriage stability A measure of the degree to which a marriage remains intact, undisturbed by divorce, separation, or desertion.

marriage success A measure of the degree to which both partners in a marriage fulfill their goals and expectations.

material means The ability to take on a financial burden; for example, one of the most obvious requirements of parenthood is the ability to cover the costs of raising a child.

material resources Goods—food, clothing, appliances, money—that families consume.

material value A belief or feeling related to possessions we treasure.

menarche First menstruation.

menstruation A monthly discharge of blood and tissue debris from the uterus of a nonpregnant, sexually mature female; a signal of sexual maturation.

mental (or cognitive) development The process by which individuals acquire the knowledge and skills that enable them to think and solve problems.

middlescence A period of questioning and self-reflection among middle-aged adults.

mitosis The process of cell division and growth.

moral value A belief or feeling based on what an individual considers to be right or wrong. A moral value is a thought or a code.

motor skills Physical abilities that permit movement and eye-hand coordination.

mutual dependency Reliance of people upon one another for support and encouragement.

myth A widely accepted belief or set of ideas which are unrealistic or unfounded.

need fulfillment Gaining confidence, assurance, respect, love, or affection in a relationship.

nonverbal communication Behaviors, gestures, actions, and ways of communicating other than the spoken word.

normal range of physical development A span of ages during which average child development takes place. Developmental changes, such as the ability to drink from a cup, do not occur "on time." They occur over an average time span, say, from age six months to age ten months.

nurture To supply with nourishment and further the development of.

obesity A physical condition marked by excessive amounts of body fat.

object permanence An important aspect of an infant's cognitive development; knowledge that an object exists even though the infant can no longer see, feel, or touch it.

ova Mature female reproductive cells.

ovaries Female reproductive organs that produce ova.

parenting family stage That stage of family life when preschoolers, schoolagers, and adolescents are present in the family.

passive listening Listening in which one's responses (gestures, body language, etc.) do not relay ideas or judgments back to the speaker. The listener sets up a climate that invites the speaker to share ideas.

peer group A group of individuals who are roughly the same age.

perceptual ability The degree to which an individual can exercise the senses of seeing, hearing, smelling, tasting, and touching.

personal distance An aspect of nonverbal communication; a distance of 20 to 38 inches that is used for private, not highly intimate, conversation.

personal reasons One of several types of motivations for working. Personal reasons for working include desire for self-expression and desire to contribute to society. *See also* economic need; social reasons.

personality The visible pattern of an individual's characteristics and behavior; the expression of one's self-concept.

personality predisposition The native or inborn tendency to behave in a certain way.

physical development The manner in which a person's body changes as he or she grows older.

physical development milestones A series of significant events that mark a child's maturation.

physical intimacy A measure of growth in a relationship characterized by physical closeness.

potential self An arena within Johari's Window; that part of the self unknown to yourself or to others.

prejudice A preconceived judgment or hostile opinion of an individual, group, or race usually without knowledge or accurate information.

prenatal stage The earliest stage of human physical development, beginning with conception and ending with birth.

preoperational stage One stage in a child's cognitive development, as defined by Jean Piaget. From 2 to 7 years, a child learns to use words and gestures to communicate and to categorize information and objects.

preventive education for marriage Courses, counseling, or other programs designed to help couples enrich their marriage and avoid problems.

principal The amount of money that is borrowed and on which interest is paid.

principle of least interest A factor that may determine who holds the most power in a relationship. Since the least interested person in a relationship does not care if the relationship ends or flounders, that person has the *power* to risk any kind of behavior, often without consequence.

priorities The set of values, interests, and goals that are of highest importance to an individual.

private self An arena within Johari's Window; that part of the self known to you but not known to others.

proactive A mode of behavior characterized by action and initiation. Leaders are usually said to exhibit proactive behaviors.

process of disenchantment The tendency for the levels of love and satisfaction in a marriage to decline over time.

propinquity Nearness to others in place or time; proximity.

prosocial behavior Behavior marked by a positive orientation toward others.

puberty When adolescence begins; the period when an individual reaches full sexual and reproductive maturity.

pubescence *See* puberty.

public distance An aspect of nonverbal communication; a distance over 13 feet that is used when making impersonal presentations, as in an assembly.

public self An arena within Johari's Window; that part of the self known to yourself and to others.

quickening Instances of fetal movement.

rapport Harmony or feelings of ease and comfort with another person.

reactive A mode of behavior that responds to rather than initiates events. Followers are usually said to exhibit reactive behaviors.

relocation A condition of employment that requires a worker (and his or her family) to uproot and move to a new location.

remedial marriage education Counseling designed to help married couples deal with major problems and concerns.

restoring workers One of several important functions of the family; the activities of the family associated with reducing worker tensions.

résumé A brief history of one's work experience and qualifications usually prepared by job applicant.

role A set of expectations or behavioral standards applied to an individual in a certain position.

self-concept The set of ideas about one's own unique being including ideas of one's own strengths and weaknesses, values, and beliefs.

self-inventory A personal description of one's interests, values, skills, abilities, and job preferences.

self-revelation Telling someone revealing information about one's self and one's feelings.

senescence The period in the life of an aging adult when the body's ability to heal and regenerate itself slows, making the body more susceptible to disease and infection.

senility A disorder, usually related to aging, marked by mental confusion and disorientation.

sensorimotor stage An aspect of an infant's cognitive development defined by Jean Piaget. At the sensorimotor stage of development an infant's knowledge is limited to knowledge and desires that can be attained through the senses.

separate property laws Laws dealing with how property is to be divided in case of divorce, which focus on what property spouses brought into the marriage and which spouse paid for property acquired during the marriage.

separation agreement A legal contract (often a forerunner of divorce) that contains terms and conditions under which marriage partners agree to live apart.

separation anxiety A common behavior of infants marked by crying and fussiness exhibited when they lose sight of their caretakers.

seriation The ability of preoperational children to arrange objects in a series; for example, in order of length, from shortest to tallest.

sex roles Patterns of behavior traditionally associated with either a male or female.

sexual identity An aspect of socialization whereby an individual acquires knowledge of his or her identity as a boy or girl.

sexually transmitted diseases (STDs) A number of diseases, such as syphilis, AIDS, and gonorrhea, that are spread from one individual to another by means of sexual contact.

shadowing A term referring to a formal means of observing a worker on the job.

short-term goal An object that can be attained rather quickly.

single parent A mother or father who assumes child-care responsibilities without a marriage partner.

small muscle coordination The ability to move and manipulate small groups of muscles permitting a child to pick up objects, eat, and drink.

social development The process of acquiring skills that allow an individual to interact, relate, and adjust to other people.

social distance An aspect of nonverbal communication; a distance of 38 inches to 13 feet used for conducting business and daily activity.

social reasons One of several types of motivations for working. Desires for social status and friendship needs are examples of social reasons for working. *See also* economic need; personal reasons.

social skills Abilities and patterns of behavior, such as listening when someone else is talking and taking turns, acquired and improved over time, that allow individuals to relate to others in considerate ways.

social status *See* status.

socialization The process of acquiring knowledge and skills in order to exist in a social setting.

sperm cells Mature male reproductive cells.

standard of living The set of all necessities, comforts, and luxuries (material resources) that a family *desires* to have.

status The relative rank or position of an individual in the eyes of others.

status quo The existing state of affairs.

STDs *See* sexually transmitted diseases.

stereotype A standardized perception of what people are and how they behave.

sterile Incapable of producing offspring.

stranger anxiety A fear of unfamiliar people often exhibited by infants.

stress The positive or negative response of the body to any demand made upon it.

stressor The stress-producing situation; may be positive or negative.

subculture A group within a culture which has characteristic patterns of behavior that distinguish the members of the group from others in the larger culture.

substitute parents Those people (teachers, ministers, coaches, etc.) in our society whom we trust to perform various parenting functions.

superficial relationship A casual, uninvolved relationship; the opposite of an intimate relationship.

symbolic play The ability of preoperational-age children to pretend that one object stands for another; for example, to pretend that blue carpet is water.

symbol An object that is used to stand for something else.

testicles Male reproductive organs that produce sperm.

thanatology The study of death.

trimester Any of the three-month periods in which a pregnancy is divided.

unaware self An arena within Johari's Window; that part of the self that is known to others but to which you are blind.

universal value A belief or feeling on which most, if not all, people can agree. Universal values include equality, justice, brotherhood, and respect for oneself and others.

uterus The female reproductive organ (also called the womb) that contains and nourishes a developing fetus.

value A belief or feeling that someone or something is worthwhile. Values can be thought of as standards or yardsticks to guide actions, judgments, and attitudes.

work ethic A term used to explain an individual's or a society's attitude and philosophy about work. The American work ethic suggests that all able-bodied people should work and that work be a major part of people's existence.

workaholic A person who works an excessive amount.

zygote A fertilized egg cell.

index

D

E

F

G